Manual of Clinical Psychopharmacology for Nurses

T0176409

Manual of Clinical Psychopharmacology for Nurses

Edited by

Laura G. Leahy, M.S.N., P.M.H.-A.P.R.N.

Associate Director and Senior Lecturer,
Psychiatric Mental Health Nurse Practitioner Program,
University of Pennsylvania School of Nursing, Philadelphia;
Family Psychiatric Nurse Practitioner,
APNSolutions, LLC,
Vineland, New Jersey

Christian G. Kohler, M.D.

Associate Professor of Psychiatry,
Hospital of the University of Pennsylvania,
Philadelphia, Pennsylvania

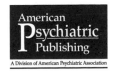

American
Psychiatric
Publishing
A Division of American Psychiatric Association

Washington, DC
London, England

Copyright © 2013 American Psychiatric Association
ALL RIGHTS RESERVED

Manufactured in the United States of America on acid-free paper
17   16   15   14   13   5   4   3   2   1
First Edition

Typeset in Adobe's AGaramond and Formata.

American Psychiatric Publishing,
a Division of American Psychiatric Association
1000 Wilson Boulevard
Arlington, VA 22209-3901
www.appi.org

Library of Congress Cataloging-in-Publication Data
Manual of clinical psychopharmacology for nurses / edited by Laura G. Leahy, Christian G. Kohler. — 1st ed.
        p. ; cm.
    Includes bibliographical references and index.
    ISBN 978-1-58562-434-8 (pbk. : alk. paper)
    I. Leahy, Laura G. II. Kohler, Christian G., 1960– III. American Psychiatric Publishing.
    [DNLM: 1. Mental Disorders—drug therapy—Nurses' Instruction. 2. Psychotropic Drugs—therapeutic use—Nurses' Instruction. WM 402]
    616.89′18—dc23

                                                                                    2012040421

British Library Cataloguing in Publication Data
A CIP record is available from the British Library.

The soul is healed by being with children.
—Dostoevsky (1821–1881)

This book is dedicated to the children who heal my soul,
Claire and Kyle,
and to the memories of my paternal grandparents,
Francis Albert Groblewski (1911–1989)
and Albertina Lugar Groblewski (1914–2005),
through whom I learned of the hidden suffering and resilience
of those with psychiatric illness
and the value of pharmacotherapeutics.

Laura G. Leahy, M.S.N., P.M.H.-A.P.R.N.

Contents

Contributors xxi

Foreword. xxv
Christian G. Kohler, M.D.

Preface xxvii
Laura G. Leahy, M.S.N., P.M.H.-A.P.R.N.

1 **Introduction to Clinical Psychopharmacology
for Nurses 1**
Laura G. Leahy, M.S.N., P.M.H.-A.P.R.N.
Psychiatric Assessment From an Advanced
   Practice Nurse's Perspective 3
Medications and the U.S. Food and Drug
   Administration 7
Neuroanatomy and Neurochemistry. 12
Genetic Markers in Psychiatry 17
Basic Pharmacological Terminology 17
Special Considerations in Psychopharmacological
   Prescribing. 18
Summary 20
References. 23
Appendix: Brain Structures and Pathways 24

PART I
Psychopharmacological Treatment
and Management of Psychiatric Disorders

2 **Anxiety Disorders. 31**
Sarah Seabrook-de Jong, M.S.N., A.P.R.N., P.M.H.-C.N.S./F.N.P., B.C.
Overview of Anxiety Disorders. 32
Neurobiology of Fear and Anxiety. 37

Medications Used to Treat Anxiety Disorders 40
Treatment of Special Populations..................... 50
Treatment Monitoring 53
Summary... 54
Clinical Pearls 54
References.. 55

3 Depressive Disorders..........................59

LaKeetra M. Josey, M.S.N., A.P.R.N., P.M.H.-F.N.P., B.C.
Elaine M. Neidert, M.S.N., A.P.R.N., P.M.H.-N.P., B.C.

Overview of Depressive Disorders 60
Neurobiology of Depression 67
Medications Used to Treat Depressive Disorders 68
U.S. Food and Drug Administration Warnings 78
Treatment of Special Populations..................... 79
Treatment Monitoring 80
Summary... 81
Clinical Pearls 82
References.. 83

4 Bipolar Disorders...........................85

Candice Knight, Ph.D., Ed.D., A.P.R.N., P.M.H.-C.N.S./N.P., B.C.

Overview of Bipolar Disorders...................... 86
Neurobiology of Bipolar Disorders 89
Treatment of Bipolar Disorders..................... 91
Medications Used to Treat Bipolar Disorders.......... 97
Treatment of Special Populations.................... 117
Summary.. 122
Clinical Pearls 122
References....................................... 124

5 **Psychotic Disorders** **129**

Serena M. Natal, M.S.N., A.P.R.N., P.M.H.-F.N.P., B.C.
Taresa Pittman, B.S.N., R.N.
Shannon Richmond, M.S.N., A.P.R.N., P.M.H.-F.N.P., B.C.
Linden Spital, M.S.N., A.P.R.N., P.M.H.-F.N.P., B.C.
Megan Walsh, M.S.N., A.P.R.N., P.M.H.-F.N.P., B.C.

Overview of Schizophrenia Spectrum and
   Other Psychotic Disorders 130
Etiology of Psychotic Disorders 133
Pathophysiology of Schizophrenia 137
Antipsychotic Medications 141
Treatment of Special Populations 149
Summary 151
Clinical Pearls 152
References 153

6 **Attention-Deficit/Hyperactivity and Autistic**
Spectrum Disorders **155**

Patti A. Varley, M.N., A.P.R.N., P.M.H.-C.N.S., B.C.
Laura G. Leahy, M.S.N., P.M.H.-A.P.R.N.

Attention-Deficit/Hyperactivity Disorder 156
Autistic Spectrum Disorders 158
Biological Underpinnings of Neurodevelopmental
   Disorders 159
Medications Used to Treat Symptoms Associated
   With Autism 165
Medications Used to Treat Symptoms of
   Attention-Deficit/Hyperactivity Disorder 165
Dosing Considerations 175
Treatment Monitoring 175
Treatment of Special Populations 177
Summary 178
Clinical Pearls 179
References 180

7   Substance Use Disorders 183
Laura G. Leahy, M.S.N., P.M.H.-A.P.R.N.
Overview of Substance Use Disorders 186
Neurobiology of Substance Abuse and Dependence ... 186
Pharmacological Properties of Agents Used to
    Treat Substance Use Disorders 190
Safety Concerns 203
Treatment of Special Populations 209
Summary 211
Clinical Pearls 212
References 212

8   Sleep-Wake Disorders 215
Elaine M. Neidert, M.S.N., A.P.R.N., P.M.H.-N.P., B.C.
Overview of Sleep-Wake Disorders 215
Neurobiology of the Human Sleep Cycle 225
Pharmacological Treatment of Insomnia 225
Pharmacological Treatment of Hypersomnia 230
Pharmacological Treatment of Parasomnias 231
Summary 232
Clinical Pearls 233
References 234

9   Trauma and Posttraumatic Stress Disorder 235
Donna Sabella, Ph.D., M.Ed., M.S.N., P.M.H.-C.N.S.
Overview of Traumatic Stress Disorders 236
Neuroanatomy and Neurochemistry of Fear and
    Response to Threat 241
Biological Underpinnings of Trauma- and
    Stressor-Related Disorders 244
Treatment Approach to Traumatic Stress Disorders 245
Treatment Issues in Specific Populations 259
Pretreatment Assessment and Treatment Monitoring .. 264
Summary 264
Clinical Pearls 265
References 266

10 Delirium and Dementia..................271

Richard Pessagno, D.N.P., A.P.R.N., P.M.H.-C.N.S./N.P., B.C.

Overview of Neurocognitive Disorders...............272
Biological Underpinnings of Neurocognitive
  Disorders.......................................278
Clinical Assessment of Delirium and Dementia........280
Medications Used to Treat Psychiatric Symptoms
  in Delirium and Dementia........................281
Dosing Guidelines.................................286
Treatment of Special Populations...................292
Nonpharmacological Treatment....................293
Summary..294
Clinical Pearls..................................294
References.......................................295

PART II
Special Issues in Clinical
Psychopharmacology

11 Psychopharmacology in Psychiatric
Emergencies..............................301

Mary Kay Dollard, M.S.N., A.P.R.N., P.M.H.-N.P., B.C.

Approach to Psychiatric Crisis Intervention...........303
Differential Diagnosis in Psychiatric Emergency
  Assessment.....................................304
Psychiatric Conditions Requiring Emergency
  Intervention....................................308
Psychotropic Medications Used in Emergency
  Settings..315
Treatment of Special Populations...................316
Treatment Monitoring............................323
Summary..324
Clinical Pearls..................................327
References.......................................327

12 Management of Metabolic Side Effects of Psychotropic Medications. 331

Barbara J. Limandri, Ph.D., A.P.R.N., P.M.H.-C.N.S., B.C.

Overview of Medication-Associated Metabolic
Side Effects 331
Features of Metabolic Syndrome. 334
Factors Associated With Metabolic Syndrome 336
Treatment Monitoring and Clinical Guidelines 338
Summary 347
Clinical Pearls 348
References. 348

13 Complementary and Alternative Pharmacotherapies 353

Bobbie Posmontier, Ph.D., C.N.M., A.P.R.N., P.M.H.-N.P., B.C.

Herbal Preparations Commonly Used to Treat
Psychiatric Symptoms 354
Summary 371
Clinical Pearls 371
References. 372

14 Culturally Sensitive Psychopharmacology. 379

Barbara Jones Warren, Ph.D., A.P.R.N., P.M.H.-C.N.S., B.C., F.A.A.N.

Role of Culture in Relation to Mental Health,
Wellness, and Illness 380
Health Care Disparities. 381
Definitions of Cultural Terms. 381
Biopsychosocial Cultural Connections 383
Drug Metabolism and the Cytochrome P450 System. . . 385
Stereotyping or Culturally Competent Care? 387
The Culturally Competent Therapeutic Relationship. . . . 387
Cultural Language and Patterns of Communication. . . . 389
Inclusion of Family, Friends, and Significant Others 392

Culturally Competent Psychiatric Assessment:
Implications for Practice. 393
Summary 398
Clinical Pearls 399
References. 399

PART III
Appendixes

**Appendix 1: Approximate Psychotropic
Drug Dose Equivalencies. 405**

**Appendix 2: Psychotropic and
Other Medications Influenced by
the Cytochrome P450 (CYP) System 411**

**Appendix 3: Psychopharmacogenetic
Variations: Implications for Practice 417**

Appendix 4: Psychiatric Rating Scales. 423
Patient Health Questionnaire: Somatic, Anxiety,
and Depressive Symptoms (PHQ-SADS) 427
Hamilton Anxiety Scale (Ham-A). 431
17-Item Hamilton Rating Scale for Depression
(Ham-D-17) 433
Edinburgh Postnatal Depression Scale (EPDS)
for Postpartum Depression 436
Parent Version of the Young Mania Rating Scale
(P-YMRS). 439
Abnormal Involuntary Movement Scale (AIMS). 443
Vanderbilt ADHD Diagnostic Parent Rating Scale
(VADPRS) 447
Vanderbilt ADHD Diagnostic Teacher Rating Scale
(VADTRS). 451

Adult ADHD Self-Report Scale—Version 1.1
  (Adult ASRS-v1.1) Symptom Checklist. 455
Clinical Institute Withdrawal Assessment of Alcohol
  Scale, Revised (CIWA-Ar). 459
Sleep Disorder Scales. 462
PTSD Checklist—Civilian Version (PCL-C) 463

Appendix 5: Online Resources 465

Index 467

List of Tables and Figures

Table 1–1   Components of pre-prescribing assessment 4

Table 1–2   Diagnostic assessment tools 6

Table 1–3   Definitions of controlled substance schedules. 10

Table 1–4   Black box warnings for psychotropic drugs. 11

Table 1–5   Endogenous neurotransmitters. 13

Table 1–6   U.S. Food and Drug Administration (FDA)
             pregnancy risk categories. 22

Figure A1–1 Brain structures and functions. 24

Figure A1–2 Neurotransmitter pathways 26

Table 2–1   Epidemiology of anxiety disorders 32

Table 2–2   DSM-IV-TR diagnostic criteria for panic disorder
             with (300.21) or without (300.01) agoraphobia . . .33

Table 2–3   DSM-IV-TR diagnostic criteria for 300.29
             specific phobia 34

Table 2–4   DSM-IV-TR diagnostic criteria for 300.23
             social phobia 35

Table 2–5   DSM-IV-TR diagnostic criteria for 300.3
             obsessive-compulsive disorder. 36

Table 2–6   DSM-IV-TR diagnostic criteria for 300.02
             generalized anxiety disorder .38

Table 2–7   DSM-IV-TR diagnostic criteria for 293.84
             anxiety disorder due to a general medical
             condition. 39

Figure 2–1   Neural pathway related to fear and autonomic
             response. 40

Table 2–8   Drugs with U.S. Food and Drug Administration–
             approved indications for anxiety disorders 43

Table 2–9   Anxiety drug dosages and side effects 44

Table 2–10   Prescribing considerations for antianxiety
             medications 46

Table 3–1	DSM-IV-TR diagnostic criteria for 296.2 major depressive disorder, single episode	61
Table 3–2	DSM-IV-TR diagnostic criteria for 296.3 major depressive disorder, recurrent	62
Table 3–3	DSM-IV-TR diagnostic criteria for 300.4 dysthymic disorder	63
Table 3–4	Key features of antidepressant medications commonly used in the treatment of depressive disorders	70
Table 3–5	Inhibition of cytochrome P450 (CYP) enzymes by antidepressants	82
Table 4–1	Mood-stabilizing agents: lithium and anticonvulsants	98
Table 4–2	Mood-stabilizing agents: antipsychotics	100
Table 4–3	Titration of lamotrigine	109
Table 5–1	Psychotic disorders at a glance	131
Table 5–2	DSM-IV-TR diagnostic criteria for schizophrenia	132
Table 5–3	DSM-IV-TR diagnostic criteria for 295.40 schizophreniform disorder	134
Table 5–4	DSM-IV-TR diagnostic criteria for 295.70 schizoaffective disorder	134
Table 5–5	DSM-IV-TR diagnostic criteria for 297.1 delusional disorder	135
Table 5–6	DSM-IV-TR diagnostic criteria for 298.8 brief psychotic disorder	136
Table 5–7	DSM-IV-TR diagnostic criteria for psychotic disorder due to a general medical condition	137
Table 5–8	Off-label uses for commonly prescribed antipsychotics	142
Table 5–9	Pharmacokinetics of antipsychotic medications	144

Table 6–1   Symptoms of attention-deficit/hyperactivity
               disorder across the life span 157

Figure 6–1   Potential areas of impairment related to
               attention-deficit/hyperactivity disorder (ADHD)
               across the life span 158

Table 6–2   DSM-IV-TR diagnostic criteria for attention-deficit/
               hyperactivity disorder. 160

Table 6–3   DSM-IV-TR diagnostic criteria for 299.00
               autistic disorder 162

Table 6–4   DSM-IV-TR diagnostic criteria for 299.80
               Asperger's disorder 163

Table 6–5   Medications commonly prescribed to treat
               symptoms associated with autism 166

Table 6–6   U.S. Food and Drug Administration (FDA)–
               approved medications used in the treatment
               of attention-deficit/hyperactivity disorder (ADHD) . . 167

Table 7–1   DSM-IV-TR diagnostic criteria for substance
               dependence. 187

Table 7–2   DSM-IV-TR diagnostic criteria for substance
               abuse188

Table 7–3   DSM-IV-TR diagnostic criteria for substance
               intoxication 190

Table 7–4   DSM-IV-TR diagnostic criteria for substance
               withdrawal 190

Table 7–5   Medications used in the treatment of alcohol
               and opioid/opiate abuse and dependence 191

Table 7–6   Medications used in the treatment of
               opioid/opiate abuse and dependence. 195

Table 7–7   Medications used in the treatment of nicotine
               dependence. 197

Table 7–8   Blood alcohol level (BAL): symptoms and
               effects. 201

Figure 7–1   Alcohol/benzodiazepine (sedative-hypnotic)
               withdrawal protocol 204

Figure 7–2   Opiate withdrawal protocol 206

Table 8–1	Age-related sleep needs across the life span..... 217
Table 8–2	Effects of disrupted sleep 217
Table 8–3	Components of a sleep evaluation............. 218
Table 8–4	Stages of healthy non–rapid eye movement (REM) sleep............................... 220
Table 8–5	DSM-IV-TR sleep disorders 221
Table 8–6	Healthy sleep habits 224
Table 8–7	Commonly used benzodiazepines and nonbenzodiazepines for sleep 228

Table 9–1	DSM-IV-TR diagnostic criteria for 309.81 posttraumatic stress disorder.................. 238
Table 9–2	DSM-IV-TR diagnostic criteria for 308.3 acute stress disorder 240
Table 9–3	Pharmacological characteristics of selective serotonin reuptake inhibitors (SSRIs)........... 248
Table 9–4	Pharmacological characteristics of non–selective serotonin reuptake inhibitor antidepressants 250
Table 9–5	Overview of antidepressants used to treat posttraumatic stress disorder (PTSD)........... 252
Table 9–6	Dosing of medications commonly used in the treatment of posttraumatic stress disorder (PTSD) 260

Table 10–1	Risk factors for delirium...................... 274
Table 10–2	Common types of dementia................... 276
Table 10–3	Side effects of medications commonly used in the treatment of delirium 282
Table 10–4	Side effects of medications commonly used in the treatment of dementia 285
Table 10–5	Acetylcholinesterase inhibitors 289

Table 11–1	Medical conditions that may present as psychiatric emergencies....................... 306
Table 11–2	Differential diagnosis of delirium............... 307

Table 11–3 Psychiatric disorders that may have acute
            manifestations 309

Table 11–4 Factors predictive of aggressive and violent
            behaviors 314

Table 11–5 Risk factors for suicide 315

Table 11–6 Medications commonly used in psychiatric
            emergencies. 318

Table 11–7 General approach to psychiatric emergency
            intervention 326

Table 12–1 Criteria for metabolic syndrome 335

Table 12–2 Recommended monitoring for metabolic
            syndrome 339

Table 12–3 Treatment recommendations for metabolic
            syndrome 340

Table 12–4 Percentage of metabolic side effects for
            selected psychotropic drugs 342

Table 13–1 Complementary and alternative
            pharmacotherapies commonly used for
            psychiatric symptoms 356

Table 14–1 Nursing cultural assessment questions. 389

Table 14–2 Cultural and psychiatric language descriptions
            of emotional symptoms 391

Table 14–3 Models of illness and disease 391

Table 14–4 Overall assessment questions. 395

Table 14–5 Questions to assess patient perceptions
            regarding causes of illness and disease 396

Table 14–6 Cultural assessment questions on medication
            treatment 397

Table 14–7 Cultural discussion areas for patient instructions . . 397

Table 14–8 Internet resources 398

Contributors

Mary Kay Dollard, M.S.N., A.P.R.N., P.M.H.-N.P., B.C.
Psychiatric Nurse Practitioner, Philadelphia Prison System, Philadelphia, Pennsylvania

LaKeetra M. Josey, M.S.N., A.P.R.N., P.M.H.-F.N.P., B.C.
Family Psychiatric Nurse Practitioner; Associate Director, PMH Nurse Practitioner Program, University of Pennsylvania, School of Nursing, Philadelphia, Pennsylvania

Candice Knight, Ph.D., Ed.D., A.P.R.N., P.M.H.-C.N.S./N.P., B.C.
Coordinator, PMH Nurse Practitioner Program, New York University, New York, New York; Psychiatric Nurse Practitioner and Licensed Psychologist, Wellspring Center for Health and Wellbeing, Flemington, New Jersey

Christian G. Kohler, M.D.
Associate Professor of Psychiatry, Hospital of the University of Pennsylvania, Philadelphia, Pennsylvania

Laura G. Leahy, M.S.N., P.M.H.-A.P.R.N.
Associate Director and Senior Lecturer, Psychiatric Mental Health Nurse Practitioner Program, University of Pennsylvania School of Nursing, Philadelphia; Family Psychiatric Nurse Practitioner, APNSolutions, LLC, Vineland, New Jersey

Barbara J. Limandri, Ph.D., A.P.R.N., P.M.H.-C.N.S., B.C.
Professor of Nursing, School of Nursing, Linfield College, Portland, Oregon

Serena M. Natal, M.S.N., A.P.R.N., P.M.H.-F.N.P., B.C.
Psychiatric Nurse Practitioner, University of Pennsylvania School of Nursing, Psychiatric Mental Health Nurse Practitioner Program, Students in Advanced Psychopharmacology Across the Lifespan, Philadelphia, Pennsylvania

Elaine M. Neidert, M.S.N., A.P.R.N., P.M.H.-N.P., B.C.
Psychiatric Nurse Practitioner, Berkshire Psychiatric and Behavioral Associates, Reading, Pennsylvania

Richard Pessagno, D.N.P., A.P.R.N., P.M.H.-C.N.S./N.P., B.C.
Clinical Assistant Professor, Rutgers, The State University of New Jersey, College of Nursing, Newark, New Jersey; Psychiatric Nurse Practitioner, Private Practice, Moorestown, New Jersey

Taresa Pittman, B.S.N., R.N.
University of Pennsylvania School of Nursing, Psychiatric Mental Health Nurse Practitioner Program, Students in Advanced Psychopharmacology Across the Lifespan, Philadelphia, Pennsylvania

Bobbie Posmontier, Ph.D., C.N.M., A.P.R.N., P.M.H.-N.P., B.C.
Family Psychiatric Nurse Practitioner; Assistant Professor and DrNP Track Coordinator, Drexel University College of Nursing and Health Professions, Philadelphia, Pennsylvania

Shannon Richmond, M.S.N., A.P.R.N., P.M.H.-F.N.P., B.C.
Psychiatric Nurse Practitioner, University of Pennsylvania School of Nursing, Psychiatric Mental Health Nurse Practitioner Program, Students in Advanced Psychopharmacology Across the Lifespan, Philadelphia, Pennsylvania

Donna Sabella, Ph.D., M.Ed., M.S.N., P.M.H.-C.N.S.
Contributing Editor, Mental Health Matters, *American Journal of Nursing;* Assistant Dean of Health Sciences, Arcadia University, College of Global Studies, Glenside, Pennsylvania

Sarah Seabrook-de Jong, M.S.N., A.P.R.N., P.M.H.-C.N.S./F.N.P., B.C.
Family Psychiatric Nurse Practitioner; Administrative Director, Behavioral Health Services, South Jersey HealthCare, Bridgeton Division, Bridgeton, New Jersey

Linden Spital, M.S.N., A.P.R.N., P.M.H.-F.N.P., B.C.
Psychiatric Nurse Practitioner, University of Pennsylvania School of Nursing, Psychiatric Mental Health Nurse Practitioner Program, Students in Advanced Psychopharmacology Across the Lifespan, Philadelphia, Pennsylvania

Patti A. Varley, M.N., A.P.R.N., P.M.H.-C.N.S., B.C.
Child and Adolescent Psychiatric Nurse Practitioner, Children's Hospital and Regional Medical Center; Clinical Faculty, University of Washington School of Nursing, Seattle, Washington

Megan Walsh, M.S.N., A.P.R.N., P.M.H.-F.N.P., B.C.
Psychiatric Nurse Practitioner, University of Pennsylvania School of Nursing, Psychiatric Mental Health Nurse Practitioner Program, Students in Advanced Psychopharmacology Across the Lifespan, Philadelphia, Pennsylvania

Barbara Jones Warren, Ph.D., A.P.R.N., P.M.H.-C.N.S., B.C., F.A.A.N.
Professor, Clinical Nursing; Director, Psychiatric Nursing Program, National Institutes of Health/American Nurses Association Ethnic/Racial Minority Fellow, The Ohio State University College of Nursing, Columbus, Ohio

Disclosure of Competing Interests

The contributors have no competing interests to report.

Foreword

Christian G. Kohler, M.D.

Over the past 30 years, a decline of psychiatrists in the United States coincided with the growing demand for mental health services (Leslie and Rosenheck 2000). This development shifted the challenge of psychiatric care to nonpsychiatrist providers. Some of these clinicians, such as primary care practitioners, are frequently challenged by constraints in time and training to provide quality mental health services. At the same time, productive efforts emerged within the field of nursing to train nurses in advanced provider-oriented roles. Because of the nationwide need for easier access to mental health services, psychiatric mental health advanced practice registered nurses (PMH-APRNs) fulfill important roles, both as independent providers of psychiatric care and as collaborative providers with other mental health professionals, such as social workers, psychologists, and psychiatrists (for further information, see www.apna.org). Specific areas of subspecialty for PMH-APRNs include child and adolescent mental health nursing, gerontological-psychiatric nursing, forensics, and substance use disorders. The core philosophy of the advanced practice nursing field is aimed at individualized mental health care with focus on patients' conditions and their effects on the lives of the patients and their families. Within the biopsychosocial model of mental health care, PMH-APRNs are uniquely qualified to offer symptom-based treatment that is attuned and tailored to the patient's medical and social circumstances because of their nursing background and their holistic approach to the individual.

Over the years, I have had the opportunity to work with many PMH-APRNs in both academic and clinical settings, and I have been impressed with their caring and knowledgeable approach to individuals with mental health disorders, combining perspectives drawn from a nursing background with multimodal therapeutic interventions. The growing field of PMH-APRNs mandates the need for a psychopharmacology textbook, lacking until now, specifically aimed at education of nursing professionals that merges the fundamentals of medication treatment in common disorders with the therapeutic approach of the nursing field in general.

It has been a pleasure to co-edit this book, *Manual of Clinical Psychopharmacology for Nurses,* under the guidance of Laura G. Leahy, M.S.N., A.P.R.N., P.M.H.-C.N.S./F.N.P., B.C. The individual chapters, authored by psychiatric nurses, are geared toward informing nursing students and practitioners in psychopharmacology, and the chapters survey the most common psychiatric conditions in which pharmacotherapy represents a major part of treatment. In particular, contents of each chapter focus on diagnostic criteria and neurobiology of the relevant disorder(s), pharmacological choices and recommendations on monitoring, side effects to consider, and treatments for special populations and those with medical illnesses.

We hope that this book fulfills the specific needs of both nurses in training and nurses in clinical practice and provides an educational and informational source of current pharmacotherapies for psychiatric disorders commonly encountered in clinical settings.

Reference

Leslie DL, Rosenheck RA: Comparing quality of mental health care for public-sector and privately insured populations. Psychiatr Serv 51:650–655, 2000

Preface

Laura G. Leahy, M.S.N.,
P.M.H.-A.P.R.N.

I suppose it was only a matter of time before I began working with pharmacotherapeutics. With three generations of pharmacists preceding me on both sides of my family, including my paternal great-grandfather, who was an international patent medicine man at the turn of the twentieth century, I am now on the prescribing side of pharmacy. As a psychiatric advanced practice nurse with a passion to impart my knowledge of psychopharmacology to the next generation of nurses, my colleagues and peers, and my patients and their families, I welcomed the opportunity to work with American Psychiatric Publishing (APP) on this text.

The *Manual of Clinical Psychopharmacology for Nurses* is an endeavor brought to life by both nursing educators and clinicians in psychiatric nursing. In guiding the reader through the most common psychiatric conditions, each chapter presents an overview of the particular disorder; the pharmacodynamics and pharmacokinetics of the psychotropic medications used to treat that disorder; relevant dosing, titration, and augmentation strategies for those medications; and clinical pearls on the prescribing of psychotropic medications from a nursing perspective. This manual is intended to serve as both an academic textbook for psychiatric advanced practice nurses and a reference book for nurses of all disciplines as well as consumers of psychiatric services who have a desire to learn more about their illness and medications.

Although the field of psychopharmacology has experienced a revolution over the past two decades, much remains unknown about the human brain, neuropathology, and neurotransmitters as they relate to an individual's thoughts, moods, and behaviors. Yet, prescribing from a symptom-based perspective and identifying the neurotransmitters that may reduce those symptoms have served as a prescribing template for many advanced practice registered nurses. The *Manual of Clinical Psychopharmacology for Nurses* will augment the knowledge base of prescribers and offer suggestions to further improve the treatment outcomes and quality of life of our patients.

This text certainly would not have been possible without the many chapter authors who tolerated the multiple e-mails regarding chapter deadlines. Over the years, I have had the opportunity to work with many of these highly respected psychiatric nurses, educators, and prescribers. Many thanks go to all of you! A load of gratitude also goes to my co-editor, Dr. Christian Kohler, who, like the chapter authors, embraced my e-mails and worked with me to make this manual a reality. John McDuffie and Dr. Robert Hales at APP placed their trust in me as a psychiatric advanced practice nurse by allowing me the opportunity to publish this textbook through the American Psychiatric Association's publishing branch. They have been most patient in offering extensions and support, and I am most grateful. Finally, I must acknowledge my amazing husband, John, and my children, Claire and Kyle, without whom I would have never completed this project. Their encouragement to "get 'er done" kept me going through many a late hour of writing and editing.

I truly hope that this manual will foster a passion for psychopharmacology in the students, clinicians, and others who read it. Most important, though, my hope is that the information shared in this text will offer new perspectives and treatment suggestions to further improve the quality of life of patients who are prescribed psychotropic medications.

1

Introduction to Clinical Psychopharmacology for Nurses

Laura G. Leahy, M.S.N., P.M.H.-A.P.R.N.

> The trained nurse has become one of the great blessings of humanity, taking a place beside the physician and the priest and not inferior to either in her mission.
>
> —Sir William Osler, Canadian physician, in his address to Johns Hopkins Hospital (1897)

Today's health care arena is rapidly changing, and nurses, as the largest group of health care professionals, will play an essential and expanded role in caring for patients. Increasing numbers of men and women are entering the field of nursing with the intent to obtain a master's degree or higher to be able to practice in an advanced role. Although psychiatric or mental health nursing remains a relatively small area of specialization within the nursing workforce as a whole, the public's need for psychiatric services and psychopharmacological services continues to increase. Thus, nurses, whether in an advanced practice role as the patient's primary psychiatric treatment provider or as a registered nurse caring for patients in the hospital or community, must remain current in the therapeutic and neuroscience advances within the field.

Advanced practice registered nurses (APRNs) serve as primary care providers, psychotherapists, and psychopharmacologists to name but a few. Nurse leader and champion for advanced nursing practice Brenda Lyon, D.N.S., R.N., F.A.A.N., characterized nursing's unique phenomena of expertise to include four constructs: 1) viewing the patient from a holistic rather than a disease-focused perspective, 2) caring, 3) connecting at some level with the subjective or lived experience of the patient, and 4) meeting patients' needs for assistance in achieving wellness and well-being (Lyon 2010). The American Association of Colleges of Nursing (1996) defined those attributes that must be cultivated within the graduate education programs of all APRNs. Included skills were critical thinking, decision making, planning, critical and accurate assessment, ability to create appropriate interventions, and evaluation of patient responses. The ability to analyze, synthesize, and use the knowledge accrued through education and patient assessment is crucial to the success of the APRN. All APRNs must be able to assess, diagnose, prescribe therapy, and maintain accountability. Finally, the skill of effective communication is an invaluable tool and prerequisite for all APRNs (National Association of Clinical Nurse Specialists 2004).

Mental illness affects the lives of men, women, children, adolescents, and the elderly. Its ramifications extend beyond the family and individual household of the patient to school settings, the workplace, communities, and entire nations across the world. Neuropsychiatric disorders are the second-leading cause of disability throughout the world (Roberts and Jain 2011). Psychiatric APRNs are uniquely positioned to work with those experiencing psychiatric symptoms because they are educated and trained to provide not only psychotherapeutic interventions but also psychopharmacological interventions. APRNs in other disciplines such as adult or pediatric primary care also may further their training to specialize in treating mental health symptoms with psychotropic medications. Given the extent to which psychiatric illness can devastate the population, the United States has a paucity of psychiatric providers—not only as prescribers but also as therapists and behavioral health specialists. As a profession, nurses approach patient care from a biological, psychological, emotional, and social perspective and tend to incorporate aspects of the same in their treatment. The *Manual of Clinical Psychopharmacology for Nurses* incorporates those fundamental treatment approaches while presenting the current neuroscience advances in the field of psychopharmacology. The *Manual of Clinical Psychopharmacology for Nurses* provides a template for nurses of all levels of practice and all disciplines to aid and treat psychiatric or mental health symptoms across the life span. This manual is not simply a re-creation of other drug and pharmacotherapy texts but rather a guide to provide insights into the ways nurses process information and use psychopharmacotherapeutics to construct their treatment plans.

Psychiatric Assessment From an Advanced Practice Nurse's Perspective

Approximately 600 million patient visits were made to APRNs in 2010 (Driscoll 2012). Many of those patients received prescriptions for medications, laboratory studies, and diagnostic testing. The primary focus of this manual is on the psychotropic medications, but some background information must be introduced before exploring the various psychiatric symptoms and the medications used to treat them. Table 1–1 indicates some of the areas to be assessed before prescribing psychotropic medications. Although Table 1–1 offers guidelines on areas to review with the patient before prescribing, the practitioner may not be able to obtain all of the information. In those cases, the practitioner's best clinical judgment and rationalizations should be used to guide the decision whether to prescribe psychotropics on the basis of the patient's current symptoms and presentation. Table 1–2 offers additional guidelines when considering the use of psychotropic medications. These laboratory and other diagnostic tests will assist the APRN in determining differential diagnoses and ruling out disorders that may mimic the psychiatric symptoms.

Table 1–1.   Components of pre-prescribing assessment

Evaluation components	Areas to explore
Identifying information	Age, marital status, ethnicity, gender, other informants
Chief complaint	Quote patient's own words verbatim
History of present illness	Recent (over past 2–6 weeks) symptoms leading to evaluation
Past psychiatric history	Symptoms, dates, hospitalizations, partial care, outpatient treatment
Psychotropic medication history	Drug, dose, time frame, effect, combinations
Family psychiatric history	Treatments, including medications
Birth/developmental history	Include maternal prenatal history, toileting, bed-wetting
Medical/surgical history	Include head trauma, loss of consciousness, concussions, seizures, menstrual/pregnancy history in females, chronic illness, pain syndromes
Medication history	Include over-the-counter medications, vitamins, herbal preparations, contraceptives, supplements
Sexual history	Sexual orientation, number of partners, masturbation, problems or concerns
Dangerous and risk-taking behaviors	Speeding, cutting (self-injurious behaviors), bingeing, overspending, promiscuity
Sleep assessment	Time to bed, time to wake, feeling rested, difficulties, dreams and nightmares, caffeine use (including energy drinks); "Who or what else is in bed?"
Appetite assessment	Weight gain or loss, dieting patterns, laxatives, vomiting, restricting
Educational history	Learning disabilities, highest level completed
Occupational history	Length of time in job, periods of unemployment, Supplemental Security Income/Social Security Disability Insurance
Social history	Marital status; "Who is in household?"

Table 1–1. Components of pre-prescribing assessment *(continued)*

Evaluation components	Areas to explore
History of abuse	Physical, sexual, emotional; "Who was perpetrator? Any criminal report?"
Substance use and abuse history	Age at first use, amounts, date of last use; "How does _____ help?"
Legal and criminal history	Whether or not caught

Mental status examination

General	Appearance, grooming
	Orientation/sensorium
Behavior	Speech (tone, rate, fluency)
	Attention span
	Motoric behaviors
	Attitude during evaluation
	Mood
	Affect
	Thought content (delusions, obsessions, paranoia, suicidality, aggressive ideations)
	Thought process (abstractions, loose associations, flight of ideas, concrete)
	Perceptual disturbances (hallucinations)
Cognition	Concentration/calculations
	Information/intellect
	Long-term memory (anniversary, where born, current events over last year)
	Short-term memory (yesterday, meals)
	Immediate memory (identify and repeat three objects now and after 5 minutes)
	Judgment
	Insight

Table 1–2.   Diagnostic assessment tools

Laboratory studies (for medication monitoring, use ICD-9-CM diagnostic code V58.69)

> Complete blood count with differential
>
> Comprehensive metabolic panel
>
> Lipid panel
>
> Triiodothyronine, thyroxine, thyroid-stimulating hormone
>
> Hemoglobin A_{1c}
>
> β-Human chorionic gonadotropin (in females of reproductive age; qualitative and quantitative)
>
> Serum toxicology (including ethanol and tetrahydrocannabinol)

Laboratory studies if clinically indicated

> Prolactin level (specify pediatric or adult)
>
> Epstein-Barr virus titer (qualitative and quantitative)
>
> HIV titer
>
> Lyme disease titer
>
> Any medication levels (lithium, valproic acid, carbamazepine)

Other studies

> Electrocardiogram
>
> Electroencephalogram
>
> Polysomnography
>
> Computed tomographic scan of brain
>
> Magnetic resonance image of brain

Note.   Prescription should include patient's diagnosis (ICD-9 [World Health Organization 1977] code) and rationale for test.

In today's society, many patients present to prescribing clinicians seeking a "quick fix" with medication. These experiences are often quite difficult for the APRN to negotiate because the patient may be demanding or directing the course of treatment to include medication, when the APRN does not believe that a psychotropic is indicated. Again, the APRN must use his or her best clinical judgment to offer the patient a sound rationale for the treatment plan being presented. The decision not to prescribe may potentially lead to the loss (to the practice, not suicide) of a patient who was solely seeking medication intervention. If the assessment and symptoms do not warrant the prescribing of a psychotropic medication, APRNs should not feel compelled to prescribe. At times, this is the most appropriate decision to protect both the APRN's practice and the patient's overall health and well-being.

Medications and the U.S. Food and Drug Administration

The U.S. Food and Drug Administration (FDA) oversees the security, safety, and efficacy of every pharmaceutical agent that finds its place on a pharmacy shelf. For the purposes of this text, three types of agents receive FDA oversight relevant to pharmacotherapy in live patients: human drugs, medical foods, and dietary supplements. The FDA is also responsible for approving bioequivalent drug products, commonly known as *generics,* before they appear on the shelves of pharmacies. Although various adverse events or side effects may come to the forefront when a patented medication is released and used within the general population, there has been much recent controversy regarding the efficacy and, to a more limited extent, safety of bioequivalent drug products. According to the U.S. Food and Drug Administration Center for Drug Evaluation and Research (2012), for a drug to be approved as a generic pharmaceutical equivalent or alternative product, "the drug must not show a significant difference from the rate and extent of absorption of the original reference drug when administered at the same dose of the therapeutic ingredient under similar experimental conditions" (p. 9). In testing bioequivalent generic pharmaceuticals, the FDA and medical experts determined that a difference of greater than 20% would be deemed significant, and the generic drug would not be approved in that case. With this in mind, the prudent practitioner will carefully monitor his or her patient for any changes in symptoms and if breakthrough symptoms occur, will question the patient about any changes to the prescription labeling and appearance of the medication.

Therapeutic Equivalence Evaluation Codes

The coding system for therapeutic equivalence evaluations is constructed to allow users to determine quickly whether the FDA has evaluated a particular approved product as therapeutically equivalent to other pharmaceutically equivalent products and to provide additional information on the basis of the FDA's evaluations.

- "A" drug products are those that the FDA considers to be therapeutically equivalent to other pharmaceutically equivalent products.
- "AB" drug products are those that the FDA determined had actual or potential bioequivalence problems, which have been resolved with adequate in vivo or in vitro evidence supporting bioequivalence.
- "B" drug products are those that the FDA considers *not* to be therapeutically equivalent to other pharmaceutically equivalent products. Often the problem is with specific dosage forms rather than with the active ingredients (U.S. Food and Drug Administration 2012).

Medical Foods

The Orphan Drug Amendments of 1988 defined *medical food* as a food that is formulated to be consumed or administered under the supervision of a physician and intended for the specific dietary management of a disease or condition for which distinctive nutritional requirements, based on recognized scientific principles, are established by medical evaluation. All ingredients must be generally recognized as safe or approved food additives. A few medical foods pertain to psychiatry: L-methylfolate (Deplin) is used in the augmentation of antidepressants, and L-methylfolate/methylcobalamin/N-acetylcysteine (CerefolinNAC) and caprylidene (Axona) are used in the treatment of cognitive decline in the elderly.

Dietary Supplements

Although dietary supplements fall under the FDA's "umbrella" of foods, they are not conventional foods and cannot constitute the sole item of a meal or diet but rather supplement one's nutrition (U.S. Food and Drug Administration 2010). Unlike medical foods, dietary supplements do not require FDA approval before becoming available to the public, so the FDA cannot guarantee the safety or efficacy of these products (U.S. Food and Drug Administration 2012).

Controlled Substances

APRNs in all but two states, Alabama and Florida, are able to prescribe some medications classified as controlled substances. Definitions and examples of drugs in each of the U.S. Drug Enforcement Administration (DEA) Controlled Substance Schedules are shown in Table 1–3. Some of these agents play a large role in the treatment of psychiatric illnesses. The psychostimulants, used in the treatment of attention-deficit/hyperactivity disorder, are primarily Schedule II controlled substances. The benzodiazepines, used in the treatment of anxiety and panic disorders, psychiatric emergencies, and detoxification from alcohol and other substances of abuse, are Schedule IV controlled substances. These are just two examples of the use of controlled substance psychotropic medications in the treatment of psychiatric symptoms. Some states require additional training before APRNs can obtain their controlled substances license or certification or their DEA certification (U.S. Department of Justice Drug Enforcement Administration Office of Diversion Control ND). As described in Table 1–3, the DEA regulates the controlled substances to guard against abuse, misuse, diversion, and dependence. With the comprehensive training and holistic approach to prescribing used by APRNs, these risk factors are seemingly quite low.

Black Box Warnings

The FDA, as the overseer of drug safety and efficacy in the United States, issues black box warnings when a drug may pose potentially serious or life-threatening adverse events. Because this list is ever-changing, readers should refer to www.FDA.gov for the most current information. Table 1–4 presents a list of the current (as of the date of publication) U.S. Food and Drug Administration black box warnings issued for psychotropic drugs.

Table 1–3.   Definitions of controlled substance schedules

Schedule I substances

Schedule I drugs, substances, or chemicals are defined as drugs with no currently accepted medical use and a high potential for abuse. Schedule I drugs are the most dangerous drugs of all the drug schedules with potentially severe psychological or physical dependence. Examples of Schedule I drugs include heroin, lysergic acid diethylamide (LSD), marijuana (cannabis), 3,4-methylenedioxymethamphetamine (ecstasy), and peyote.

Schedule II substances

Schedule II drugs, substances, or chemicals are defined as drugs with a high potential for abuse, less abuse potential than Schedule I drugs, with use potentially leading to severe psychological or physical dependence. These drugs are also considered dangerous. Examples of Schedule II drugs include cocaine, methamphetamine, methadone, hydromorphone (Dilaudid), meperidine (Demerol), oxycodone (OxyContin), fentanyl, Dexedrine, Adderall, and Ritalin.

Schedule III substances

Schedule III drugs, substances, or chemicals are defined as drugs with a moderate to low potential for physical and psychological dependence. The abuse potential of Schedule III drugs is less than that of Schedule I and Schedule II drugs but more than that of Schedule IV drugs. Examples of Schedule III drugs include combination products with less than 15 milligrams of hydrocodone per dosage unit (e.g., Vicodin), products containing less than 90 milligrams of codeine per dosage unit (e.g., Tylenol with codeine), ketamine, anabolic steroids, and testosterone.

Schedule IV substances

Schedule IV drugs, substances, or chemicals are defined as drugs with a low potential for abuse and low risk of dependence. Examples of Schedule IV drugs include alprazolam (Xanax), diazepam (Valium), lorazepam (Ativan), zolpidem (Ambien), modafinil (Provigil), and carisoprodol (Soma).

Schedule V substances

Schedule V drugs, substances, or chemicals are defined as drugs with lower potential for abuse than Schedule IV drugs and consist of preparations containing limited quantities of certain narcotics. Schedule V drugs are generally used for antidiarrheal, antitussive, and analgesic purposes. Examples of Schedule V drugs include cough preparations with less than 200 milligrams of codeine or per 100 milliliters (e.g, Robitussin AC), Lomotil, pregabalin (Lyrica), and Parapectolin.

Source.   Adapted from U.S. Drug Enforcement Administration ND.

Table 1-4.   Black box warnings for psychotropic drugs

Increased risk of suicidality (suicidal thinking and behavior) in children, adolescents, and young adults

Selective serotonin reuptake inhibitor antidepressants

Citalopram, escitalopram, fluoxetine, fluvoxamine, paroxetine, sertraline, vilazodone

Tri- and heterocyclic antidepressants

Amitriptyline, clomipramine, desipramine, doxepin, imipramine, nortriptyline, trazodone

Monoamine oxidase inhibitor antidepressants

Isocarboxazid, phenelzine, selegiline, tranylcypromine

Other antidepressants

Bupropion hydrobromide, bupropion hydrochloride, desvenlafaxine, duloxetine, mirtazapine, nefazodone, venlafaxine

Second-generation (atypical) antipsychotics

Aripiprazole, olanzapine/fluoxetine, quetiapine

Other agents

Atomoxetine

Increased risk of mortality in elderly with dementia-related psychosis

All first-generation (typical) antipsychotics

Chlorpromazine, fluphenazine, haloperidol, loxapine, perphenazine, pimozide, thioridazine, thiothixene, trifluoperazine

All second-generation (atypical) antipsychotics

Aripiprazole, asenapine, clozapine, iloperidone, lurasidone, olanzapine, paliperidone, quetiapine, risperidone, ziprasidone

High potential for abuse and dependence with misuse; and misuse may lead to sudden death or serious cardiovascular events

All formulations of psychostimulant medications

Dexmethylphenidate, dextroamphetamine, dextroamphetamine/amphetamine, lisdexamfetamine, methylphenidate

Table 1–4.   Black box warnings for psychotropic drugs *(continued)*

Life-threatening hepatic failure/potential for severe liver injury
Atomoxetine (bolded,* not black box), nefazodone
Serious dermatological reaction, including toxic epidermal necrolysis and Stevens-Johnson syndrome
Carbamazepine, lamotrigine
Aplastic anemia and agranulocytosis
Carbamazepine, clozapine
Orthostatic hypotension, seizures, and convulsions
Clozapine

*Bolded warnings are significant but not as serious as black box warnings.

Neuroanatomy and Neurochemistry

The brain is arguably the most complex and least understood organ in the human body (see Figure A1–1 in the appendix to this chapter). Because no serum diagnostic tests offer definitive information about the origin or extent of the various psychiatric symptoms and diagnoses, much of the treatment process is trial and error. Through the "decade of the brain" in the 1990s, the field of psychiatry experienced its first real period of growth with the advent of a new class of antidepressants, the selective serotonin reuptake inhibitors. The field of psychopharmacology expanded with more discussion of the neuroscience behind the prescription medications. Although the monoamine hypothesis of mental illness was presented many decades earlier, in the 1990s serotonin, norepinephrine, and dopamine became common language in the field. Figure A1–2 in the appendix at the end of this chapter depicts these three major neuropathways, which are influential in regulating our mood, thoughts, and behaviors. Finally, in addition to the three major neurotransmitters, a number of other psychoactive neurotransmitters (Table 1–5) are discussed throughout this text. Information about these neurotransmitters, their pathways, and the brain structures from which they originate, in addition to their influence on the mood, thought patterns, and behavioral symptoms presented by patients, will serve as a guide for prudent prescribing of psychotropic medications.

Table 1–5.   Endogenous neurotransmitters

Neurotransmitter	Receptor binding	Distribution	Neuronal effects	Influences and effects
Serotonin (5-HT)	5-HT$_1$, 5-HT$_{1A}$, 5-HT$_{1B}$, 5-HT$_{1D}$, 5-HT$_{1E}$, 5-HT$_{1F}$	Brain, GI system, blood vessels	Inhibitory	Deficiency may contribute to mood dysregulation, sexual dysfunction, increased impulsivity, aggression and anxiety, sleep and appetite disturbance, addiction, problems with memory and learning
	5-HT$_2$, 5-HT$_{2A}$, 5-HT$_{2B}$, 5-HT$_{2C}$	Brain, GI system, blood vessels, heart, lungs, smooth muscles	Excitatory	Deficiency may contribute to mood dysregulation, increased anxiety, sleep and appetite disturbance, addiction, sexual dysfunction
	5-HT$_3$	Limbic system, CNS, PNS, GI system	Excitatory	Deficiency may contribute to increased anxiety, addiction, problems with learning and memory
	5-HT$_4$	CNS, GI system, smooth muscles	Excitatory	Deficiency may contribute to increased anxiety, mood dysregulation, learning and memory deficits, changes in appetite
	5-HT$_5$, 5-HT$_{5A}$	Brain	Inhibitory	Deficiency may contribute to sleep disturbances

Table 1–5. Endogenous neurotransmitters (*continued*)

Neurotransmitter	Receptor binding	Distribution	Neuronal effects	Influences and effects
Serotonin (5-HT) (*continued*)	5-HT$_6$	CNS	Inhibitory	Deficiency may contribute to mood dysregulation; increased anxiety; problems with memory, cognition, and learning
	5-HT$_7$	CNS, GI system, blood vessels	Excitatory	Deficiency may contribute to mood dysregulation, sleep disturbances, increased anxiety, memory deficits
Norepinephrine	α_1	Brain, heart, smooth muscles	Excitatory	Deficiency may contribute to disruption of sleep-wake cycle, increased dreaming and arousal, increased depression and suicidality, deficits in attention and concentration, psychomotor agitation or retardation
	α_2	Presynaptic neurons, smooth muscles, pancreas	Inhibitory	
	β_1	Brain, heart	Excitatory	
	β_2	Brain, lungs, skeletal muscles	Excitatory	
	β_3	Adipose tissue	Excitatory	

Table 1–5. Endogenous neurotransmitters *(continued)*

Neurotransmitter	Receptor binding	Distribution	Neuronal effects	Influences and effects
Dopamine	D_1, D_5	Brain, smooth muscles	Excitatory	Deficiency may contribute to positive symptoms of schizophrenia, deficits in memory Excess may contribute to movement disorders (e.g., Parkinson's)
	D_2, D_3, D_4	Brain, presynaptic terminals, cardiovascular system	Inhibitory	Deficiency may contribute to addiction, apathy, psychosis, attention and behavioral disorders, diminished concentration, decreased appetite
Glutamate	AMPA, NMDA, kainate	CNS	Excitatory	Deficiency may contribute to disrupted sleep-wake cycle, deficits in memory and learning, low energy, addiction Excess may contribute to increased anger, aggression, and impulsivity; potential disorders such as Parkinson's and multiple sclerosis
γ-Aminobutyric acid (GABA)	$GABA_A$	CNS	Inhibitory	Deficiency may contribute to sedation, sleep disturbance, increased psychosis
	$GABA_B$	ANS	Excitatory	Excess may contribute to increased anxiety and agitation, euphoria, perceptual disturbances, ataxia and tremor

Table 1–5.   Endogenous neurotransmitters (continued)

Neurotransmitter	Receptor binding	Distribution	Neuronal effects	Influences and effects
Histamine	H_1, H_2, H_3	Hypothalamus	Excitatory	Deficiency may contribute to sedation, somnolence, cognitive dulling, increased appetite/weight gain Excess may contribute to restlessness, insomnia, enhanced mental clarity, improved attention and concentration
Acetylcholine	Muscarinic (M)			Deficiency may contribute to cognitive deficits, dementia Excess may contribute to increased anxiety, parasympathetic overactivity
	M_1	CNS, ganglia, secretory glands	Excitatory	
	M_2	Nerves, heart, smooth muscle	Inhibitory	
	M_3	Endothelium smooth muscle, secretory glands	Excitatory	
	M_4	CNS, PNS, smooth muscles, secretory glands	Inhibitory	
	M_5	CNS	Inhibitory	

Table 1–5. Endogenous neurotransmitters *(continued)*

Neurotransmitter	Receptor binding	Distribution	Neuronal effects	Influences and effects
Acetylcholine *(continued)*	Nicotinic (N)			Deficiency may contribute to cognitive deficits, decreases in attention and concentration
	N_1	Neuromuscular junctions, skeletal muscles	Excitatory	Excess may contribute to increased attention, decreased impulsivity, addiction
	N_2	Adrenal medulla, ganglia, CNS	Excitatory	

Note. AMPA = α-amino-3-hydroxy-5-methyl-4-isoxazolepropionic acid; ANS = autonomic nervous system; CNS = central nervous system; GI = gastrointestinal; NMDA = *N*-methyl-D-aspartate; PNS = peripheral nervous system.

Genetic Markers in Psychiatry

One of the newest areas of discovery in psychiatry involves the use of genotyping, which serves to offer information related to an individual's ability to synthesize and use the various neurotransmitters and enzymes related to drug metabolism. Psychiatric pharmacogenomics can reduce the trial-and-error prescribing used by many clinicians, which may reduce the number of medication trials for the patient and improve patient outcomes and mental well-being. (Refer to Appendix 3, "Psychopharmacogenetic Variations: Implications for Practice," for further information on genetic markers.) Pharmacogenetics may reduce the incidence of drug adverse events through the provision of data related to a drug's metabolism or its interactions with other drugs the patient may be prescribed. Possibly one of the most important aspects of the use of genetic testing in psychiatry is the validation our patients experience when their genotype supports their symptoms and experiences with the psychotropics, and the patient subsequently realizes "it hasn't all been in my head." Genotyping in psychiatry serves to validate the psychiatric disorders as medical in origin! This is a relatively new science in the field of psychiatry, but it is the closest we have come to being able to offer patients a meaningful test on an outpatient basis that will offer concrete data on the innermost workings of our patients' bodies and minds.

Basic Pharmacological Terminology

Pharmacokinetics is what the body does to a drug, resulting in a concentration of the drug in the body. This process is accomplished through four mechanisms: absorption, distribution, metabolism, and excretion.

1. *Absorption* is the process by which a substance enters the circulatory system.
2. *Distribution* is the dispersion of a substance throughout the body's fluids and tissues.
3. *Metabolism* is sometimes referred to as *biotransformation,* which is the irreversible transformation of a parent compound into its metabolites mostly through the liver. Major forms of hepatic metabolism include oxidation via various cytochrome P450 enzymes or conjugation reactions.
4. *Excretion* is the elimination of the substance from the body.

Both metabolism and excretion are dependent on the functioning of the liver and kidneys. A medication's *half-life* also plays an important role in the metabolism and excretion of the medication. The half-life refers to the amount of time it takes for 50% of the drug to be eliminated from the body. A medication's half-life may contribute to overdose or toxicity if the half-life is considerably long, as is the case with fluoxetine. Half-life is also critical in determining the dosing frequency and time to achieve steady state.

Pharmacodynamics is what the drug does to the body. Pharmacodynamics determine the potential therapeutic benefit or adverse events the drug may produce in the body.

Titration is the process by which the drug is increased to achieve therapeutic benefits without adverse events. Nurses have historically learned to "start low and go slow" when titrating their patients' medication dosages.

Augmentation refers to the addition of a drug to the current regimen to improve the therapeutic benefits of the original compound. The process of augmentation has been used to improve the outcomes of patients with treatment-resistant depression. Agents such as lithium, levothyroxine, alternative antidepressant drugs, and, more recently, atypical antipsychotics have been used to augment antidepressant pharmacotherapies.

Discontinuation refers to the stopping of a psychotropic medication because of adverse events, remission, or other reasons. For most psychotropic medications, the process of discontinuation is essentially the reverse of the initial drug titration process. A gradual reduction in the medication dosage over time typically allows the patient to stop the medication safely and comfortably. At times, patients may decide to abruptly discontinue their medications. They should be cautioned against this practice because of potential adverse events, including, in the extreme, death, depending on the psychotropic medication.

Special Considerations in Psychopharmacological Prescribing

In the field of psychiatric nursing, clinicians approach patients from a holistic perspective. Each patient is unique and requires careful consideration of his or her own specific characteristics. This is commonly accepted among APRNs, but a few patient populations require further expansion: children, elderly patients, medically fragile patients, and women who are pregnant or nursing.

For many decades, psychiatric prescribers have written prescriptions for children and adolescents despite the lack of FDA indications and approvals. Much of the evidence related to prescribing psychotropics to children is anecdotal. It is well known that children manifest symptoms of psychiatric illnesses, but only a small minority of these children ever receive treatment—medication or therapy. Most of the psychotropics prescribed to children and adolescents are considered "off-label," and this fact should be disclosed to the parents or guardians and noted in the medical record when prescribing. Despite the lack of FDA approval for use in children and adolescents, many of the psychotropics have improved their symptoms and overall quality of life. Additionally, for the most part, children are able to metabolize medications with great efficiency. This idea needs to be taken into consideration when prescribing to this population. In any case, however, the psychiatric APRN must use his or her own best clinical judgment in deciding to prescribe to children and adolescents.

The elderly also present unique challenges to the prescribing psychiatric APRN. Unlike children, older individuals may metabolize medications less efficiently and be more prone to adverse effects of the psychotropic medications. Dosing of the psychotropics often requires downward adjustment to avoid side effects and potential toxicity. The aging population in the United States also may have multiple medical comorbidities and thus multiple medications, which may induce side effects that mimic the symptoms of psychiatric illness. As "scientists," psychiatric APRNs need to thoroughly investigate the origin of psychiatric symptoms in the elderly so as not to complicate the clinical picture further by adding medication when the symptoms may warrant medication discontinuation. Another consideration in prescribing for this population is the potential for inadvertent abuse. Because it may not always be clear which medications are current and which have been discontinued, the patient may unknowingly be taking more medication than prescribed. The elderly patient also may have forgotten if he or she took the medication, which may lead to additional dosing. Psychiatric APRNs provide education to patients and their caregivers, and these scenarios should not be overlooked.

Patients who are medically compromised certainly offer a challenge to the prescriber. When a patient is already taking a medication, the addition of a psychotropic medication, with its own constellation of potential side effects and unique metabolism, may potentiate a drug-drug interaction. Whenever possible, it is best to delay use of the psychotropics until the patient is deemed medically stable. When the medically compromised patient has a comorbid psychiatric illness, polypharmacy may be unavoidable. Again, exploring the metabolics of all pharmaceutical agents, including over-the-counter medications and supplements, and their potential interactions is imperative before prescribing.

Women who are pregnant, attempting to become pregnant, or breast-feeding an infant present with their own set of advisements. The psychiatric APRN must be cognizant that he or she is now prescribing for two individuals—mother and infant. Most clinicians attempt to avoid prescribing to women during this period; however, the potential risks and benefits of the effect of the woman's symptoms on both herself and her fetus/newborn need to be considered. Untreated mental illness during pregnancy may lead to premature labor and lower-birth-weight infants, greater risk for postpartum depression, and potentially postpartum psychosis. Although most psychotropic medications are Category C for pregnancy (Table 1–6), many studies have documented the safety and efficacy in pregnant and nursing women. Psychiatric APRNs are known to collaborate with professionals of other disciplines, and this would be a prime time to collaborate with the woman's obstetrical provider.

Summary

Each chapter in the *Manual of Clinical Psychopharmacology for Nurses* offers an overview of the symptoms and disorders that the various psychotropic agents are intended to treat. A review of the specific neurochemistry and neuropathways provides the scientific basis to aid the psychiatric APRN in making appropriate prescribing choices. The pharmacokinetics and pharmacodynamics of each drug class are explored and provide the APRN with guidelines on how the drug will affect the patient and how the patient's body will metabolize the psychotropic agent. Because psychiatric APRNs view patients from a holistic perspective, the unique characteristics of the various patient populations are identified, and treatment monitoring guidelines are provided. Finally, clinical pearls are offered by APRNs clinically working with and prescribing to patients across the life span with symptoms of psychiatric illness.

Table 1–6. U.S. Food and Drug Administration (FDA) pregnancy risk categories

Category A

Adequate and well-controlled studies have failed to show a risk to the fetus in the first trimester of pregnancy (and no evidence of risk is seen in later trimesters).

Category B

Animal reproduction studies have failed to show a risk to the fetus, and no adequate and well-controlled studies have been done in pregnant women.

Category C

Animal reproduction studies have shown an adverse effect on the fetus, and no adequate and well-controlled studies have been done in humans, but potential benefits may warrant use of the drug in pregnant women despite potential risks.

Category D

Positive evidence of human fetal risk is based on adverse reaction data from investigational or marketing experience or studies in humans, but potential benefits may warrant use of the drug in pregnant women despite potential risks.

Category X

Studies in animals or humans have reported fetal abnormalities, or positive evidence of human fetal risk is based on adverse reaction data from investigational or marketing experience, and the risks involved in use of the drug in pregnant women clearly outweigh the potential benefits.

Source.   Adapted from U.S. Food and Drug Administration ND.

References

American Association of Colleges of Nursing: The Essentials of Master's Education for Advanced Practice Nursing (task force report). 1996. Available at: http://www.aacn.nche.edu/education-resources/MasEssentials96.pdf. Accessed March 3, 2012.

Driscoll B: Are APPs just as capable? QuantiaMD. February 2012. Available at: https://secure.quantiamd.com/player/tdgdkget?cid=53. Accessed March 20, 2012.

Lyon BL: Clinical reasoning model: a clinical inquiry guide for solving problems in the nursing domain, in Foundation of Clinical Nurse Specialist Practice. Edited by Fulton JS, Lyon BL, Goudreau KA. New York, Springer, 2010, pp 61–76

National Association of Clinical Nurse Specialists: Statement on Clinical Nurse Specialist Practice and Education, 2nd Edition. Harrisburg, PA, NACNS, 2004. Available at: http://journals.lww.com/cns-journal/Documents/CNS%20Statement%202004.pdf. Accessed March 3, 2012.

Roberts LW, Jain S: Ethical issues in psychopharmacology. Psychiatric Times 28(5):1–10, 2011

U.S. Department of Justice Drug Enforcement Administration Office of Diversion Control: Definition of controlled substance schedules. ND. Available at: http://www.deadiversion.usdoj.gov/schedules/index.html#define. Accessed January 2, 2013.

U.S. Food and Drug Administration: FDA Pregnancy Categories. ND. Available at: http://depts.washington.edu/druginfo/Formulary/Pregnancy.pdf. Accessed January 14, 2012.

U.S. Food and Drug Administration: Dietary supplements. 2010. Available at: http://www.fda.gov/AboutFDA/Transparency/Basics/ucm193949.htm. Accessed January 14, 2012.

U.S. Food and Drug Administration Center for Drug Evaluation and Research: Orange Book Preface (from Approved Drug Products With Therapeutic Equivalence Evaluations, 32nd Edition. 2012). Available at: http://www.fda.gov/Drugs/DevelopmentApprovalProcess/ucm079068.htm#Bioequivalent%20Drug%20Products. Accessed January 14, 2012.

World Health Organization: International Classification of Diseases, 9th Revision. Geneva, World Health Organization, 1977

World Health Organization: International Classification of Diseases, 9th Revision, Clinical Modification. Ann Arbor, MI, Commission on Professional and Hospital Activities, 1978

Appendix: Brain Structures and Pathways

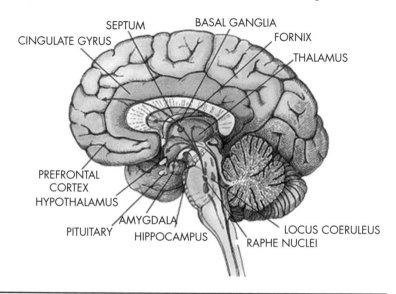

Figure A1–1.   Brain structures and functions.

Amygdala—activates fight-or-flight response arousal, emotional regulation, hormonal secretion; links memories with emotional relevance

Basal ganglia—composed of striatum, pallidum, substantia nigra, and subthalamic nucleus; modulates goal-directed motoric behaviors, coordination, procedural memory, cognition

Cingulate gyrus—coordinates sensory input with emotions, regulates aggressive behaviors, controls emotional responses to pain

Fornix—connects hippocampus to mammillary bodies, regulates episodic memory

Hippocampus—consolidates new memories; stores long-term memories; regulates navigation and spatial orientation; vulnerable to aging, stress, disease

Hypothalamus—regulates sleep-wake cycle, food and water intake, temperature, blood pressure, rage, libido

Figure A1–1.   Brain structures and functions *(continued).*

Locus coeruleus—mediates sympathetic response to stress/panic; regulates depression and anxiety; activated during opiate withdrawal

Pituitary—"master gland" that regulates endocrine function; stores hormones produced by hypothalamus; produces growth hormone and hormones that act on muscles, kidneys, and other endocrine glands

Prefrontal cortex—dorsal lateral prefrontal cortex ("executive functioning," judgment, problem solving, analysis, motor functioning), orbital prefrontal cortex (attention and impulse inhibition), ventral medial prefrontal cortex (emotional processing)

Raphe nucleus—regulates homeostasis; part of endogenous opiate system; regulates pain, especially in the spinal cord

Septum—part of limbic system, no particular functional effects on its own

Thalamus—major relay station for motor control, auditory, visual, and somatosensory signals and sensory perception; mediates sleep-wake cycle

Source.   Image ©Carol Donner. Used with permission.

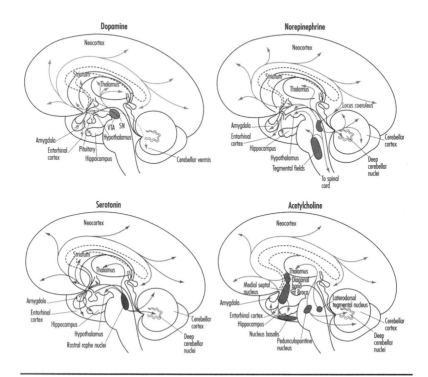

Figure A1–2.   Neurotransmitter pathways.

Dopamine pathways

Mesolimbic pathway—ventral tegmental area (VTA), nucleus accumbens, amygdala, and hippocampus; involved in regulating pleasure, reward, and addiction

Mesocortical pathway—VTA, prefrontal cortex, and frontal lobe; regulates motivation and emotional responses

Nigrostriatal pathway—substantia nigra (SN), caudate nucleus, putamen, and striatum; involved in movement via basal ganglia motor loop

Tuberoinfundibular pathway—hypothalamus to pituitary gland; regulates secretion of prolactin

Figure A1–2. Neurotransmitter pathways *(continued)*.

Serotonin pathways

Caudal pathway—raphe nucleus, medulla, and spinal cord; regulates muscle contractions, stimulates release of endorphins, and may trigger emesis
Middle pathway—raphe nucleus to cerebral cortex and basal ganglia; regulates mood and affect
Rostral pathway—raphe nucleus to one of five areas: raphe nuclei (self-inhibits), sensory cortex (perceptual disturbances and hallucinations), limbic system (pleasure and anxiety), hypothalamus and thalamus (thermoregulation), or suprachiasmatic nucleus (sleep-wake cycle)

Norepinephrine pathways

Locus coeruleus—spinal cord, thalamus, hypothalamus, striatum, cingulate gyrus, cingulum, hippocampus, and amygdala; regulates arousal, vigilance, and reward
Lateral tegmental area—extends to hypothalamus; regulates arousal and reactivity to stimuli

Acetylcholine pathways

Dorsolateral tegmental nuclei—Muscarinic M_1 receptors in brain stem, cerebellum, raphe nucleus, lateral reticular nucleus, thalamus, basal ganglia, and basal forebrain; regulates learning, short-term memory, arousal, and reward
Basal optic nucleus of Meynert—Muscarinic M_1 receptors in neocortex; regulates learning and short-term memory
Medial septal nuclei—Muscarinic M_1 receptors in neocortex and hippocampus; regulates learning and memory

Histamine pathways (not shown in figure)

Tuberomammillary nucleus of the hypothalamus—extends to prefrontal cortex, thalamus, and brain stem; regulates sleep-wake cycle, thermoregulation, motor activity, learning, self-stimulation, pain perception, stress, and aggression and modulates blood pressure

Source. Image caption adapted from Heimer L: *The Human Brain and Spinal Cord: Functional Neuroanatomy and Dissection Guide,* 2nd Edition. New York, Springer-Verlag, 1995.
Image reprinted from Melchitzky DS, Lewis DA: "Chemical Neuroanatomy of the Primate Brain," in *The American Psychiatric Publishing Textbook of Psychopharmacology,* 4th Edition. Edited by Schatzberg AF, Nemeroff CB. Washington, DC, American Psychiatric Publishing, 2009, pp. 105–134 (Figure 4–1; p. 107). Used with permission.

PART I

Psychopharmacological
Treatment and Management
of Psychiatric Disorders

2

Anxiety Disorders

Sarah Seabrook-de Jong, M.S.N., A.P.R.N., P.M.H.-C.N.S./F.N.P., B.C.

Heavy thoughts bring on physical maladies;
when the soul is oppressed, so is the body.

—Martin Luther

Anxiety disorders affect about 40 million adult Americans (about 18%) in a given year (National Institute of Mental Health 2009). Anxiety is a state of arousal or feeling of fear or uncertainty that occurs in response to a threatening event or situation. The threat can be real or perceived. Anxiety disorders are diagnosed when the state of anxiety persists over time and when the threat or perceived threat is no longer present (Cabrera and Schub 2011). The onset of anxiety disorders often occurs by early adulthood and is more common in women than in men.

Table 2–1. Epidemiology of anxiety disorders

Panic disorder	Affects 6 million adult Americans
	Appears to be inherited
	Begins in late adolescence or early adulthood
	Twice as common in women as in men
Specific phobia	Affects 19.2 million adult Americans
	Tends to run in families
	Twice as common in women as in men
	Appears in childhood or adolescence; persists into adulthood
Social phobia	Affects 15 million adult Americans
	Evidence supports genetic involvement
	Affects men and women equally
	Usually develops in childhood or early adolescence
Obsessive-compulsive disorder (OCD)	Affects 2.2 million adult Americans
	May run in families
	Affects men and women equally
	One-third of adults with OCD develop symptoms as children
Generalized anxiety disorder	Affects 6.8 million adult Americans
	Can develop at any point in the life cycle
	Twice as common in women as in men
	Highest risk is between childhood and middle age

Source. Adapted from National Institute of Mental Health 2009.

Overview of Anxiety Disorders

Symptoms frequently associated with anxiety disorders include feelings of doom, fear, worry, restlessness, insomnia, irritability, impaired concentration, sweating, tachycardia, tremors, and dyspnea (Cabrera and Schub 2011). Notably, these symptoms appear not only in other mental disorders but also in medical conditions; this overlap can significantly complicate the diagnostic picture and subsequent treatment options. Table 2–1 offers an overview of the epidemiology of common anxiety disorders.

Table 2–2.   DSM-IV-TR diagnostic criteria for panic disorder with (300.21) or without (300.01) agoraphobia

A.   Both (1) and (2):

   (1)   recurrent unexpected panic attacks

   (2)   at least one of the attacks has been followed by 1 month (or more) of one (or more) of the following:

      (a)   persistent concern about having additional attacks

      (b)   worry about the implications of the attack or its consequences (e.g., losing control, having a heart attack, "going crazy")

      (c)   a significant change in behavior related to the attacks

B.   Presence (300.21) or absence (300.01) of agoraphobia

C.   The panic attacks are not due to the direct physiological effects of a substance (e.g., a drug of abuse, a medication) or a general medical condition (e.g., hyperthyroidism).

D.   The panic attacks are not better accounted for by another mental disorder, such as social phobia (e.g., occurring on exposure to feared social situations), specific phobia (e.g., on exposure to a specific phobic situation), obsessive-compulsive disorder (e.g., on exposure to dirt in someone with an obsession about contamination), posttraumatic stress disorder (e.g., in response to stimuli associated with a severe stressor), or separation anxiety disorder (e.g., in response to being away from home or close relatives).

DSM-IV-TR (American Psychiatric Association 2000) includes criteria for the following anxiety disorders:

- Panic disorder with or without agoraphobia (Table 2–2)
- Agoraphobia without history of panic disorder
- Specific phobia (Table 2–3)
- Social phobia (Table 2–4)
- Obsessive-compulsive disorder (Table 2–5)
- Posttraumatic stress disorder (see Chapter 9, "Trauma and Posttraumatic Stress Disorder")
- Acute stress disorder (see Chapter 9, "Trauma and Posttraumatic Stress Disorder")
- Generalized anxiety disorder (Table 2–6)
- Anxiety disorder due to a general medical condition (Table 2–7)
- Substance-induced anxiety disorder
- Anxiety disorder not otherwise specified

Table 2–3.   DSM-IV-TR diagnostic criteria for 300.29 specific phobia

A.   Marked and persistent fear that is excessive or unreasonable, cued by the presence or anticipation of a specific object or situation (e.g., flying, heights, animals, receiving an injection, seeing blood).

B.   Exposure to the phobic stimulus almost invariably provokes an immediate anxiety response, which may take the form of a situationally bound or situationally predisposed panic attack.   **Note:** In children, the anxiety may be expressed by crying, tantrums, freezing, or clinging.

C.   The person recognizes that the fear is excessive or unreasonable.   **Note:** In children, this feature may be absent.

D.   The phobic situation(s) is avoided or else is endured with intense anxiety or distress.

E.   The avoidance, anxious anticipation, or distress in the feared situation(s) interferes significantly with the person's normal routine, occupational (or academic) functioning, or social activities or relationships, or there is marked distress about having the phobia.

F.   In individuals under age 18 years, the duration is at least 6 months.

G.   The anxiety, panic attacks, or phobic avoidance associated with the specific object or situation are not better accounted for by another mental disorder, such as obsessive-compulsive disorder (e.g., fear of dirt in someone with an obsession about contamination), posttraumatic stress disorder (e.g., avoidance of stimuli associated with a severe stressor), separation anxiety disorder (e.g., avoidance of school), social phobia (e.g., avoidance of social situations because of fear of embarrassment), panic disorder with agoraphobia, or agoraphobia without history of panic disorder.

   Specify type:

   Animal Type

   Natural Environment Type (e.g., heights, storms, water)

   Blood-Injection-Injury Type

   Situational Type (e.g., airplanes, elevators, enclosed places)

   Other Type (e.g., fear of choking, vomiting, or contracting an illness; in children, fear of loud sounds or costumed characters)

Table 2–4.   DSM-IV-TR diagnostic criteria for 300.23 social phobia

A. A marked and persistent fear of one or more social or performance situations in which the person is exposed to unfamiliar people or to possible scrutiny by others. The individual fears that he or she will act in a way (or show anxiety symptoms) that will be humiliating or embarrassing.   **Note:** In children, there must be evidence of the capacity for age-appropriate social relationships with familiar people and the anxiety must occur in peer settings, not just in interactions with adults.

B. Exposure to the feared social situation almost invariably provokes anxiety, which may take the form of a situationally bound or situationally predisposed panic attack.   **Note:** In children, the anxiety may be expressed by crying, tantrums, freezing, or shrinking from social situations with unfamiliar people.

C. The person recognizes that the fear is excessive or unreasonable.   **Note:** In children, this feature may be absent.

D. The feared social or performance situations are avoided or else are endured with intense anxiety or distress.

E. The avoidance, anxious anticipation, or distress in the feared social or performance situation(s) interferes significantly with the person's normal routine, occupational (academic) functioning, or social activities or relationships, or there is marked distress about having the phobia.

F. In individuals under age 18 years, the duration is at least 6 months.

G. The fear or avoidance is not due to the direct physiological effects of a substance (e.g., a drug of abuse, a medication) or a general medical condition and is not better accounted for by another mental disorder (e.g., panic disorder with or without agoraphobia, separation anxiety disorder, body dysmorphic disorder, a pervasive developmental disorder, or schizoid personality disorder).

H. If a general medical condition or another mental disorder is present, the fear in criterion A is unrelated to it, e.g., the fear is not of stuttering, trembling in Parkinson's disease, or exhibiting abnormal eating behavior in anorexia nervosa or bulimia nervosa.

Specify if:

Generalized: if the fears include most social situations (also consider the additional diagnosis of avoidant personality disorder)

Table 2–5. DSM-IV-TR diagnostic criteria for 300.3 obsessive-compulsive disorder

A. Either obsessions or compulsions:

Obsessions as defined by (1), (2), (3), and (4):

(1) recurrent and persistent thoughts, impulses, or images that are experienced, at some time during the disturbance, as intrusive and inappropriate and that cause marked anxiety or distress

(2) the thoughts, impulses, or images are not simply excessive worries about real-life problems

(3) the person attempts to ignore or suppress such thoughts, impulses, or images, or to neutralize them with some other thought or action

(4) the person recognizes that the obsessional thoughts, impulses, or images are a product of his or her own mind (not imposed from without as in thought insertion)

Compulsions as defined by (1) and (2):

(1) repetitive behaviors (e.g., hand washing, ordering, checking) or mental acts (e.g., praying, counting, repeating words silently) that the person feels driven to perform in response to an obsession, or according to rules that must be applied rigidly

(2) the behaviors or mental acts are aimed at preventing or reducing distress or preventing some dreaded event or situation; however, these behaviors or mental acts either are not connected in a realistic way with what they are designed to neutralize or prevent or are clearly excessive

B. At some point during the course of the disorder, the person has recognized that the obsessions or compulsions are excessive or unreasonable. **Note:** This does not apply to children.

C. The obsessions or compulsions cause marked distress, are time consuming (take more than 1 hour a day), or significantly interfere with the person's normal routine, occupational (or academic) functioning, or usual social activities or relationships.

D. If another Axis I disorder is present, the content of the obsessions or compulsions is not restricted to it (e.g., preoccupation with food in the presence of an eating disorder; hair pulling in the presence of trichotillomania; concern with appearance in the presence of body dysmorphic disorder; preoccupation with drugs in the presence of a substance use disorder; preoccupation with having a serious illness in the presence of hypochondriasis; preoccupation with sexual urges or fantasies in the presence of a paraphilia; or guilty ruminations in the presence of major depressive disorder).

Table 2–5. DSM-IV-TR diagnostic criteria for 300.3 obsessive-compulsive disorder *(continued)*

E. The disturbance is not due to the direct physiological effects of a substance (e.g., a drug of abuse, a medication) or a general medical condition.

Specify if:

With Poor Insight: if, for most of the time during the current episode, the person does not recognize that the obsessions and compulsions are excessive or unreasonable

Neurobiology of Fear and Anxiety

The functional anatomy of anxiety involves amygdala-based neurocircuits with critical reciprocal connections to the medial prefrontal cortex. Traumatic experiences leave emotional imprints involving the amygdala, with facilitated fear-conditioned associations involving declarative memory traces. Avoidance conditioning is an additional component (Ninan 1999). Continued stressful circumstances can potentiate amygdala functioning, allowing it to become more powerful, at times exerting subcortical control over human cortical reasoning. This potentiated activity can exacerbate symptoms of mental illness. Chronic stress through kindling can create hard-wired, hypersensitive neural networks capable of directing and automating instinctual behavioral patterns. Kindling rewires the brain's circuitry, thus making permanent pathways that deviate from the typical route (Ninan 1999). Emotional memories are stored in the central part of the amygdala, where it is suggested that distinct fears (e.g., dogs, spiders, flying) are created. The hippocampus encodes threatening events into memories. Studies have shown that the hippocampus in some victims of child abuse and military combat appears smaller (National Institute of Mental Health 2009). Figure 2–1 illustrates the neuropathways associating fear and autonomic responses.

In a brain imaging study (Indovina et al. 2011), researchers from University of California–Berkeley and Cambridge University discovered two distinct neural pathways that play a role in whether we develop and overcome fears. The first involves an overactive amygdala, home to the brain's primal fight-or-flight reflex, which plays a role in developing phobias. The second involves activity in the ventral prefrontal cortex, a neural region that helps us to over-

Table 2–6.   DSM-IV-TR diagnostic criteria for 300.02 generalized anxiety disorder

A.   Excessive anxiety and worry (apprehensive expectation), occurring more days than not for at least 6 months, about a number of events or activities (such as work or school performance).

B.   The person finds it difficult to control the worry.

C.   The anxiety and worry are associated with three (or more) of the following six symptoms (with at least some symptoms present for more days than not for the past 6 months).   **Note:** Only one item is required in children.

   (1)   restlessness or feeling keyed up or on edge

   (2)   being easily fatigued

   (3)   difficulty concentrating or mind going blank

   (4)   irritability

   (5)   muscle tension

   (6)   sleep disturbance (difficulty falling or staying asleep, or restless unsatisfying sleep)

D.   The focus of the anxiety and worry is not confined to features of an Axis I disorder, e.g., the anxiety or worry is not about having a panic attack (as in panic disorder), being embarrassed in public (as in social phobia), being contaminated (as in obsessive-compulsive disorder), being away from home or close relatives (as in separation anxiety disorder), gaining weight (as in anorexia nervosa), having multiple physical complaints (as in somatization disorder), or having a serious illness (as in hypochondriasis), and the anxiety and worry do not occur exclusively during posttraumatic stress disorder.

E.   The anxiety, worry, or physical symptoms cause clinically significant distress or impairment in social, occupational, or other important areas of functioning.

F.   The disturbance is not due to the direct physiological effects of a substance (e.g., a drug of abuse, a medication) or a general medical condition (e.g., hyperthyroidism) and does not occur exclusively during a mood disorder, a psychotic disorder, or a pervasive developmental disorder.

Table 2–7. DSM-IV-TR diagnostic criteria for 293.84 anxiety disorder due to a general medical condition

A.   Prominent anxiety, panic attacks, or obsessions or compulsions predominate in the clinical picture.

B.   There is evidence from the history, physical examination, or laboratory findings that the disturbance is the direct physiological consequence of a general medical condition.

C.   The disturbance is not better accounted for by another mental disorder (e.g., adjustment disorder with anxiety in which the stressor is a serious general medical condition).

D.   The disturbance does not occur exclusively during the course of a delirium.

E.   The disturbance causes clinically significant distress or impairment in social, occupational, or other important areas of functioning.

Specify if:

   With Generalized Anxiety: if excessive anxiety or worry about a number of events or activities predominates in the clinical presentation

   With Panic Attacks: if panic attacks predominate in the clinical presentation

   With Obsessive-Compulsive Symptoms: if obsessions or compulsions predominate in the clinical presentation

   Coding note: Include the name of the general medical condition on Axis I, e.g., 293.84 anxiety disorder due to pheochromocytoma, with generalized anxiety; also code the general medical condition on Axis III (see DSM-IV-TR Appendix G for codes).

come our fears and worries. Researchers used functional magnetic resonance imaging to examine the brains of adults and were able to view two separate routes in brain circuitry that predicted anxiety responses. Perhaps in the future, knowing which type of neural vulnerabilities a person has may predict the type of treatment that will be most effective—for example, either cognitive therapy or medication (Indovina et al. 2011; Nauert 2011).

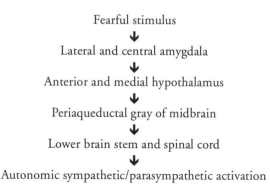

Fearful stimulus
↓
Lateral and central amygdala
↓
Anterior and medial hypothalamus
↓
Periaqueductal gray of midbrain
↓
Lower brain stem and spinal cord
↓
Autonomic sympathetic/parasympathetic activation

Figure 2–1. Neural pathway related to fear and autonomic response.

Medications Used to Treat Anxiety Disorders

Pharmacodynamics and Pharmacokinetics

The selective serotonin reuptake inhibitors (SSRIs), including fluoxetine, fluvoxamine, paroxetine, sertraline, escitalopram, and citalopram, have similar pharmacodynamics. Generally, they block the reuptake of serotonin in the presynaptic neuron allowing for increased serotonin in the synapse. They do, however, differ in pharmacokinetic properties. Their steady-state half-lives vary from 21 hours for paroxetine to potentially days for fluoxetine. SSRIs undergo extensive metabolism by the liver's cytochrome P450 (CYP) system, with a high degree of variability between individuals. The most serious difference among the SSRIs is their potential for drug-drug interactions resulting from inhibition of CYP enzymes, including CYP2D6, CYP1A2, CYP2C19, and CYP3A4 (Hiemke and Härtter 2000).

By combining the actions of serotonin and norepinephrine in the serotonin-norepinephrine reuptake inhibitors (SNRIs), the serotonin and adrenergic systems are synergistically amplified. They are rapidly absorbed after oral administration, with relatively short half-lives (8–12 hours) (Stahl et al. 2005). Norepinephrine action is greater at higher doses, leading to the potential for increased efficacy. The SNRIs can be effective in patients who are responders but not remitters to SSRIs (Dwivedi 2006).

The primary target of the benzodiazepines is the γ-aminobutyric acid (GABA) receptor. Benzodiazepine medications share a common template (binding to the $GABA_A$ receptor), but they differ in physiochemical properties, including lipid solubility, which influences their pharmacokinetics and their rate of absorption and diffusion (McDonagh et al. 2011).

Safety and Precautions

The SSRIs have been closely scrutinized as a result of the U.S. Food and Drug Administration (FDA) black box warning. After initiation of the antidepressant medications, reports of increased suicidal ideation in some children, adolescents, and young adults arose and caused a public outcry. The FDA investigated, and the outcome was a 2004 directive requiring manufacturer labeling to display a black box warning about increased risk of suicidality in young people (see Table 1–4 in Chapter 1, "Introduction to Clinical Psychopharmacology for Nurses"). These at-risk patients should be monitored closely and regularly to assess for suicide concerns. Other safety concerns with SSRIs include taking them during pregnancy, potential drug interactions (especially with blood-thinning medication), serotonin syndrome (cumulative effect of serotonergic medications, which increases availability of serotonin and contributes to potentially life-threatening consequences), and discontinuation syndrome (when an SSRI is abruptly stopped, flulike symptoms can occur) (Mayo Clinic 2010). SSRIs are effective and well tolerated in patients with anxiety disorders (Schmitt et al. 2005; Van der Linden et al. 2000).

Venlafaxine was found to be more lethal than other SNRIs in overdose. The SNRI medications have an unpredictable degree of efficacy and tolerability. They do, however, appear to be effective in a wide range of anxiety disorders, with efficacy equal to or greater than that of the SSRIs (Stahl et al. 2005).

For decades, the benzodiazepines have been used extensively for the treatment of anxiety disorders and remain a mainstay as both monotherapy and adjunctive therapy. These medications have varying degrees of efficacy, with advantages of a quick onset of action and being well tolerated. However, factors that require consideration include the patient's diagnoses, medication's characteristics, potential for drug interactions, risk of dependence and withdrawal, and frequency of dosing (Kaplan and DuPont 2005). Hesitation and caution should be exercised because dependence, abuse, and physiological tolerance must be considered when prescribing and monitoring patients taking this class of medication. Short-term use is ideal yet because of the immediate response and efficacy, patients continue to desire them without contemplating the risks.

U.S. Food and Drug Administration–Approved Indications and Warnings

The FDA has approved several psychotropic medications for use in the various anxiety disorders (refer to Table 2–8). In addition to those drugs that are FDA approved, clinicians have historically used others within the same classes in an off-label capacity to treat the symptoms of anxiety. It is important to remember that clinicians who prescribe medications off-label must inform the patient of the use, rationale, and potential risks and benefits so that an informed decision can be made about treatment. It is also imperative that this conversation with the patient and family be documented in the patient's medical record.

Dosing for Titration, Augmentation, and Discontinuation

In this section, I offer dosing suggestions and considerations for specific psychotropic medications used in the treatment of anxiety disorders. Tables 2–9 and 2–10 list information regarding drug dosages, potential side effects, and considerations regarding specific antianxiety medications. Also, the specific medication's package insert provides comprehensive prescribing, precautionary, and side-effect data, which the advanced practice registered nurse (APRN) should incorporate into his or her repertoire.

Selective Serotonin Reuptake Inhibitors

Paroxetine (Paxil, Paxil CR).
- When paroxetine is discontinued, withdrawal effects may be more likely than with other SSRIs (especially akathisia, restlessness, gastrointestinal symptoms, dizziness, tingling, dysesthesias, nausea, and stomach cramps).
- Paroxetine has mild anticholinergic actions that can enhance the rapid onset of anxiolytic and hypnotic efficacy but also cause mild anticholinergic side effects. It can cause cognitive and affective flattening and may be less activating than other SSRIs.
- For sexual dysfunction, the psychiatric APRN can augment with bupropion to facilitate the action of dopamine, "the pleasure-enhancing neurochemical," or switch to a non-SSRI such as bupropion or mirtazapine.
- Nonresponse to paroxetine in elderly patients may require consideration of mild cognitive impairment or Alzheimer's disease as potential causes of anxiety symptoms.

Table 2–8. Drugs with U.S. Food and Drug Administration–approved indications for anxiety disorders

Drug	Panic disorder	Social phobia	Obsessive-compulsive disorder	Generalized anxiety disorder	Anxiety disorder not otherwise specified
Paroxetine	X	X	X	X	
Fluvoxamine		X	X		
Sertraline	X	X	X (ages 6+)	X	
Fluoxetine	X	X	X (ages 7+)		
Escitalopram				X	
Buspirone	X			X	X
Venlafaxine	X	X		X	
Duloxetine				X	
Alprazolam	X			X	
Diazepam	X			X	
Lorazepam	X			X	

Table 2–9. Anxiety drug dosages and side effects

Drug	Daily dosage range (mg)	Weight gain	Sedation	Sexual dysfunction	GI distress	CNS effects	Comments
Paroxetine (Paxil; Paxil CR)	20–50; 12.5–75	+	+	+	+/–	+	Increases effects of tricyclics
Fluvoxamine (Luvox; Luvox CR)	100–300; 150–300	–	+	+/–	+/–	+	Non-CR: divide dose; CR: once per day
Sertraline (Zoloft)	25–200	+/–	+/–	+	+	+	Approved for obsessive-compulsive disorder in ages 6+
Fluoxetine (Prozac; Prozac Weekly)	10–60; 90–180 weekly	+/–	–	+	+/–	+	Long half-life; weekly formulation may be activating
Escitalopram (Lexapro)	10–30	–	–	+/–	+	+	Few drug-drug interactions

Table 2–9. Anxiety drug dosages and side effects *(continued)*

Drug	Daily dosage range (mg)	Weight gain	Sedation	Sexual dysfunction	GI distress	CNS effects	Comments
Buspirone (BuSpar)	5–60 (divided doses)	–	+/–	+	+	+	May take 6+ weeks for effect
Venlafaxine (Effexor XR)	37.5–375 (may divide dose)	–	–	+	+	+	Potential for discontinuation syndrome
Duloxetine (Cymbalta)	30–120	+/–	+/–	+/–	+	+	Potential for discontinuation syndrome

Note.   CNS=central nervous system; CR=controlled release; GI=gastrointestinal; XR=extended release. – = negative; + = positive; +/– = intermediate.

Table 2–10.   Prescribing considerations for antianxiety medications

Drug	Pros	Cons
Paroxetine (Paxil, Paxil CR)	Preferred for comorbid anxiety and depression; calming and sedating effects due to histamine agonism; less activating	Short half-life; high incidence of sexual dysfunction; monitor for discontinuation syndrome (headaches, "shocklike" sensations); pregnancy Category D
Fluvoxamine (Luvox, Luvox CR)	May provide early relief of insomnia and anxiety	Immediate-release formulation may require divided daily doses
Sertraline (Zoloft)	Works well with female hormonal system; approved for children ages 6 years and older	Can require titration; may contribute to gastrointestinal distress; may exacerbate insomnia
Fluoxetine (Prozac, Prozac Weekly)	"Energizing," weekly formulation useful in decreasing discontinuation syndrome with other SSRIs; weekly form convenient for adolescent population	Long half-life (up to 5 weeks with active metabolites) may delay ability to start other medications; side effects may persist longer; potential for agitation
Escitalopram (Lexapro)	Few drug-drug interactions; rapid onset of action	Like other antidepressants, may increase suicidality in children through young adults
Buspirone (BuSpar)	Favorable safety profile; nonaddicting; few side effects	Extended time to onset of action; may reduce aggression in patients with autism
Venlafaxine (Effexor XR)	Effective for patients with broad array of anxiety symptoms; wide dose range	Monitor for hypertension, especially at higher doses; discontinue slowly to reduce potential side effects

Table 2–10. Prescribing considerations for antianxiety medications *(continued)*

Drug	Pros	Cons
Duloxetine (Cymbalta)	Works well for patients with comorbid anxiety, depression, and pain symptoms	May contribute to nausea if not taken with small amount of food
Clonazepam (Klonopin—tabs and wafers)	Less euphoria, dependence, withdrawal, and abuse potential than other benzodiazepines	Physiological dependence increases with longer duration of treatment and higher doses; may cause CNS changes (confusion)
Alprazolam (Xanax, Xanax XR)	Rapid onset of action; XR formulation beneficial for panic prophylaxis	Immediate-release formulation may cause euphoria; high abuse potential
Diazepam (Valium)	Inexpensive; long half-life; useful adjunct to SSRIs and SNRIs	Long half-life may cause cumulative effect; avoid alcohol; risk of respiratory depression
Lorazepam (Ativan)	Frequently used in hospital settings; rapid onset of action; available in oral and injectable forms	Possibly more sedating than other benzodiazepines; may cause euphoria

Note. CNS = central nervous system; SNRI = serotonin-norepinephrine reuptake inhibitor; SSRI = selective serotonin reuptake inhibitor.

Fluvoxamine (Luvox).

• Fluvoxamine should be given once a day at night; splitting doses asymmetrically, with the larger dose taken at night, can improve tolerability with the immediate-release formulation.

Sertraline (Zoloft).

• Many patients will require a higher dosage than 50 mg/day of sertraline.
• The more anxious and agitated the patient, the lower the starting dose, the slower the titration, and the higher the chances of needing polypharmacy.

Fluoxetine (Prozac).

- Fluoxetine can cause serotonin syndrome when combined with a monoamine oxidase inhibitor (MAOI); 2–5 weeks must pass after discontinuing fluoxetine before starting an MAOI.
- Using lower doses and titrating slowly may have beneficial effects for the more anxious patient; augmentation with a benzodiazepine may be necessary to manage symptoms.
- Fluoxetine may increase levels of alprazolam, buspirone, and triazolam.
- Generally, fluoxetine is not well tolerated by patients with panic and other anxiety disorders unless combined with a benzodiazepine.
- Fluoxetine has a long half-life, so tapering is generally not necessary.

Nonbenzodiazepine Anxiolytic

Buspirone (BuSpar).

- Chronic anxiety disorders may require long-term maintenance with buspirone to control symptoms.
- Buspirone may raise levels of nordiazepam, an active metabolite of diazepam, which may cause increased symptoms of dizziness, headache, or nausea.

Serotonin-Norepinephrine Reuptake Inhibitors

Venlafaxine (Effexor XR).

- Lower doses of venlafaxine are usually serotonergic, and higher doses are noradrenergic (>225 mg).
- If response is inadequate at lower doses, try a higher dose.
- Hypertension may be an adverse event at higher doses. Periodic blood pressure monitoring is recommended when higher doses are prescribed.
- Discontinue very slowly because withdrawal effects include dizziness, nausea, tingling, and sweating. Discomfort can be reduced by adding an SSRI, such as fluoxetine, before initiating discontinuation of venlafaxine.

Duloxetine (Cymbalta).

- Patients may need to take duloxetine indefinitely to maintain remission of anxiety symptoms.
- Cigarette smoking induces CPY1A2 and may reduce plasma levels of duloxetine, but dosage changes are not recommended for smokers.

- Inhibitors of CYP2D6 (paroxetine, fluoxetine) may increase plasma levels and require lower dose of duloxetine.
- Duloxetine usually should not be prescribed to patients with substantial alcohol use or evidence of chronic liver disease (Eli Lilly 2007).

Benzodiazepines

Clonazepam (Klonopin)

- If anxiety symptoms are experienced during interdose periods, clonazepam can be divided into more frequent doses, or the dose can be increased.
- Risk of dependence increases with longer duration (>12 weeks) and higher doses; patients with severe panic disorder may require more than 4 mg/day.
- A longer half-life makes clonazepam easier to taper than some benzodiazepines.

Alprazolam (Xanax, Xanax XR)

- Alprazolam increases inhibitory effects of $GABA_A$ by binding to benzodiazepine receptors in the ligand-gated chloride channel complex.
- Alprazolam inhibits neuronal activity in amygdala-centered fear circuits to reduce anxiety.
- Long-term adaptations in benzodiazepine receptors may explain development of dependence, tolerance, potential for rebound anxiety, and withdrawal.
- The lowest possible dose should be used for the shortest duration. The need to continue treatment should be assessed on a regular basis.
- Frequency of dosing in practice can be predicted from half-life because duration of biological activity is often shorter than pharmacokinetic terminal half-life.
- Fatalities have been reported both when alprazolam is used as monotherapy and when it is combined with alcohol. Overdose symptoms include sedation, confusion, poor coordination, diminished reflexes, and coma.

Lorazepam (Ativan)

- Lorazepam is the primary benzodiazepine administered in hospital settings on both medical and psychiatric units.
- Lorazepam has a rapid onset of action and treats acute anxiety symptoms.

Management of benzodiazepine withdrawal.   A general rule of thumb in discontinuing the benzodiazepines on an outpatient basis is to reduce the total daily dose by 25% every 1–2 weeks. The active doses may need to be readjusted (further divided) to provide optimal symptom relief and reduce withdrawal effects. It may take months to comfortably withdraw patients from the benzodiazepines in an outpatient setting.

Psychiatric APRNs need to collaborate with their patients to ensure optimal symptom relief with minimal side effects.

Treatment of Special Populations

Children and Adolescents

Clinicians must regularly monitor patients face to face, particularly during the first several weeks of treatment. Use antidepressants with caution, observing for activation of known or unknown bipolar disorder and suicidal ideation, and inform parents or guardians of this risk so that they can help observe the child or adolescent patients. Anyone considering the use of an antidepressant in a child, an adolescent, or a young adult must balance this risk with the clinical need. In small studies, investigators found that the risk of suicidal ideation, suicidal behavior, or a suicide attempt was approximately twice as high among children and adolescents receiving one of the newer antidepressants (non–tricyclic antidepressants [non-TCAs]) as among those receiving placebo (Hammad et al. 2006). However, large studies have shown that the risk of a suicide attempt decreases after patients begin psychopharmacological treatment (Simon et al. 2006). Communities with higher rates of antidepressant use have lower rates of suicide (Gibbons et al. 2006).

It is most important for clinicians to observe the following guidelines (Simon 2006):

- Increase the frequency of follow-up visits with the pediatric population.
- Make recommendations regarding the risks of this method of treatment.
- Obtain informed consent for off-label use.
- Recognize that suicide attempts are unpredictable, so patients must be monitored for agitation and restlessness.
- Consider regular and possibly active outreach as essential.

Elderly Patients

Late-life anxiety symptoms may be a manifestation of stressors or losses, depression, coexisting medical problems, substance abuse, medication or herb side effects, withdrawal syndromes, or general disability. The physiological changes that occur during aging may influence the effects of psychotropic medications in older adults. Increased distribution and decreased metabolism and clearance of medication result in higher medication plasma levels and longer elimination half-lives. Medication compliance in older patients may be complicated by sensitivity to anticholinergic side effects; coexisting medical illnesses; polypharmacy, particularly in institutionalized settings; and sensory and cognitive deficits.

SSRIs and SNRIs generally are safe and produce fewer side effects and drug-drug interactions compared with TCAs, especially in geriatric patients (Newhouse 1996). SSRIs and SNRIs may be useful for generalized anxiety disorder, panic disorder, and obsessive-compulsive disorder in older patients. Benzodiazepines often are used for acute or short-term anxiety management, but chronic use in geriatric patients can cause cognitive impairment, falls, and other serious side effects. Buspirone may be beneficial for generalized anxiety disorder and is well tolerated in older persons but may take 2–4 weeks to be effective. Nonresponse to paroxetine in elderly patients may indicate mild cognitive impairment or Alzheimer's disease.

Pharmacotherapy for anxiety disorders in geriatric patients often is used in conjunction with psychotherapy, including cognitive-behavioral therapy (CBT), exposure therapy, dialectical behavioral therapy, and interpersonal therapy. Increasing evidence supports the effectiveness of psychotherapy in treating anxiety disorders in younger adults and in older patients, often in combination with pharmacotherapy. In older patients with generalized anxiety disorder, CBT is associated with a greater improvement in worry severity, depressive symptoms, and overall mental health compared with usual care. Complementary and alternative therapies can be used in late-life anxiety, including biofeedback; progressive relaxation; acupuncture; yoga; massage therapy; art, music, or dance therapy; meditation; prayer; and spiritual counseling (Bassil et al. 2011). In elderly patients age 65 and older, antidepressants reduced the risk of suicidal thoughts and actions compared with placebo (Gibbons et al. 2012).

Medically Compromised Patients

Cardiovascular Impairment

Fluvoxamine has been widely studied in patients with cardiovascular impairment, and evidence suggests that it has no effect on cardiovascular function in physically healthy patients and is safe in patients with cardiovascular disease (Prager et al. 1991). Treating depression with SSRIs in patients with acute angina or following myocardial infarction may reduce cardiac events and improve survival and mood.

Buspirone enhances the acceleration of the evoked cardiac component, which may reflect an increase in cognitive effort directed to the performance of task-relevant behavior (Unrug et al. 1997).

Renal Impairment

The dosing recommendations for buspirone in patients with compromised renal or hepatic function are not conclusive because of high intra- and intersubject variability. Initial doses of buspirone in these patients must be administered cautiously (Barbhaiya et al. 1994).

Dose adjustments for duloxetine are not necessary for patients with mild or moderate renal impairment. For patients with end-stage renal disease or severe renal impairment, exposure to duloxetine and its metabolites would be expected to increase; therefore, duloxetine use is not recommended for these patients (Lobo et al. 2010).

Hepatic Impairment

Because of its short half-life and inactive metabolites, lorazepam may be the preferred benzodiazepine in patients with liver disease (Stahl 2008).

Duloxetine should be avoided in patients with substantial alcohol use or evidence of chronic liver disease (Eli Lilly 2012).

Pregnant Women

Information on the various FDA pregnancy categories is available in Table 1–6 in Chapter 1, "Introduction to Clinical Psychopharmacology for Nurses."

Paroxetine has been changed to pregnancy risk Category D and is generally not recommended for use during pregnancy, especially during the first trimester. Epidemiological data have shown an increased risk of cardiovascular malformations (primarily ventricular and atrial septal defects) in infants whose mothers took paroxetine during the first trimester. Paroxetine use late in pregnancy may be associated with a higher risk of neonatal complications, including respiratory distress (U.S. Food and Drug Administration 2005).

One reason to select an SSRI or SNRI over a benzodiazepine for pregnant patients is that the benzodiazepines are Category D medications. An increased risk of birth defects is possible when the benzodiazepines are taken during pregnancy (Tuke 2006). The risk-benefit ratio, as it pertains to both the woman and her unborn child, must be thoroughly discussed and determined, a responsibility of the APRN prescriber.

Treatment Monitoring

Medications prescribed for symptoms of anxiety should be very closely monitored for several reasons. First is the heightened risk of suicidal ideation associated with the SSRIs and SNRIs and other antidepressants. The time of greatest concern may be the month before the initiation of medication, but data do not indicate a significant increase in risk of suicide or attempts after starting treatment with newer antidepressant drugs (Simon et al. 2006). The presence of suicidal ideation, the availability of responsible family members or supports, and any evidence of activation are critical to explore and document. In patients age 24 or younger, informed consent should take these concerns into account, and detailed education should be provided.

When prescribing benzodiazepines, clinicians must continually assess the use and response reported by the patient. Because of the potential for addiction, this class of medication is listed among the controlled and dangerous substances by the Drug Enforcement Administration. The quick mechanism of action of the benzodiazepines also produces nearly immediate relief, but the benefit and risk, as well as reliability and symptom report of the patient, must be assessed, with expectations of duration of use identified early on in treatment.

Other reasons for frequent and regular treatment monitoring are to evaluate the adherence and side effects of the prescribed medication. If the anticipated side effects are identified before initiation of psychopharmacology, patients can be better prepared for when to expect relief, what potential side effects may surface, and which ones must be reported to the prescriber. Most side effects of SSRIs, SNRIs, and benzodiazepines dissipate over time, so patience is encouraged.

The final item to keep in mind is the patient's reaction to therapy. As noted earlier, therapy can rewire the neurotransmitters, which will modify the patient's response to anxiety. Therefore, the need for psychotropic medication may be reduced if the therapy modality can provide coping skills, increased awareness, behavior changes, and reduction of anxiety. Medications, particularly SSRIs and SNRIs, should be continued for some time (up to 6 months) after symptoms abate.

Summary

Anxiety disorders are increasingly common in today's society. This is likely in part due to increased daily stress and heightened expectations as well as improved diagnostic skills and testing, increased knowledge of the psychiatric disorders, enhanced public education via the Internet, and increased reliance on medications for the "quick fix." This set of disorders poses treatment challenges for the APRN because of the noted comorbidities and ever-evolving patient presentation. Completion of a specific, detailed evaluation will begin the diagnostic process, after which additional questions must be answered before initiating psychopharmacological treatment. Factors including clinical severity and medication indication require further patient education and informed consent. Medication choices and the following must be taken into account when considering psychopharmacological therapy: class of anxiolytic medication, comorbid medical or psychiatric conditions, side-effect profile, anticipated patient adherence, cost, feasibility, and patient agreement with overall treatment monitoring. As symptoms and presentation evolve and change, the prescribing APRN must continue to assess and modify the regimen, while continuing to meet the patient's current and future psychiatric needs.

Clinical Pearls

- Anxiety is often complicated by the presence of alcohol or drug abuse and depression.
- Anxiety may result from many factors, including stressful circumstances; drugs that affect the nervous system, including caffeine, alcohol, cocaine, nicotine, amphetamines, and some herbal medications;

biological factors, including brain chemistry imbalances (serotonin and norepinephrine); personality traits; faulty perceptions and irratio- nal beliefs; and unresolved emotional conflicts.

• According to Cabrera and Schub (2011), risk factors for anxiety include being female, having a family member with anxiety disorders, experi- encing stressful life events, using ineffective coping strategies, and having a history of physical or psychological trauma.

References

American Psychiatric Association: Diagnostic and Statistical Manual of Mental Disor- ders, 4th Edition, Text Revision. Washington, DC, American Psychiatric Associ- ation, 2000

Barbhaiya RH, Shukla UA, Pfeffer M, et al: Disposition kinetics of buspirone in pa- tients with renal or hepatic impairment after administration of single and mul- tiple doses. Eur J Clin Pharmacol 46:41–47, 1994

Bassil N, Ghandour A, Grossberg GT: How anxiety presents differently in older adults: age-related changes, medical comorbidities alter presentation and treatment. Cur- rent Psychiatry 10(3):65–71, 2011. Available at: http://www.currentpsychiatry. com/pdf/1003/1003CP_Article3.pdf. Accessed February 6, 2013.

Cabrera G, Schub T: Substance Abuse and Anxiety Disorders. Glendale, CA, Cinahl Information Systems, September 2, 2011

Dwivedi Y: Pharmacodynamics of antidepressants, mood stabilizing agents, anxiolyt- ics, sedative-hypnotics. Department of Psychiatry Lecture, University of Illinois, Chicago, 2006. Available at: http://www.uic.edu/classes/pcol/pcol331/ dentalpharmhandouts2006/lecture48.pdf. Accessed February 6, 2013.

Eli Lilly: FDA approves Cymbalta for treatment of generalized anxiety disorder. February 26, 2007. Available at: newsroom.lilly.com/releasedetail.cfm?releaseid=231196. Accessed February 6, 2013.

Eli Lilly: Highlights of prescribing information: Cymbalta (duloxetine delayed-release capsules) for oral use. PV 9474 AMP. Literature revised November 9, 2012. Avail- able at: http://pi.lilly.com/us/cymbalta-pi.pdf. Accessed February 6, 2013.

Gibbons RD, Hur K, Bhaumik DK, et al: The relationship between antidepressant prescription rates and rate of early adolescent suicide. Am J Psychiatry 163:1898– 1904, 2006

Gibbons RD, Brown CH, Hur K, et al: Suicidal thoughts and behavior with antide- pressant treatment: reanalysis of the randomized placebo-controlled studies of fluoxetine and venlafaxine. Arch Gen Psychiatry 69:580–587, 2012]

Hammad TA, Laughren T, Racoosin J: Suicidality in pediatric patients treated with antidepressant drugs. Arch Gen Psychiatry 63:332–339, 2006

Hiemke C, Härtter S: Pharmacokinetics of selective serotonin reuptake inhibitors. Pharmacol Ther 85:11–28, 2000

Indovina I, Robbins T, Nunez-Elizalde A, et al: Fear conditioning mechanisms associated with trait vulnerability to anxiety in humans. Neuron 69:563–571, 2011

Kaplan ME, DuPont RL: Benzodiazepines and anxiety disorders: a review for the practicing physician. Curr Med Res Opin 21:941–950, 2005

Lobo ED, Heathman M, Kuan HY, et al: Effects of varying degrees of renal impairment on the pharmacokinetics of duloxetine: analysis of single-dose phase I study and pooled steady-state data from phase II/III trials. Clin Pharmacokinet 49:311–321, 2010

Mayo Clinic: Depression (major depression). December 9, 2010. Available at: www.mayoclinic.com/health/ssris/MH00066/NSECTIONGROUP=2. Accessed February 6, 2013.

McDonagh EM, Whirl-Carrillo M, Garten Y, et al: From pharmacogenomic knowledge acquisition to clinical applications: the PharmGKB as a clinical pharmacogenomic biomarker resource. Biomark Med 5:795–806, 2011

National Institute of Mental Health: Anxiety Disorders (NIH Publ No 09 3879). Bethesda, MD, National Institute of Mental Health, 2009

Nauert R: Defects in brain pathways linked to anxiety. February 11, 2011. Available at: http://psychcentral.com/news/2011/02/11/defects-in-brain-pathways-linked-to-anxiety/23420.html. Accessed February 6, 2013.

Newhouse PA: Use of serotonin selective reuptake inhibitors in geriatric depression. J Clin Psychiatry 57:12–22, 1996

Ninan PT: The functional anatomy, neurochemistry, and pharmacology of anxiety. J Clin Psychiatry 60:12–17, 1999

Panksepp J: Affective Neuroscience: The Foundations of Human and Animal Emotions. New York, Oxford University Press, 1998

Prager G, Stollmaier W, Parger R, et al: Safety and tolerance of fluvoxamine in cardiac patients. TW Neurologie Psychiatrie 5:548–562, 1991

Schmitt R, Gazalle FK, Lima MS, et al: The efficacy of antidepressants for generalized anxiety disorder: a systematic review and meta-analysis. Rev Bras Psiquiatr 27(1):18–24, 2005

Simon GE: The antidepressant quandary—considering suicide risk when treating adolescent depression. N Engl J Med 355:2722–2723, 2006

Simon GE, Savarino J, Operskalski B, et al: Suicide risk during antidepressant treatment. Am J Psychiatry 163:41–47, 2006

Stahl SM: Stahl's Essential Psychopharmacology: Neuroscientific Basis and Practical Applications, 3rd Edition. New York, Cambridge University Press, 2008

Stahl SM, Grady MM, Moret C, et al: SNRIs: their pharmacology, clinical efficacy, and tolerability in comparison with other classes of antidepressants. CNS Spectr 10:732–747, 2005

Tuke S: Benzodiazepine use in pregnancy. 2006. Available at: www.bcnc.org.uk/BZ_pregnancy.pdf. Accessed February 6, 2013.

Unrug A, Bener J, Barry RJ, et al: Influence of diazepam and buspirone on human heart rate and the evoked cardiac response under varying cognitive load. Int J Psychophysiol 25:177–184, 1997

U.S. Food and Drug Administration: Updated product labeling warns of birth defect risk with Paxil. FDA Release P05-97, December 8, 2005

Van der Linden GJ, Stein DJ, van Balkom AJ: The efficacy of the selective serotonin reuptake inhibitors for social anxiety disorder (social phobia): a meta-analysis of randomized controlled trials. Int Clin Psychopharmacol 15:S15–23, 2000

3

Depressive Disorders

LaKeetra M. Josey, M.S.N., A.P.R.N., P.M.H.-F.N.P., B.C.

Elaine M. Neidert, M.S.N., A.P.R.N., P.M.H.-N.P., B.C.

When you're surrounded by all these people, it can be lonelier than
when you're by yourself. You can be in a huge crowd, but if you don't
feel like you can trust anyone or talk to anybody, you feel like you're
really alone.

—Fiona Apple, singer/songwriter

In 2011, the Centers for Disease Control and Prevention (CDC) estimated
that 1 in 10 adults experience depression. Depression is a psychiatric illness
that is both common and treatable but can be both costly and debilitating to
its patients. The diagnosis of major depression requires a significant change in

a person's level of functioning. This significant change in the individual's level of functioning contributes to exacerbations of chronic illnesses, poor work productivity and absenteeism, disability, and disrupted relationships with family and friends. According to the Behavioral Risk Factor Surveillance System (BRFSS), a division of the CDC (2010), the following groups are at risk for depression:

- Individuals with chronic medical conditions and unhealthy behaviors (e.g., smoking, physical inactivity, binge drinking)
- Women
- Persons ages 45–64 years
- Black, Hispanic, and non-Hispanic individuals of other or multiple races

Protective factors for depression include

- Post–high school education
- Marriage or current significant relationship
- Current employment and health insurance

Depression can be particularly debilitating if the symptoms include decreased motivation and feelings of hopelessness because these symptoms can lead an individual to feel alone and desperate and may lead to suicidality. Additionally, motivation and hope are the key factors for executing change in one's life. Without hope and motivation, a vicious cycle can ensue and worsen depressive symptoms. As a whole, regardless of practice setting, nurses can be helpful in providing a source of hope and motivation for those struggling with depressive symptoms.

Overview of Depressive Disorders

Refer to Tables 3–1, 3–2, and 3–3 for DSM-IV-TR (American Psychiatric Association 2000) criteria for depressive disorders and related mood disorders.

Table 3–1. DSM-IV-TR diagnostic criteria for 296.2 major depressive disorder, single episode

A. Presence of a single major depressive episode.

B. The major depressive episode is not better accounted for by schizoaffective disorder and is not superimposed on schizophrenia, schizophreniform disorder, delusional disorder, or psychotic disorder not otherwise specified.

C. There has never been a manic episode, a mixed episode, or a hypomanic episode. **Note:** This exclusion does not apply if all of the manic-like, mixed-like, or hypomanic-like episodes are substance or treatment induced or are due to the direct physiological effects of a general medical condition.

If the full criteria are currently met for a major depressive episode, *specify* its current clinical status and/or features:

Mild, Moderate, Severe Without Psychotic Features/Severe With Psychotic Features

Chronic

With Catatonic Features

With Melancholic Features

With Atypical Features

With Postpartum Onset

If the full criteria are not currently met for a major depressive episode, *specify* the current clinical status of the major depressive disorder or features of the most recent episode:

In Partial Remission, In Full Remission

Chronic

With Catatonic Features

With Melancholic Features

With Atypical Features

With Postpartum Onset

Table 3–2.   DSM-IV-TR diagnostic criteria for 296.3 major depressive disorder, recurrent

A.   Presence of two or more major depressive episodes.

    Note: To be considered separate episodes, there must be an interval of at least 2 consecutive months in which criteria are not met for a major depressive episode.

B.   The major depressive episodes are not better accounted for by schizoaffective disorder and are not superimposed on schizophrenia, schizophreniform disorder, delusional disorder, or psychotic disorder not otherwise specified.

C.   There has never been a manic episode, a mixed episode, or a hypomanic episode.   **Note:** This exclusion does not apply if all of the manic-like, mixed-like, or hypomanic-like episodes are substance or treatment induced or are due to the direct physiological effects of a general medical condition.

If the full criteria are currently met for a major depressive episode, *specify* its current clinical status and/or features:

    Mild, Moderate, Severe Without Psychotic Features/Severe With Psychotic Features

    Chronic

    With Catatonic Features

    With Melancholic Features

    With Atypical Features

    With Postpartum Onset

If the full criteria are not currently met for a major depressive episode, *specify* the current clinical status of the major depressive disorder or features of the most recent episode:

    In Partial Remission, In Full Remission

    Chronic

    With Catatonic Features

    With Melancholic Features

    With Atypical Features

    With Postpartum Onset

    Specify:

    Longitudinal Course Specifiers (With and Without Interepisode Recovery)

    With Seasonal Pattern

Table 3–3.   DSM-IV-TR diagnostic criteria for 300.4 dysthymic disorder

A.   Depressed mood for most of the day, for more days than not, as indicated either by subjective account or observation by others, for at least 2 years.   **Note:** In children and adolescents, mood can be irritable and duration must be at least 1 year.

B.   Presence, while depressed, of two (or more) of the following:

   (1)   poor appetite or overeating

   (2)   insomnia or hypersomnia

   (3)   low energy or fatigue

   (4)   low self-esteem

   (5)   poor concentration or difficulty making decisions

   (6)   feelings of hopelessness

C.   During the 2-year period (1 year for children or adolescents) of the disturbance, the person has never been without the symptoms in criteria A and B for more than 2 months at a time.

D.   No major depressive episode has been present during the first 2 years of the disturbance (1 year for children and adolescents); i.e., the disturbance is not better accounted for by chronic major depressive disorder, or major depressive disorder, in partial remission.

   Note: There may have been a previous major depressive episode provided there was a full remission (no significant signs or symptoms for 2 months) before development of the dysthymic disorder. In addition, after the initial 2 years (1 year in children or adolescents) of dysthymic disorder, there may be superimposed episodes of major depressive disorder, in which case both diagnoses may be given when the criteria are met for a major depressive episode.

E.   There has never been a manic episode, a mixed episode, or a hypomanic episode, and criteria have never been met for cyclothymic disorder.

F.   The disturbance does not occur exclusively during the course of a chronic psychotic disorder, such as schizophrenia or delusional disorder.

G.   The symptoms are not due to the direct physiological effects of a substance (e.g., a drug of abuse, a medication) or a general medical condition (e.g., hypothyroidism).

H.   The symptoms cause clinically significant distress or impairment in social, occupational, or other important areas of functioning.

Table 3–3.   DSM-IV-TR diagnostic criteria for 300.4 dysthymic disorder *(continued)*

Specify if:

Early Onset: if onset is before age 21 years

Late Onset: if onset is age 21 years or older

Specify (for most recent 2 years of dysthymic disorder):

With Atypical Features

Major Depressive Disorder

Symptoms of a major depressive episode must include five or more of the following symptoms, including depressed mood for at least a 2-week period:

1. Depressed or sad mood most of the day, nearly every day
2. Markedly diminished interest or pleasure in all or almost all activities most of the day, nearly every day
3. Significant weight loss (not dieting) or weight gain
4. Insomnia or excessive sleeping nearly every day
5. Psychomotor retardation or agitation observed by others
6. Fatigue or loss of energy nearly every day
7. Feelings of worthlessness or excessive or inappropriate guilt nearly every day
8. Decreased concentration or indecisiveness nearly every day
9. Recurrent thoughts of death or suicidal ideation without a specific plan, or a suicide attempt or specific plan for committing suicide

The symptoms cause significant impairment and distress in the patient's life and are not better accounted for by the loss of loved one, psychotic symptoms, or the direct physiological effects of a substance or a general medical condition (e.g., hypothyroidism). Major depressive disorder (MDD) often can be described along with specifics such as postpartum onset, with psychotic features, or other identifiers, which indicate acuity, type of onset, or features (American Psychiatric Association 2000). Depression in children and adolescents often looks more like irritability than depression. The elderly should always be evaluated thoroughly because depression often can be confused with cognitive disorders such as Alzheimer's disease. Mood symptoms may be less apparent than cognitive symptoms in elderly individuals.

Dysthymic Disorder

Patients who have dysthymic disorder struggle with symptoms of "low-grade" depressed mood for most days for at least 2 years. During this time, they also share similar symptoms with MDD of poor sleep or hypersomnia, poor appetite or overeating, and poor concentration and indecisiveness. They also report poor self-esteem, self-criticism, and hopelessness, and clinicians, when consulted, will hear the individual report that "I'm always like this." Individuals with dysthymic disorder often present with superimposed MDD and are at higher risk for episodes of MDD in the future (American Psychiatric Association 2000).

Depressive Disorder Not Otherwise Specified

Depressive disorder not otherwise specified includes depressive disorders that do not meet the criteria for a diagnosis of MDD, dysthymic disorder, or adjustment disorder with depressed mood, or other depressive disorders that clinicians cannot categorize as primary, substance induced, or due to a general medical condition (American Psychiatric Association 2000). Premenstrual dysphoric disorder (PMDD) is an example of depressive disorder not otherwise specified and is discussed separately later in this chapter.

Mood Disorder Due to a General Medical Condition (With Depressive Features)

Individuals who have a depressed mood and related symptoms but do not qualify for a diagnosis of MDD, and whose symptoms are directly related to a medical diagnosis, proven by physical and laboratory findings, are given the diagnosis of mood disorder due to a general medical condition. Common medical issues related but not limited to this diagnosis are hypothyroidism, stroke, Parkinson's disease, vitamin B_{12} deficiency, post–myocardial infarction events, and other central nervous system (CNS) diseases (American Psychiatric Association 2000).

Premenstrual Dysphoric Disorder

PMDD is another debilitating disorder that affects a woman's personal, social, and occupational worlds. During more months of the year than not, the woman experiences a constellation of symptoms that contribute to changes in mood, typically of a depressive nature. Irritability and anger are also common manifestations. Additionally, the woman may experience physiological symptoms such as bloating, breast tenderness, headaches, joint or muscle pain, and weight gain. The symptoms typically occur during the late luteal phase of the menstrual cycle and tend to remit with the onset of menstruation. This cycle can last anywhere from 2 to 14 days, depending on the woman and her cycle.

Preliminary research suggests that abnormalities in the orbitofrontal cortex and the amygdala may contribute to symptoms of PMDD (Protopopescu et al. 2008). Recent neuroimaging studies in Korea indicated that gray matter abnormalities in the limbic and paralimbic cortices may be associated with PMDD, suggesting a neurobiological basis for the disorder (Jeong et al. 2012). Additionally, it has long been believed that PMDD is caused by a complex set of interactions between the woman's reproductive hormones (progesterone and estrogen) and the brain's neurotransmitters, especially serotonin. Because the selective serotonin reuptake inhibitor (SSRI) antidepressants have been used to treat PMDD and have shown efficacy, this would seem to hold true; however, this interaction is not yet fully understood (Stoppler 2009).

Postpartum Depression

Postpartum depression is a very real and concerning disorder, not only for the woman but also for the relationship between the mother and her infant. Our society views the postpartum period as a time to be filled with excitement and joy, but for women whose "baby blues" progress to postpartum depression or the extreme, postpartum psychosis, this time can be devastating. The stress, hormonal fluctuations, discomfort from childbirth, lack of supports, and potential financial hardship all increase a woman's risk for developing postpartum depression. The Edinburgh Postnatal Depression Scale, a 10-item tool identifying women at risk, is typically used to screen for postpartum depression (Cox et al. 1987; a copy of this screening instrument is provided in Appendix 4, "Psychiatric Rating Scales"). This screening is conducted during the woman's hospital stay for the birth of her infant, which offers limited time to arrange psychiatric follow-up for those women who are found to be at risk. Note that despite screenings and the presentation of symptoms of postpartum depression, a very low percentage of depressed women ever receive treatment during the postpartum period (Vesga-Lopez et al. 2008).

Although a definitive cause of postpartum depression has yet to be determined, numerous risk factors may predispose a woman to this disorder. Many women conceive while taking prescribed medications, including oral contraceptives; nearly 50% of all pregnancies are unplanned; and woman do have psychiatric disorders before, during, and after pregnancy (Cooper et al. 2007). Although no psychotropic agents are currently approved for use during pregnancy, antidepressant use during pregnancy has markedly increased over the past decade to about 1 in 10 women (Cooper et al. 2007). Although taking an antidepressant during pregnancy may prophylactically protect against the development of postpartum depression, it is not a cure.

Neurobiology of Depression

The primary neurotransmitters implicated in depression are serotonin, dopamine, and norepinephrine. Serotonin is a neurotransmitter involved in depression and anxiety symptoms, whereas dopamine is involved in feelings of pleasure, motivation, thought disturbances, and cognition. Norepinephrine is involved in relation to attention, concentration, and anxiety (Stahl 2008). SSRIs are generally the first line of treatment when a person presents with depressive symptoms. SSRIs work by blocking the reuptake of serotonin into the presynaptic neuron. This allows for it to remain in the postsynaptic cleft longer and to bind to the postsynaptic neuron, thus creating the desired effect. Serotonin-norepinephrine reuptake inhibitors (SNRIs) work by blocking the reuptake of serotonin and norepinephrine into the presynaptic neuron. The addition of the norepinephrine action can help relieve issues with concentration and focus, increase motivation, reduce anhedonia (lack of pleasure) symptoms, and relieve neuropathic pain symptoms. Bupropion (is the only norepinephrine-dopamine reuptake inhibitor. The effect of the dopamine action can further reduce symptoms of anhedonia. The norepinephrine action can help with attention, focus, concentration, and motivation. Thus, augmentation of the SSRI antidepressants with a norepinephrine or dopamine agent may further improve symptoms, especially in those with treatment-resistant depression.

Medications Used to Treat Depressive Disorders

Choice of medication treatment for depression is based on history of response and weighing potential side effects associated with specific antidepressants and their classes. In general, many clinicians favor serotonin reuptake inhibitors as the first-line medication treatment, despite the fact the these agents may take 4–6 weeks to be fully efficacious. In the past 10 years, algorithms have been established for antidepressant treatment, such as those based on the Sequenced Treatment Alternatives to Relieve Depression (STAR*D; e.g., Trivedi et al. 2006), a large-scale clinical National Institute of Mental Health–funded trial, and the Texas Medication Algorithm Project (TMAP; e.g., Trivedi et al. 2004). However, the clinician should be aware that for a variety of reasons, outcomes of clinical trials and their participants may not reflect efficacy in the field, especially in the individual patient with depression. The sections below provide a synopsis of first- and second-line antidepressants, followed by medications used for augmentation in treatment-resistant depression, older classes of antidepressants, and complementary and alternative agents. Table 3–4 provides an overview of the most commonly prescribed antidepressants and their key features.

Selective Serotonin Reuptake Inhibitors

When fluoxetine (Prozac) hit the market in the late 1980s, it revolutionized the way clinicians conceptualized and treated depressive disorders. Until that time, the antidepressant agents were fraught with a myriad of undesirable side effects that often contributed to lack of adherence on the patient's part and a paucity of treatment options on the part of the prescriber. Additionally, the antidepressants used before fluoxetine also contributed to the potential for overdose and suicide. When the SSRIs became available with their improved tolerability and low incidence of overdose, they rapidly became the drug of choice for treating depression and other disorders. Today, most SSRIs are available in a generic form, and they are relatively inexpensive in comparison to other medications. Serotonin is involved in depression and anxiety symptoms, so the SSRIs can be helpful for those patients who may have anxiety and depressive symptoms. The SSRIs are also prescribed for treatment of PMDD and postpartum depression. The SSRIs include the following psychotropic agents: fluoxetine (Prozac), sertraline (Zoloft), paroxetine (Paxil, Paxil CR), citalopram (Celexa), escitalopram (Lexapro), and fluvoxamine (Luvox, Luvox CR), although fluvoxamine is primarily used in the treatment of obsessive-compulsive disorder.

Given the high visibility of SSRIs in the media and public marketplace over the past few decades, nurses have treated patients who have been prescribed the SSRIs for any number of "off-label" conditions. Over the years, patients have reported being prescribed fluoxetine for "high blood pressure," sertraline for "stomach issues," citalopram for "diabetes," and paroxetine "to prevent a heart attack." Typically, the prescribing for these conditions originates in the primary care offices. It is imperative for nurses in all practice settings to be certain that the patient is informed of the labeled or off-label use of the medication and the risks and benefits.

Medication side effects for the SSRI class of antidepressants include headache, upset stomach, sleep disturbances, induction of mania symptoms if an underlying bipolar disorder is present, feelings of restlessness or agitation, increasing suicidal ideation, and sexual side effects such as inability to achieve or maintain an erection in males or difficulty achieving orgasm in females. SSRIs generally do not have an effect on sexual desire. Side effects tend to present on initiation of medication and with dosage increases. They often remit with time. Sometimes decreasing the dosage and then titrating up more slowly can alleviate side effects. Side effects and dosages of the SSRIs can be found in Table 3–4.

Serotonin Partial Agonist and Reuptake Inhibitor

Vilazodone (Viibryd) is the newest antidepressant agent on the market. It not only blocks the reuptake of serotonin at the presynaptic neuron but also stimulates the serotonin transporter to augment the serotonin available in the synaptic cleft. This mechanism of action may potentially improve symptoms that have only partially responded to the SSRIs. Its side-effect profile is similar to that of the SSRIs as well.

Serotonin-Norepinephrine Reuptake Inhibitors

The SNRIs include duloxetine (Cymbalta), venlafaxine (Effexor, Effexor XR), and desvenlafaxine (Pristiq). Medication side effects include headache, nausea, irritability or agitation, jitteriness or restlessness, dizziness on standing, sedation, increased suicidal thoughts, and sleep disturbances. Similar to other

Table 3–4. Key features of antidepressant medications commonly used in the treatment of depressive disorders

Drug	Dosage	Anticho-linergic effects	Sedation	Sexual effects	Gastro-intestinal upset	Agitation/ Insomnia	Weight gain	Half-life (hours)	Comments
SSRIs									
Citalopram (Celexa)	20–60 mg/day	None	None	+++	+++	+	+	24–48	Low drug-drug interactions
Escitalopram (Lexapro)	10–20 mg/day	None	None	+	++	+	+	27–32	Generic now available; tends to work more rapidly than other SSRIs
Fluoxetine (Prozac, Prozac Weekly, Sarafem)	20–80 mg/day or 90 mg/week	None	None	++++	+++	+++	+	48–216	Can be too activating for some patients; Serafem indicated for PMDD
Paroxetine (Paxil, Paxil CR, Pexeva)	20–60 mg/day or 12.5–75 mg/day (CR)	++	++	++++	+++	+	++	10–24	Contraindicated in pregnancy (Category D)

Table 3–4. Key features of antidepressant medications commonly used in the treatment of depressive disorders *(continued)*

Drug	Dosage	Anticho-linergic effects	Sedation	Sexual effects	Gastro-intestinal upset	Agitation/ Insomnia	Weight gain	Half-life (hours)	Comments
SSRIs *(continued)*									
Sertraline (Zoloft)	50–200 mg/day	None	None	++++	+++	+	++	26	Works well with female cycle; indicated for luteal-phase dosing for PMDD
Fluvoxamine (Luvox, Luvox CR)	50–300 mg/day	None	None	++	++	+	+	16 (up to 26 in elderly)	Indicated for OCD
Vilazodone (Viibryd; brand only)	10–40 mg/day	None	None	++	+	+	+	25	Also a serotonin agonist

Table 3–4. Key features of antidepressant medications commonly used in the treatment of depressive disorders (*continued*)

Drug	Dosage	Anticholinergic effects	Sedation	Sexual effects	Gastrointestinal upset	Agitation/Insomnia	Weight gain	Half-life (hours)	Comments
SNRIs									
Venlafaxine hydrochloride (Effexor, Effexor XR)	37.5–375 mg/day	+	+	+++	+++	++	None	5–11	Serotonergic action to 150 mg Noradrenergic to 300 mg Possibly dopaminergic at >300 mg
Desvenlafaxine (Pristiq; brand only)	50–400 mg/day	None	+	+	++	+	+	11 (up to 23 in ESRD)	
Duloxetine (Cymbalta; brand only)	20–120 mg/day	None	+	+	+++	+	+	12	

Table 3–4. Key features of antidepressant medications commonly used in the treatment of depressive disorders *(continued)*

Drug	Dosage	Anticho-linergic effects	Sedation	Sexual effects	Gastro-intestinal upset	Agitation/ Insomnia	Weight gain	Half-life (hours)	Comments
NDRIs									
Bupropion hydrochloride (Wellbutrin, Wellbutrin SR and XL, Budeprion SR and XL)	150–450 mg/day	None	None	None	+	+++	None	8–24	Contraindicated with seizures
Bupropion hydrobromide (Aplenzin; brand only)	174–522 mg/day	None	None	None	+	+++	None	21	Hydrobromide 174, 348, and 522 mg equivalent to Hydrochloride 150, 300, and 450 mg, respectively

Table 3–4. Key features of antidepressant medications commonly used in the treatment of depressive disorders (*continued*)

Drug	Dosage	Anticho-linergic effects	Sedation	Sexual effects	Gastro-intestinal upset	Agitation/ Insomnia	Weight gain	Half-life (hours)	Comments
SARI									
Trazodone (Desyrel, Oleptro)	50–600 mg/day or 150–375 mg/day (Oleptro)	+++	++++	None	+	None	++	4–9	Used primarily as sedative-hypnotic
NaSSA									
Mirtazapine (Remeron/ SolTab)	7.5–45 mg	+++	++++	None	+	None	+++	20–40	Often used for insomnia

Note. ESRD=end-stage renal disease; GI=gastrointestinal; NaSSA=noradrenergic and specific serotonergic antidepressant; NDRI=norepinephrine-dopamine reuptake inhibitor; OCD=obsessive-compulsive disorder; PMDD=premenstrual dysphoric disorder; SARI=serotonin antagonist and reuptake inhibitor; SNRI=serotonin-norepinephrine reuptake inhibitor; SSRIs=selective serotonin reuptake inhibitor. +=minimal to none; ++=mild; +++=moderate; ++++=high.

medications, side effects tend to present on initiation of the medication and then again with dosage increases.

Because most of these medications are available only as brand names, they can be more expensive. Patients' insurance companies may require a preauthorization for these medications to cover them. This should not be a deterrent to initiating the medication if it is the most appropriate agent on the basis of the symptom presentation. Patients may need to be educated that a delay in filling their prescription is possible because of the need for prior authorization from their insurance carriers. Table 3–4 offers more information on the SNRIs.

Norepinephrine-Dopamine Reuptake Inhibitor

Bupropion hydrochloride (Wellbutrin) is available in three formulations: immediate release, sustained release, and extended release (24-hour delivery). Bupropion hydrobromide (Aplenzin) is an extended-delivery formulation with U.S. Food and Drug Administration–approved bioequivalence to bupropion hydrochloride; it is not a generic. Bupropion is sometimes used as an adjunct to treatment with an SSRI if the depressive symptoms are not reduced with the SSRI alone. It can also help reduce the sexual side effects of the SSRIs. The norepinephrine action can be stimulating to people and, therefore, may not be the best choice when concurrent anxiety issues exist because the stimulation can increase feelings of anxiety. Common side effects include headache, upset stomach, appetite changes, sleep disturbances, agitation, increased anxiety, dizziness, and seizures. Refer to Table 3–4 for more information.

Serotonin Antagonist and Reuptake Inhibitors and Noradrenergic and Specific Serotonergic Antidepressants

Mirtazapine (Remeron) and trazodone (Desyrel and Oleptro) are generally used more for the side effect of sedation than as a primary treatment for depression. Their serotonin action can make them helpful as adjuncts to SSRIs and help reduce sleep disturbances because they also target histamine receptor blockade. Side effects are sedation, headache, dizziness, dry mouth, increased suicidal thoughts, and weight gain.

Atypical Antipsychotics Used for Augmentation

Atypical antipsychotics such as aripiprazole (Abilify) and quetiapine (Seroquel) primarily work with dopamine, but they also have serotonergic actions, which can make them helpful to treat depressive symptoms or depression with psychotic features. Although atypical antipsychotics generally are not approved as first-line treatments, they can be helpful adjuncts to an SSRI or other antidepressant, especially if the patient is struggling with a poor response to treatment. Side effects include headache, nausea, dizziness, involuntary muscle movements, metabolic disturbances, weight gain, and increased risk of death in elderly dementia patients (black box warning). Additionally, the prudent psychiatric advanced practice registered nurse (APRN) will monitor even more closely for the potential of "flipping" the patient into mania and the increased risk for serotonin syndrome, which are discussed later in the chapter. More information about the dosing and side effects of the second-generation (atypical) antipsychotics is available in Chapter 4, "Bipolar Disorders," and Chapter 5, "Psychotic Disorders."

Lithium Used for Augmentation

Lithium (Eskalith, Lithobid), the most common choice for mood stabilization in bipolar disorder, is sometimes used for augmentation in treatment-resistant depression. Its mechanism of action in depression and mood stabilization is unknown, but it has been proved highly effective. It is used in low (subtherapeutic) doses for adjunctive therapy with antidepressants (<900 mg/day). It is one of the few agents available to aid in alleviating suicidal ideation. Major side effects include weight gain, diarrhea, nausea, increased thirst and urination, tremor, and changes to the kidneys and thyroid over time. Thyroid and renal function studies, as well as a baseline electrocardiogram for anyone older than 50 and a pregnancy test for any woman of childbearing age, should be ordered before starting lithium and periodically monitored during ongoing treatment. More information on the dosing and side effects of lithium can be found in Chapter 4, "Bipolar Disorders."

Tricyclic Antidepressants and Monoamine Oxidase Inhibitors

Because of their less favorable side-effect profile and potential for lethality in overdose, the tricyclic antidepressants (TCAs) are rarely used in practice today, especially given the new and safer choices of medications available. They still, however, have their place if used wisely among patients whose symptoms do not respond to the newer classes of medications. TCAs remain the gold standard for some disorders—such as obsessive-compulsive disorder, for which clomipramine (Anafranil) is still used as a first-line agent, or enuresis in children, for which imipramine (Tofranil) is used. Amitriptyline (Elavil) is often used for patients who have both depression and chronic pain states or may be used in lower doses for migraine. TCAs such as amitriptyline or doxepin (Sinequan; Silenor) are frequently used in low doses at bedtime for comorbid treatment of insomnia.

The monoamine oxidase inhibitors (MAOIs) are less frequently used because of their potential interactions with most medications and the rare but potential risk for life-threatening hypertensive crisis if specific dietary restrictions are not followed. A transdermal formulation of selegiline (Emsam), an irreversible MAOI with relative selectivity for the MAO type B isoenzyme, is currently available, which has fewer dietary restrictions in the lower doses, but it has not been widely used.

Complementary and Alternative Medications

Folate, or folic acid, is a water-soluble essential vitamin that has been linked to multiple CNS disorders, including depression. Several studies have shown that as many as 56% of those who are depressed have an inability to metabolize folate into its most usable form, L-methylfolate, which can cross the blood-brain barrier. Folate deficiency also has been linked to later onset of action and lesser improvements in those taking antidepressants (Roman and Bembry 2011).

The metabolite L-methylfolate is the end product of folate or folic acid that is consumed by an individual through foods or folic acid supplementation. However, if the patient lacks the enzyme to convert folic acid to L-methylfolate, the patient may not enjoy the benefits of enhanced mood and reduced depressive symptoms associated with the trimonoamines. L-Methylfolate acts as a regulator of a critical cofactor for trimonoamine neurotransmitter synthesis. Defects in any step of the conversion result in the vitamin being unavailable to the CNS. L-Methylfolate is classed as a trimonoamine modulator and a medical food, used in the treatment of depression. It is commonly prescribed as an adjunctive therapy to an antidepressant therapy. It is well tolerated. and side effects in clinical trials were similar or favorable to those caused by placebo. As with all of the antidepressants, L-methylfolate should be used with caution in anyone with a history of bipolar disorder.

U.S. Food and Drug Administration Warnings

Whereas the primary U.S. Food and Drug Administration (FDA)–approved indication for all antidepressants is treatment of major depressive disorder in adults older than 18 years, a few antidepressant drugs have been approved for the treatment of depression in children and adolescents. Although many of the antidepressants have extensive data regarding their use in treating depression in children and adolescents, the FDA has formally approved only two agents for the treatment of major depressive disorder in individuals younger than 18 years. Fluoxetine (Prozac) is approved for the treatment of major depressive disorder in children age 8 years and older, and escitalopram (Lexapro) is approved for the treatment of depression in youth ages 12–17 years (Iannelli 2011). Additionally, many of the antidepressants have been used off-label for the treatment of other psychiatric and medical conditions. The alternative FDA-approved indications (i.e., anxiety, posttraumatic stress disorder, smoking cessation, insomnia, and nocturnal enuresis, among others) and off-label uses of antidepressant drugs are discussed in other chapters in this manual.

In 2004, the FDA issued an advisory warning for *all* antidepressant medications regarding "the increased risk of suicidal thinking and behavior, known as suicidality, in children, adolescents, and young adults ages 18 to 24 during the initial treatment (generally the first 1 to 2 months)" (U.S. Food and Drug Administration 2004, 2007). The psychiatric APRN should closely monitor patients receiving antidepressants, especially during titration, dosage changes, and discontinuation. Black box warnings have also been issued for nefazodone (a serotonin antagonist and reuptake inhibitor that is rarely used today) regarding hepatotoxicity and for bupropion (when prescribed for smoking cessation under the trade name Zyban) regarding neuropsychiatric symptoms and suicidality.

Treatment of Special Populations

Elderly and Medically Compromised Patients

Drug treatment should begin at 50% of the typical starting dose start in elderly patients, with the dosage titrated upward if tolerated. The elderly may require subtherapeutic doses because of the high comorbidity of medical conditions and polypharmacy as well as decreased liver and kidney function.

Dosage adjustments may be necessary in patients with medically compromised states. Check individual medications for dosage reductions as needed.

Children, Adolescents, and Young Adults

Similar to initial dosing in the elderly, drug treatment should begin at 50% of the recommended starting dose in children, with the dosage titrated upward if tolerated. Children can sometimes require dosages equivalent to therapeutic adult dosing because of their higher rate of metabolism.

Given the black box warning for the increased risk of suicidal thoughts and behaviors in children, adolescents, and young adults, the risks and benefits of psychopharmacological treatment need to be carefully considered and discussed with parents or guardians. Written consent also should be obtained before initiation of treatment.

Women

Paroxetine is contraindicated in pregnancy (Category D) because it has been implicated in cardiac defects in the infant. It is important for the prescribing APRN to discuss sexual habits and contraception practices with patients before they become pregnant.

Prescribing of any medication during pregnancy is typically contraindicated; however, the risks and benefits must be carefully considered for the woman at risk for postpartum depression.

PMDD is a debilitating disorder that can reduce a woman's quality of life on a monthly basis. Although only two antidepressants (fluoxetine and sertraline) are indicated for the treatment of PMDD, other antidepressants have shown anecdotal efficacy.

Treatment Monitoring

As with all medications, treatment monitoring is an ongoing process. A few unique treatment-emergent adverse events can occur with the antidepressants.

Serotonin Syndrome

Serotonin syndrome is a potentially life-threatening adverse drug event that causes the body to have too much serotonin. The most common cause of serotonin syndrome is when two serotonergic drugs are taken together. Drugs such as the SSRIs, SNRIs, MAOIs, triptans used for management of migraine headaches, meperidine (Demerol) used for pain management, dextromethorphan found in cough medications, Ecstasy, LSD, and St. John's wort can all potentially contribute to serotonin syndrome (Perez and Zieve 2012).

Symptoms of serotonin syndrome can occur within minutes to hours. They can variably include restlessness, tachycardia, agitation, hyperthermia, ataxia, hyperactive reflexes and myoclonus, variable blood pressure, nausea, vomiting, diarrhea, and hallucinations. This syndrome is considered a medical emergency requiring immediate intervention. Treatments may include cyproheptadine (Periactin), which blocks production of serotonin; benzodiazepines to reduce agitation, muscle stiffness, and seizurelike activity; intravenous fluids; and discontinuation of serotonergic medications. Observation should occur over the course of at least 24 hours, during which time the symptoms should subside with treatment. Without treatment, serotonin syndrome can lead to death from hyperthermia, seizures, rhabdomyolysis, renal failure, or shock (Perez and Zieve 2012). The presentation is similar to neuroleptic malignant syndrome and is differentiated by the presence of rigidity in neuroleptic malignant syndrome and hyperreflexia and myoclonus in serotonin syndrome.

Switch to Mania

In addition to serotonin syndrome, the antidepressants have been known to "flip" patients into previously unrecognized mania. In children, this phenomenon may present with symptoms of agitation, defiance, irritability, sleep disturbance, and hypersexual behaviors. In adults, the symptoms of grandiosity, out-of-character behaviors, rapid and pressured speech, agitation, excitability, sleep disruption, and poor impulse control are not uncommon. The APRN should closely monitor the patient during medication initiation and dose changes; the patient typically is scheduled in 2-week increments during the titration phase, and children are monitored more often.

Drug-Drug Interactions

Finally, given the extent to which the antidepressant medications affect the cytochrome P450 (CYP) enzymes, they present substantial risk for drug-drug interactions. Table 3–5 illustrates some interactions between antidepressants and the CYP enzymes.

More information on the various drugs that affect the CYP enzymes is available in Appendix 2, "Psychotropic and Other Medications Influenced by the Cytochrome P450 (CYP) System," at the end of this manual. It is imperative that the APRN collect a comprehensive medication history, inclusive of over-the-counter agents, herbal supplements, and vitamins, from the patient before initiating any antidepressant or other psychotropic agent and at each appointment to reduce the potential for drug-drug interactions and the potential for adverse events.

Summary

Depressive episodes can be debilitating to not only the patient but also his or her family and friends. The depressed individual may withdraw from involvement in family and social functions, work performance may be reduced, and (of particular concern) the patient may be at increased risk for suicidal thoughts or actions. Several effective psychopharmacological treatment regimens are available to patients to help relieve some of their symptoms. In general, psychotherapy is recommended in addition to medication to assist with building coping and problem-solving skills. Nurses need to be alert to the prevalence of depression and intervene as quickly as possible to assist the patient in obtaining the most appropriate treatments. It is also important for the nurse to offer the patient hope because symptoms of depression, when identified and treated, are generally reduced, and the individual's quality of life can markedly improve.

Table 3–5.   Inhibition of cytochrome P450 (CYP) enzymes by antidepressants

Drug	CYP2D6	CYP3A3/4	CYP1A2	CYP2C19
Bupropion	+	–	–	–
Citalopram	+	–	–	–
Duloxetine	+	–	–	–
Escitalopram	–	–	–	–
Fluoxetine	+	–	–	+
Fluvoxamine	–	+	+	+
Mirtazapine	–	–	–	–
Nefazodone	–	+	–	–
Paroxetine	+	–	–	–
Selegiline	–	–	–	–
Sertraline	+	–	–	–
Tricyclics (all)	–	–	–	–
Venlafaxine	–	–	–	–

Note.   + = inhibition; – = no inhibition.

Source.   Adapted from Nemeroff et al. 2007.

Clinical Pearls

- Generic SSRIs are generally less expensive than the newer antide-pressants.
- Most of the SNRIs are available only as brand names and tend to be more expensive.
- Time to efficacy is generally 4–6 weeks, and some antidepressants may take that long or longer to be effective.
- Although most side effects are dose dependent, many can be allevi-ated by titrating slowly or by simply changing the time of day at which the antidepressant is taken.

- Treatment-resistant conditions may require combination therapy or augmentation of the antidepressant.

- Sometimes a patient may be in a depressive phase of an unknown bipolar disorder; clinicians must watch for elevated mood early in treatment with antidepressants.

- Augmentation of the antidepressants with L-methylfolate, a medical food, or lithium may benefit the patient who does not achieve remission.

- Maximizing one agent is typically the best course of action prior to changing to a different agent or augmenting the medication therapy.

- If the patient fails to respond to two adequate trials within one class of antidepressants, a change of class is generally recommended.

References

American Psychiatric Association: Diagnostic and Statistical Manual of Mental Disorders, 4th Edition, Text Revision. Washington, DC, American Psychiatric Association, 2000

Centers for Disease Control and Prevention: Current depression among adults—United States, 2006 and 2008. MMWR Morb Mortal Wkly Rep 59:1229–1235, 2010

Centers for Disease Control and Prevention: An estimated 1 in 10 US adults report depression. 2011. Available at: http://www.cdc.gov/Features/dsDepression/. Accessed April 20, 2012.

Cooper WO, Willy ME, Pont SJ, et al: Increasing use of antidepressants in pregnancy. Am J Obstet Gynecol 196:544–548, 2007

Cox JL, Holden JM, Sagovsky R: Detection of postnatal depression: development of the 10-item Edinburgh Postnatal Depression Scale. Br J Psychiatry 150:782–786, 1987

Iannelli V: Antidepressants for children: antidepressant black box warnings. Updated October 11, 2011. Available at: http://pediatrics.about.com/od/depression/a/04_andep_suicde.htm. Accessed January 7, 2013.

Jeong HG, Ham BJ, Yeo HB, et al: Gray matter abnormalities in patients with premenstrual dysphoric disorder: an optimized voxel-based morphometry. J Affect Disord 140:260–267, 2012

Nemeroff CB, Preskorn SH, DeVane CL: Antidepressant drug-drug interactions: clinical relevance and risk management. CNS Spectr 12 (5 suppl 7):1–16, 2007

Perez E, Zieve D: Serotonin syndrome (article in MedlinePlus medical encyclopedia). Updated July 8, 2012. Available at: www.nlm.nih.gov/medlineplus/ency/article/007272.htm. Accessed February 6, 2013.

Protopopescu X, Pan H, Tuescher O, et al: Toward a functional neuroanatomy of premenstrual dysphoric disorder: differential amygdala, orbitofrontal and ventral striatal activity. J Affect Disord 108:87–94, 2008

Roman MW, Bembry FH: L-Methylfolate (Deplin): a new medical food therapy as adjunctive treatment for depression. Issues Ment Health Nurs 32(2):142–143, 2011

Stahl SM: Stahl's Essential Psychopharmacology: Neuroscientific Basis and Practical Applications, 3rd Edition. New York, Cambridge University Press, 2008

Stoppler MC: Premenstrual dysphoric disorder (PMDD). 2009. Available at: http://www.emedicinehealth.com/premenstrual_dysphoric_disorder_pmdd/article_em.htm. Accessed March 30, 2012.

Trivedi MH, Rush AJ, Crismon ML, et al: Clinical results for patients with major depressive disorder in the Texas Medication Algorithm Project. Arch Gen Psychiatry 61:669–680, 2004

Trivedi MH, Rush AJ, Wisniewski SR, et al: Evaluation of outcomes with citalopram for depression using measurement-based care in STAR * D: implications for clinical practice. Am J Psychiatry 163:28–40, 2006

U.S. Food and Drug Administration: FDA launches a multi-pronged strategy to strengthen safeguards for children treated with antidepressant medications. FDA Release P04-97, October 15, 2004. Available at: http://www.fda.gov/NewsEvents/Newsroom/PressAnnouncements/2004/ucm108363.htm. Accessed February 6, 2013.

U.S. Food and Drug Administration: FDA proposes new warnings about suicidal thinking, behavior in young adults who take antidepressant medications. FDA Release P07-77, May 2, 2007. Available at: http://www.fda.gov/NewsEvents/Newsroom/PressAnnouncements/2007/ucm108905.htm. Accessed February 6, 2013.

Vesga-Lopez O, Blanco C, Keyes K, et al: Psychiatric disorders in pregnant and postpartum women in the United States. Arch Gen Psychiatry 65:805–815, 2008

4

Bipolar Disorders

Candice Knight, Ph.D., Ed.D., A.P.R.N.,
P.M.H.-C.N.S./N.P., B.C.

> I thought how unpleasant it is to be locked out;
> and I thought how it is worse, perhaps, to be locked in.
>
> —Virginia Woolf (1882–1941)

In recent years, many developments in diagnosing and treating bipolar disorder have emerged. These developments are accompanied by many questions. For example, should bipolar disorder be diagnosed as a discrete category, as currently described in DSM-IV-TR (American Psychiatric Association 2000), or should it be defined as a spectrum disorder? Has lithium (Eskalith, Lithobid), once the gold standard for treating bipolar mania, ceded to the second-generation antipsychotics (SGAs)? Furthermore, should antidepressants ever be used to treat bipolar depression, given the potential for switching patients into bipolar mania? In this chapter, I offer answers to these questions as well as provide the psychiatric advanced practice registered nurse (APRN) with up-to-date information on the most efficacious pharmacological approaches for treating bipolar disorder.

Overview of Bipolar Disorders

Bipolar disorder refers to a group of cyclical, lifelong syndromes characterized by recurrent episodes of elevated mood and recurrent episodes of depressed mood with intervening periods of normality. DSM-IV-TR defines bipolar disorder by four discrete diagnostic categories: bipolar I disorder, bipolar II disorder, cyclothymic disorder, and bipolar disorder not otherwise specified (NOS). These categories include a configuration of four different mood episodes, including manic episode, depressive episode, hypomanic episode, and mixed episode (American Psychiatric Association 2000).

A *manic episode* is a period lasting at least 1 week (or any duration if hospitalized) of abnormally and persistently elevated, expansive, or irritable mood in which three or more of the central manic symptoms have persisted (four if the mood is only irritable) and have been present to a significant degree to cause marked impairment in functioning, produce psychosis, or require hospitalization. A *hypomanic episode* is a period of at least 4 days of persistently elevated, expansive, or irritable mood that is different from the usual nondepressed mood in which three or more of the central manic symptoms (four if the mood is only irritable) have been present to a significant degree to cause an unequivocal, uncharacteristic change in functioning that is observable by others. The hypomanic episode does not cause a marked impairment in social or occupational functioning or necessitate hospitalization, and no psychotic features are present. The central symptoms of both manic and hypomanic episodes (American Psychiatric Association 2000, pp. 362, 368) include

- Inflated self-esteem or grandiosity
- Decreased need for sleep (e.g., feels rested after only 3 hours of sleep)
- More talkative than usual or pressure to keep talking
- Flight of ideas or subjective experience that thoughts are racing
- Distractibility (i.e., attention too easily drawn to unimportant or irrelevant external stimuli)

- Increase in goal-directed activity (either socially, at work or school, or sexually) or psychomotor agitation
- Excessive involvement in pleasurable activities that have a high potential for painful consequences (e.g., engaging in unrestrained buying sprees, sexual indiscretions, or foolish business investments)

The symptoms and number required are the same for both types of episodes; the main distinction between them is in the duration and the degree of severity. The manic episode requires a duration of at least 1 week and a marked impairment in functioning that may have psychotic features and require hospitalization, whereas the hypomanic episode requires a duration of at least 4 days and a change in functioning (American Psychiatric Association 2000).

In contrast, a *depressive episode* is defined as a 2-week period during which either depressed mood or loss of pleasure is present with five or more of the following central symptoms (American Psychiatric Association 2000, p. 356):

- Depressed mood most of the day, nearly every day, as indicated by either subjective report (e.g., feels sad or empty) or observation made by others (e.g., appears tearful); children and adolescents may have irritable mood.
- Markedly diminished interest or pleasure in all, or almost all, activities most of the day, nearly every day (as indicated by either subjective account or observation made by others)
- Significant weight loss when not dieting or weight gain (e.g., a change of more than 5% of body weight in a month), or decrease or increase in appetite nearly every day. In children, consider failure to make expected weight gains.
- Insomnia or hypersomnia nearly every day
- Psychomotor agitation or retardation nearly every day (observable by others, not merely subjective feelings of restlessness or being slowed down)
- Fatigue or loss of energy nearly every day
- Feelings of worthlessness or excessive or inappropriate guilt (which may be delusional) nearly every day (not merely self-reproach or guilt about being sick)
- Diminished ability to think or concentrate, or indecisiveness, nearly every day (either by subjective account or as observed by others)

- Recurrent thoughts of death (not just fear of dying), recurrent suicidal ideation without a specific plan, or a suicide attempt or a specific plan for committing suicide

A *mixed episode* is defined as a 1-week period during which the central symptoms are met for both a manic episode and a major depressive episode nearly every day. This type of episode causes impairment in occupational or social functioning, produces psychosis, or requires hospitalization (American Psychiatric Association 2000).

Bipolar disorder is associated with high levels of impairment in social, occupational, and physical functioning and a high degree of burden and human suffering. The disorder affects approximately 2.6% of the U.S. population age 18 and older in a given year. The average age at onset tends to be mid-teens to early 20s. Bipolar disorder tends to be highly recurrent, and following the first manic episode, 90% of individuals go on to develop future episodes. The lifetime risk of suicide for patients with bipolar disorder is 19%, the highest of any mental disorder. Bipolar disorder tends to occur equally among men and women, although female patients are at a greater risk for depressive episodes, rapid cycling, and bipolar II disorder, and male patients are at a greater risk for manic episodes (National Institute of Mental Health 2008).

The diagnosis of *bipolar I disorder* requires the occurrence of one or more manic episodes or mixed episodes. Thus, a patient with a manic episode who has never shown evidence of a depressive episode is still given the diagnosis. The diagnosis of *bipolar II disorder* requires the occurrence of one or more major depressive episodes and at least one hypomanic episode. Unlike bipolar I disorder, in which the patient may be given the diagnosis with only one manic episode, the patient with bipolar II disorder must have had at least one major depressive episode and one hypomanic episode. Both bipolar I and bipolar II disorder may be further defined as mild, moderate, or severe; with or without psychotic features; and with unique specifiers such as with atypical or melancholic features, postpartum onset, rapid cycling, or seasonal pattern (American Psychiatric Association 2000). Bipolar disorder with rapid cycling may be more treatment refractory and difficult to treat with medication successfully (Suppes et al. 2000).

Cyclothymic disorder is characterized by numerous periods of hypomanic and depressive symptoms for at least 2 years in adults and 1 year in children and adolescents. Also, the patient has not been without the symptoms for more than 2 months at a time (American Psychiatric Association 2000). Bipolar disorder NOS is characterized by bipolar features that do not meet the criteria for any other bipolar disorder (American Psychiatric Association 2000).

About 69% of all patients with bipolar disorder are inaccurately diagnosed, usually with major depressive disorder, and 35% of all patients are symptomatic for more than 10 years before the correct diagnosis is made (Hirschfeld et al. 2003). Complicating diagnosis is the occurrence of several comorbid conditions with overlapping symptoms, including anxiety disorders, substance abuse disorders, attention-deficit/hyperactivity disorder, and disruptive behavior disorders (Sadock and Sadock 2007).

Whether to maintain the current categorical method of diagnosing bipolar disorder as described in DSM-IV-TR or to move to a dimensional perspective that encompasses a wide range of symptoms described as bipolar spectrum disorder has been the subject of considerable debate. By broadening the definition to a spectrum disorder, many at-risk patients could be provided with early identification and psychopharmacological treatment. However, by broadening the definition, many patients may be given the diagnosis and medication who do not actually have the disorder. Ruggero et al. (2010) found that patients with borderline personality disorder are already frequently misdiagnosed with bipolar disorder, which leads to the excessive use of medication when therapy such as dialectical behavior therapy would be more effective. Strakowski et al. (2011) determined that much of the neurocognitive, neuroimaging, and genetic research to date provides no evidence for broadening the bipolar diagnosis. At this time, the evidence is too limited to conclude that broadening the definition would result in improvement in treatment.

Neurobiology of Bipolar Disorders

Although the neurochemistry of bipolar disorder is not completely understood, studies have provided data indicating that bipolar disorder is a multifactorial disorder with genetic, neurobiological, and environmental causes. Family studies provided strong evidence of a genetic factor by reporting that first-degree relatives of bipolar patients have an elevated risk for developing bipolar disorder (4%–24%); twin studies indicate a concordance rate of 60%–80% among monozygotic twins compared with 10%–20% in dizygotic twins (Dubovsky et al. 2003).

Structurally, patients with bipolar disorder have smaller prefrontal lobe volumes and enlargement of the basal ganglia, thalamus, hippocampus, and amygdala. Volumetric decreases have indicated a loss of gray matter in the left dorsolateral, ventral, and orbital prefrontal cortex as well as the anterior cingulate cortex (Martinowich et al. 2009). Functionally, virtually every imaging study has identified complex networks of activity characterized by global changes throughout the nervous system, especially within the limbic structures and prefrontal cortex (Altshuler et al. 1998). The dorsolateral prefrontal cortex has been identified as having decreased metabolism and blood flow as well as altering functions in attention, working memory, conflict monitoring, reward valuation, and response inhibition (Berns and Nemeroff 2003).

Neurotransmitter dysregulation of norepinephrine, dopamine, serotonin, γ-aminobutyric acid (GABA), and glutamate has been a central theory in bipolar disorder. The first-messenger system, the binding of the neurotransmitter to one or more receptor subtypes, has been the target for pharmacological agents (Goodwin and Jamison 2007). It also has been hypothesized that G proteins, which modulate intracellular activity, may be hyperfunctional in manic patients, causing dysregulation in the downstream effects of the cyclic adenosine monophosphate (cAMP) system and the phosphoinositide system (Manji and Lenox 2000). The second-messenger system and the sequence of intracellular events, initiated by first-messenger neurotransmitter binding, are now understood to be key factors in the neurochemistry of bipolar disorder. Second messengers transmit signals from the receptors to target molecules inside the cell, causing intracellular changes that stimulate or inhibit signaling transduction cascades. Some second-messenger molecules important in bipolar disorder are cyclic nucleotides (e.g., cAMP and cyclic guanosine monophosphate), ions (e.g., calcium^{2+} or Ca^{2+}), phospholipid-derived molecules (e.g., phosphatidylinositol), and nitric oxide. These second messengers mediate downstream events to specific protein targets, such as ion channels, that may change their conformation and function (Manji and Lenox 2000). Abnormalities have been found in the regulation of calcium signaling and neural plasticity with mitochondrial dysfunction (Martinowich et al. 2009).

Other factors recognized in the etiology of bipolar disorder include perinatal insult, head trauma, desynchronization of circadian or seasonal rhythms, psychosocial stressors and traumatic experiences, deficiency of essential amino acid precursors in the diet causing dysregulation of neurotransmitter activity, hypothalamic-pituitary-thyroid axis dysregulation, and kindling theories (Martinowich et al. 2009).

Treatment of Bipolar Disorders

The most effective treatment for bipolar disorder combines psychotherapeutic approaches with psychopharmacology (American Psychiatric Association 2002). Psychotherapeutic approaches include psychoeducation (e.g., adaptation to a chronic illness, lifestyle changes, early detection of prodromal symptoms, medication adherence) and individual, group, and family psychotherapy to identify psychosocial factors that trigger episodes, engage family members in treatment, enhance social and occupational functioning, and modulate heightened levels of expressed emotion, especially hostility. Interpersonal and social rhythm therapy, a hybrid therapy approach that combines interpersonal therapy with a variety of psychoeducational management techniques, has been highly successful in the treatment of bipolar disorder (Frank et al. 2005). The Systematic Treatment Enhancement Program for Bipolar Disorder (STEP-BD) found that patients receiving medication and intensive psychotherapy had fewer relapses, were better able to maintain their treatment, and were more likely to get well faster and stay well longer (Miklowitz et al. 2007).

Psychopharmacological treatment for bipolar disorder offers various monotherapy and combination options and includes the use of lithium, anticonvulsants, first-generation antipsychotics (FGAs), SGAs, benzodiazepines, and antidepressants. Selection is guided by illness severity, associated features (e.g., agitation, rapid cycling, psychosis), and side-effect profiles as well as cost and patient preferences.

Acute Bipolar Mania

The U.S. Food and Drug Administration (FDA) has approved four medication categories to treat acute mania: lithium, anticonvulsants (valproate [Depakote], carbamazepine [Tegretol]), FGAs (chlorpromazine [Thorazine]), and SGAs (olanzapine [Zyprexa], risperidone [Risperdal], quetiapine [Seroquel], ziprasidone [Geodon], aripiprazole [Abilify], and asenapine [Saphris]). Treatment of acute bipolar mania often necessitates a combination of these medications.

The *Practice Guideline for the Treatment of Patients With Bipolar Disorder* of the American Psychiatric Association (2002) advocates lithium or valproate in combination with an antipsychotic as the first-line treatment for severe manic episodes and monotherapy with lithium, valproate, or an SGA for less severe mania. SGAs are recommended over FGAs because of more benign side effects. Carbamazepine or oxcarbazepine (Trileptal) may be used in place of lithium or valproate. The short-term adjunctive use of benzodiazepines is also recommended to target symptoms of insomnia, anxiety, and agitation, and antidepressants should be tapered and discontinued.

Several older studies support the use of lithium and valproate and are cited in the American Psychiatric Association (2002) guideline. More recent studies have been carried out with the use of SGAs as compared with placebo, lithium, or anticonvulsants as well as various combination therapies.

In 2005, an American Psychiatric Association guideline watch was published, describing additional, evidence-based studies that used SGAs as well as extended-release carbamazepine for the acute treatment of bipolar mania. Hirschfeld (2005) concluded that these psychopharmacological agents are efficacious as both monotherapy and combination therapy and provide new treatment options.

Later, a systematic review and meta-analysis examined eight randomized controlled trials (RCTs) that compared monotherapy with combination therapy in adult and adolescent patients with acute bipolar mania and found that haloperidol (Haldol), olanzapine, risperidone, and quetiapine in combination with a traditional mood stabilizer were more efficacious than monotherapy with a mood stabilizer. However, significant weight gain occurred with the SGA combination therapy compared with monotherapy with a mood stabilizer (Smith et al. 2006).

In a recent meta-analysis, Cipriani et al. (2011) analyzed 68 RCTs that compared a mood stabilizer, FGA, or SGA with another or with a placebo. The results indicated that in the acute treatment of bipolar mania in adults, haloperidol, risperidone, olanzapine, lithium, quetiapine, aripiprazole, carbamazepine, asenapine, valproate, and ziprasidone were significantly more effective than placebo but that gabapentin (Neurontin), lamotrigine (Lamictal), and topiramate (Topamax) were not. The top five superior drugs, in order of efficaciousness, were haloperidol, risperidone, olanzapine, lithium, and quetiapine.

Clinicians often initiate combination treatment for an acutely manic patient with both lithium or valproate and an FGA or SGA for rapid control of symptoms. Some clinicians taper the antipsychotic when improvement occurs. Starting with monotherapy is also acceptable. For patients started on an SGA monotherapy, the SGA is usually continued for maintenance therapy; if the patient's symptoms are unresponsive after 3–7 days, the addition of lithium or valproate is recommended. For those started on lithium or valproate as monotherapy, an SGA is usually added after 1 or 2 weeks if the manic symptoms are unresponsive. Another approach is to add a benzodiazepine (e.g., lorazepam [Ativan] or clonazepam [Klonopin]) for insomnia and agitation. Schatzberg et al. (2010) noted that triple therapy with a benzodiazepine, an antipsychotic, and lithium allows smaller doses of the first two agents during an acute episode.

Bipolar Depression

Bipolar depression, the predominant mood state of bipolar disorder, may be associated with more severe symptoms, greater impairment, and more treatment resistance than bipolar mania. Bipolar depression is also less researched and underdiagnosed, with patients frequently receiving a diagnosis of major depressive disorder (Hirschfeld 2004). Unlike bipolar mania, the practice guidelines for treating bipolar depression vary greatly from country to country, with European practice guidelines advocating the use of more antidepressants and the United States advocating more mood stabilizers and SGAs, although controversy over the use of antidepressants also exists within the United States (Nivoli et al. 2012).

The American Psychiatric Association (2002) practice guideline supports the use of lithium or lamotrigine monotherapy as the first-line psychopharmacological treatment for bipolar depression. Antidepressants as monotherapy are not recommended. For more severely ill patients, the guideline does recommend combination treatment with lithium and an antidepressant.

Although lithium monotherapy is recommended by the American Psychiatric Association (2002) guideline, more recent research has shown that it is more effective in acute bipolar mania than in bipolar depression (Calabrese et al. 2003). Some studies indicated that lithium exerts significant antidepressant activity when prescribed at the higher therapeutic dose range (Keck et al. 2003b) and that a positive link exists between lithium use and lowering suicidal rates in patients with bipolar depression (Tondo et al. 1998).

Lamotrigine is indicated for maintenance treatment of bipolar I disorder to delay the occurrence of mood episodes. However, a recent meta-analysis found that lamotrigine was effective in treating bipolar depression as monotherapy (Geddes et al. 2009). Lamotrigine is recommended as a first-line treatment for acute bipolar depression in not only the American Psychiatric Association (2002) guideline but also other guidelines, including those of the International Consensus Group on the Evidence-Based Pharmacologic Treatment of Bipolar I and II Depression (Kasper et al. 2008), the International Society for Bipolar Disorders (Ghaemi et al. 2008), and the British Association for Psychopharmacology (Goodwin et al. 2009).

Since the American Psychiatric Association (2002) guideline was published, Symbyax, a combination of olanzapine and fluoxetine, and quetiapine have been approved by the FDA for the treatment of bipolar depression. Quetiapine was found efficacious in the treatment of bipolar depression at dosages of 300–600 mg/day (Bogart and Chavez 2009).

Whether to use antidepressants in treating bipolar depression has been controversial. Results from the STEP-BD project suggested that using antidepressants does not result in switching patients into a manic or rapid-cycling condition (Sachs et al. 2007). Several studies cited in the American Psychiatric Association (2002) guideline indicated that adding antidepressants as an augmentation strategy to lithium, valproate, or carbamazepine has been successful and resulted in no or a very low number of patients switching to hypomania or mania. Paroxetine (Paxil, Paxil CR) has been found to be particularly efficacious for augmentation. In a long-term, 68-week study by Van der Loos et al. (2011), lithium augmented by lamotrigine and paroxetine was significantly efficacious in bipolar depressed patients. Lithium is also an excellent choice for patients experiencing suicidal ideation. Other practice guidelines advocate treatment of bipolar depression with lithium or valproate in combination with bupropion (Wellbutrin), mirtazapine (Remeron), and venlafaxine (Effexor, Effexor XR) (Nivoli et al. 2012).

The American Psychiatric Association guideline watch stated that lithium, lamotrigine, olanzapine-fluoxetine combination, and quetiapine showed the strongest evidence for treating bipolar depression (Hirschfeld 2005). Other choices recommended by treatment guidelines include valproate, oxcarbazepine (Trileptal), and topiramate as well as aripiprazole, risperidone, ziprasidone, and clozapine (Clozaril) (Nivoli et al. 2012).

Whether antidepressants can cause the development of bipolar disorder in someone who did not have it prior to taking an antidepressant is also part of an ongoing debate. Stahl (2008) stated that antidepressants could activate bipolar disorder in patients known to have a bipolar spectrum disorder. However, it is likely that a patient who develops manic symptoms after taking an antidepressant already has bipolar disorder that has been undiagnosed or wrongly diagnosed, which then is unmasked—but not caused—by antidepressant treatment.

The successful treatment of bipolar depression demands early recognition of the condition and typically an arduous course of exploring different psychopharmacological treatments. In general, patients with bipolar depression may be prescribed lithium, an anticonvulsant such as lamotrigine, an SGA such as quetiapine, or a combination drug such as olanzapine-fluoxetine as first-line treatments. Patients without positive effects should then be considered for a second psychopharmacological agent. For example, if the patient with bipolar depression remains resistant to lamotrigine treatment, then the addition of quetiapine might benefit, and similarly, if the patient is prescribed quetiapine without effect, then the addition of lamotrigine might be advantageous. Patients who fail to respond to these combinations, which is common, might benefit from a third agent, such as another anticonvulsant or an antidepressant.

Mixed States of Bipolar Disorder

Mixed states of bipolar disorder are difficult to treat. Patients with mixed episodes often have accompanying symptoms of psychosis, anxiety, agitation, and mood lability. Limited studies have been conducted with these patients alone because they are frequently part of studies with bipolar manic patients (Schatzberg et al. 2010).

Although the American Psychiatric Association (2002) practice guideline supports the use of lithium or valproate plus an antipsychotic for first-line psychopharmacological treatment of mixed states, the most current evidence suggests that valproate combined with an atypical antipsychotic should be considered the first-line treatment, with lithium or carbamazepine regarded as second-line treatments (McIntyre and Yoon 2012). Lamotrigine also has been successful in patients with mixed states and predominantly depressive symptoms (Krüger et al. 2006); however, the necessity of slow titration limits its use in acute situations. Studies also have found quetiapine, ziprasidone, and clozapine to be efficacious as monotherapy in patients with mixed states in lessening both the manic and the depressed symptoms (Schatzberg et al. 2010), but most patients require combination therapy for the treatment of mixed states (McIntyre and Yoon 2012). Antidepressants should be avoided with this population.

Mixed episodes are characterized by recurrent depression more frequently than by recurrent mania. The American Psychiatric Association (2002) practice guideline suggests that the initial intervention should be to identify and treat any condition that may be contributing to rapid cycling such as hypothyroidism and substance abuse and to taper or discontinue any medication that may be a contributing factor such as antidepressants and stimulants. The efficacy of mood-stabilizing medication improves if contributory conditions and offending medications are removed.

Rapid Cycling

The American Psychiatric Association (2002) practice guideline recommends the use of lithium, valproate, or lamotrigine as first-line agents for patients with rapid cycling. Studies have shown that these agents are effective (Tondo et al. 2003). Studies that used SGAs with the olanzapine-fluoxetine combination, olanzapine alone, aripiprazole, and quetiapine also have suggested efficacy in reducing manic and depressive episodes in rapid-cycling patients (Sanger et al. 2003; Schatzberg et al. 2010). The combination of several medications is usually required because monotherapy is typically inadequate.

Maintenance Treatment

Maintenance treatment is standard protocol for patients with bipolar disorder because patients have a very high rate of relapse. According to the American Psychiatric Association (2002) practice guideline, the best evidence supports the use of lithium and valproate for maintenance treatment, with the possible alternatives of lamotrigine, carbamazepine, or oxcarbazepine. The guideline also supports optimizing the dose of maintenance medication for break-through depressive episodes; if symptoms do not respond, lamotrigine or an antidepressant such as bupropion or paroxetine should be added. Lithium, the first maintenance medication approved by the FDA in 1974, is effective in preventing both poles of bipolar disorder, but the effects are more pronounced in preventing manic recurrences, whereas lamotrigine, approved by the FDA for maintenance treatment in 2003, has greater efficacy in preventing depressive episodes (Calabrese et al. 2003). Since the 2002 guideline was published, the FDA has approved lamotrigine, olanzapine, risperidone, quetiapine, aripiprazole, and ziprasidone for maintenance treatment.

Lithium, a mood stabilizer, or an SGA is generally recommended as initial maintenance treatment for all patients with bipolar disorder. If the patient experiences a breakthrough episode of mania or depression, the dose of the first-line intervention should be optimized; if that fails, another first-line medication category should be added. For example, if the patient is taking lithium, valproate, or lamotrigine and the dose has been optimized, an SGA may be added; if an SGA is already prescribed at the optimal dose, a mood stabilizer may be added. Additional alternatives include augmenting with carbamazepine or oxcarbazepine in lieu of an additional first-line medication or changing from one mood stabilizer or antipsychotic to another.

Medications Used to Treat Bipolar Disorders

Tables 4–1 and 4–2 provide an overview of the mood-stabilizing agents prescribed to patients with bipolar disorder.

Table 4–1. Mood-stabilizing agents: lithium and anticonvulsants

Drug	Therapeutic indications	Daily dosage	Dosing tips
Antimanic agents			
Lithium carbonate (Lithobid) Lithium citrate	Bipolar mania (FDA) Bipolar maintenance (FDA) Bipolar mixed Bipolar depression	Adults: Acute mania: 1,800–2,400 mg/day Maintenance: 900–1,200 mg/day	Start at 300 mg; ↑ 300 mg every 3 days Measure serum lithium level with each change Maintenance serum level = 0.6–1.2 mEq/L
		Adolescents >12 years: Acute mania: 900–1,200 mg/day Maintenance: 600–900 mg/day	Start at 300 mg once daily; ↑ 300 mg every 3 days until serum level of 0.6–1.2 mEq/L is reached
Anticonvulsants			
Valproic acid (Depakote) (Depakote ER) (Depakene)	Bipolar mania (FDA) Bipolar mixed Bipolar maintenance Bipolar depression	Adults: Acute mania: 1,200–1,500 mg/day Maintenance: 15–60 mg/kg	Start at 15 mg/kg twice a day until serum level of 50–125 µg/mL is reached; ↑ every 3 days For ER, start at 25 mg/kg once daily until serum level of 50–100 mEq/L is reached
Oxcarbazepine (Trileptal)	Off-label	Adults: 1,200–2,400 mg/day	Start at 200 mg twice a day; ↑ 300 mg every 3 days

Table 4–1. Mood-stabilizing agents: lithium and anticonvulsants *(continued)*

Drug	Therapeutic indications	Daily dosage	Dosing tips
Anticonvulsants *(continued)*			
Carbamazepine (Equetro) (Tegretol)	Bipolar mania (XR only FDA)	Adults: 400–1,000 mg/day	Start at 200 mg twice a day; ↑ 200 mg/day until serum level of 4–12 μg/mL is reached
Lamotrigine (Lamictal)	Bipolar maintenance (FDA) Bipolar depression	Adults: 100–200 mg/day	Refer to Table 4–3
Gabapentin (Neurontin)	Off-label	Adults: 900–1,800 mg/day	Start at 100–300 mg three times a day; ↑ 300 mg every 3 days
Topiramate (Topamax)	Off-label	Adults: 50–300 mg/day	Start at 25–50 mg/day; ↑ 25–50 mg every 3 days

Note. ↑=increase; CR=controlled release; ER=extended release; FDA=approved by the U.S. Food and Drug Administration; XR=extended release.

Table 4–2. Mood-stabilizing agents: antipsychotics

Drug	Therapeutic indications	Daily dosage	Dosing tips
Chlorpromazine (Thorazine)	Bipolar mania (FDA) Acute agitation	Adults: 50–800 mg	Start at 10–25 mg po bid–qid or 25–50 mg/kg im
		Children <5 years: maximum 50 mg Children 5–10 years: maximum 200 mg	Start at 2.5 mg/kg every 4–6 hours po or 0.5 mg/kg every 6–8 hours im; titrate slowly
Olanzapine (Zyprexa)	Bipolar mania (FDA) Bipolar mixed (FDA) Bipolar maintenance (FDA) Bipolar depression Acute agitation	Adults: 5–20 mg	Start at 5–10 mg once daily; ↑ 5 mg/day; 10–20 mg/week; im start at 10 mg
		Adolescents >13 years: 5–20 mg	Start at 2.5 mg (po only)
Olanzapine-fluoxetine combination (Symbyax)	Bipolar depression (FDA)	Adults: 6 mg/25 mg – 18 mg/75 mg	Start at 6 mg/25 mg at bedtime; 6–12 mg olanzapine/25–50 mg fluoxetine; ↑ to 18 mg/75 mg
Risperidone (Risperdal)	Bipolar mania (FDA) Bipolar maintenance (FDA)	Adults: 1–6 mg	Start at 1 mg bid; ↑ 1 mg/day po until desired efficacy is attained
		Children >10 years: 0.5–6.0 mg/day divided qd–tid	Start at 0.5–2.0 mg in divided doses

Table 4–2. Mood-stabilizing agents: antipsychotics (continued)

Drug	Therapeutic indications	Daily dosage	Dosing tips
Quetiapine (Seroquel)	Bipolar mania (FDA) Bipolar maintenance (FDA) Bipolar depression (FDA)	Adults: 200–800 mg Children >10 years: 200–800 mg	Start at 50 mg/day bid; ↑ to 400 mg/day on day 4 Target daily dose: 400–800 mg For bipolar depression, 50 mg at bedtime; titrate as needed to 300 mg/day (maximum) Start at 25 mg/day bid; titrate by 50–100 mg/ day to 200 mg/day by day 5; may then increase by 50–100 mg/day to maximum dose
Ziprasidone (Geodon)	Bipolar mania (FDA) Bipolar maintenance (FDA)	Adults: 40–160 mg	Start with 40 mg bid; day 2 ↑ to 80 mg bid Target daily dose: 80–160 mg Intramuscular dose: 20 mg every 4 hours; maximum daily dose: 40 mg
Aripiprazole (Abilify)	Bipolar mania (FDA) Bipolar maintenance (FDA)	Adults: 15–30 mg Children >10 years: 2–30 mg	Start at 5–15 mg/day Start at 1–5 mg/day
Asenapine (Saphris)	Bipolar mania (FDA) Bipolar mixed (FDA)	Adults: 10–40 mg	Start with 10 mg sublingually Monotherapy: 10–20 mg bid Adjunctive therapy: 5 mg bid

Note. ↑=increase; bid=twice a day; FDA=approved by the U.S. Food and Drug Administration; im=intramuscular; po=by mouth; qid=four times a day; tid=three times a day.

Lithium

Lithium modulates the balance between excitatory and inhibitory neurotransmitter effects by increasing dopamine turnover and decreasing its synthesis, enhancing serotonin and acetylcholine neurotransmission, increasing norepinephrine and glutamate reuptake, and increasing GABA (Lenox and Hahn 2000). Lithium alters sodium transport across the cell membrane, adjusts signaling activity by affecting second-messenger systems, and modulates G proteins that function as signal transducers. Lithium also influences gene expression for growth factors and neuronal plasticity through its effects on glycogen synthetase kinase-3β, cAMP-dependent kinase, and protein kinase C (Schatzberg et al. 2010).

Lithium is completely absorbed after oral administration and is excreted entirely unchanged by the kidneys. It has a narrow therapeutic window, requiring close monitoring of plasma drug levels. It has an onset of 5–7 days, a peak of 10–21 days, and a half-life of 20–27 hours, and it takes 3–5 days to achieve a steady state. Once a therapeutic level is reached, it may take 1–2 weeks for symptom improvement (Pedersen and Leahy 2010; Stahl 2011).

Before initiating treatment, patients should have a complete blood count (CBC), a comprehensive metabolic profile, and thyroid and renal function tests. A baseline electrocardiogram should be obtained for patients older than 50 or those with suspected cardiac dysfunction. Weight and body mass index of the patient should be assessed. Caution is advised when the patient is also prescribed diuretics or nonsteroidal anti-inflammatory agents because they will markedly increase the risk for toxicity. Three days after treatment begins, a lithium level should be obtained and the dose increased by 300 mg every 3 days until the appropriate serum concentration is reached (Stahl 2011). Once the manic episode has abated, the lithium requirement often decreases. Patients should continue taking a maintenance dose to prevent recurrences. Abrupt discontinuation after long-term treatment significantly increases the rate of relapse and the risk for suicide; stopping the medication should be done gradually over a 3-month period (Schatzberg et al. 2010).

Trough serum lithium levels are monitored and should be between 1.0 and 1.5 mEq/L for acute treatment, 0.6 and 1.2 mEq/L for maintenance, and 0.4 and 0.8 mEq/L for augmentation. Levels should be checked after each dose increase or sooner if toxicity is suspected. Levels for maintenance should be checked every 6 months or whenever the health status changes. The blood sample should be drawn early in the morning, prior to the first dose, or at least 12 hours after the last dose. Patients should undergo a CBC, comprehensive metabolic profile, and renal and thyroid function tests every 3 months during the first 6 months of treatment and then every 12 months, if stable. Weight and body mass index should be monitored frequently (American Psychiatric Association 2002).

Common side effects of lithium may contribute to nonadherence. The most common adverse events include tremor, fatigue, headache, impaired memory, ataxia, sedation, dizziness, abdominal pain, anorexia, bloating, nausea, diarrhea, acne, rash, electrocardiogram changes, edema, and weight gain. Measures can be taken to reduce side effects, such as taking lithium at night or with food, changing to a controlled-release preparation, or prescribing medication to alleviate specific symptoms, such as propranolol to alleviate tremor. Hypothyroidism occurs in 5%–35% of female patients, generally after 6–18 months of treatment; it is not a contraindication to continuing lithium and is easily treated by the administration of levothyroxine (Levothroid, Synthroid) (American Psychiatric Association 2002).

Life-threatening lithium toxicity may occur when serum levels are higher than 1.5 mEq/L. Symptoms include marked tremor, drowsiness, slurred speech, blurred vision, confusion, hyperactive deep tendon reflexes, and ataxia that can progress to cardiac dysrhythmia, seizures, coma, and permanent neurological impairment. Any value greater than 2 mEq/L is considered a medical emergency and may indicate a need for hemodialysis.

Prescribing lithium for those younger than 12 should be done with caution and close monitoring. In general, children have more severe and frequent side effects. The American Psychiatric Association (2002) guideline recommends a range between 0.4 and 0.6 mEq/L when prescribing lithium to the elderly. Frequent monitoring of lithium levels is also recommended for patients who are medically compromised (Kennedy 2008). Lithium is a Category D pregnancy risk and should not be taken during pregnancy because of the increased risk of birth defects and cardiac anomalies, especially Ebstein's anomaly. Women should not breast-feed while taking lithium.

Anticonvulsant Mood Stabilizers

Anticonvulsants represent an important medication category for the treatment of bipolar disorder. Several of them are FDA approved, including valproate, carbamazepine extended-release, and lamotrigine, and others such as oxcarbazepine, gabapentin, and topiramate are used off-label.

Valproate

Valproate is available in different formulations—divalproex sodium (first FDA-approved anticonvulsant to treat acute mania in 1995), valproate sodium (Depacon), and valproic acid (Depakene)—that have been found to be as effective as lithium for treating acute mania and more effective in treating rapid cycling and mixed states (American Psychiatric Association 2002). These medications have a fast therapeutic action and reduce symptoms within a few days. For maintenance therapy, they may be used as monotherapy or in combination with lithium, other mood stabilizers, or antipsychotics. They are well tolerated, have a side-effect profile that is more favorable than lithium, and have a superior therapeutic index and less toxicity, contributing to better compliance rates (Macritchie et al. 2003).

The valproate formulations are believed to increase GABA activity by increasing its synthesis, inhibiting its degradation, and possibly potentiating GABA-mediated postsynaptic inhibition. They also regulate downstream signal transduction cascades by interacting with G proteins to exert effects on components of the cAMP-signaling system (Manji and Lenox 2000) and block voltage-sensitive sodium channels (Stahl 2011). Valproate products are well absorbed following oral administration and are rapidly distributed into plasma and extracellular fluid. They are metabolized by the liver; approximately 25% of active drug is dependent on the cytochrome P450 (CYP) system. Minimal amounts are excreted unchanged in the urine. Protein binding is 80%–90% (Pedersen and Leahy 2010; Stahl 2011).

The potential for drug interactions between valproate and other medications is high, and valproate displaces highly protein-bound drugs from their protein binding sites. If augmenting with lamotrigine, the dose of lamotrigine should be reduced by 50% because valproate inhibits the metabolism of lamotrigine and raises plasma levels, increasing the possibility of rash. All forms of valproate should be tapered slowly when discontinuing.

Valproate serum levels are checked frequently until the therapeutic range of 50–125 µg/mL is reached. Levels for maintenance should be checked every 6 months or whenever the health status changes. Patients require regular liver function tests and platelet counts, especially during the initial 6 months of therapy, and then once or twice a year. Rash and changes in the white blood cell count or liver function may necessitate a permanent or temporary discontinuation. Life-threatening pancreatitis has been reported; thus, symptoms for this disorder should be monitored via serum amylase and lipase levels.

Common side effects of the valproate formulations include sedation, tremor, ataxia, headache, dizziness, visual disturbances, abdominal pain, anorexia, nausea, vomiting, diarrhea, constipation, dyspepsia, increased appetite, weight gain, alopecia, rash, benign hepatic transaminase elevations, and osteoporosis. Measures can be taken to reduce these side effects such as taking a higher dose at night or prescribing medication to reduce specific symptoms, such as taking multivitamins fortified with zinc and selenium to help reduce alopecia (Stahl 2011). Mild thrombocytopenia and leukopenia are less frequent, and, unless severe, a dose reduction will restore blood counts to normal. Polycystic ovaries are less common but possible.

Life-threatening or dangerous side effects include hepatotoxicity (malaise, weakness, anorexia, vomiting), pancreatitis (abdominal pain, nausea, vomiting, anorexia), hyperammonemia (lethargy, vomiting, change in mental status), and suicidality (American Psychiatric Association 2002).

Valproate is a Category D pregnancy risk and should not be taken during pregnancy because of the increased risk of congenital anomalies and neural tube defects, especially if taken during the first trimester. Women should not breast-feed while taking valproate (American Psychiatric Association 2002).

Carbamazepine

Carbamazepine has been used to treat bipolar disorder for many years, but it was not until 2004 that Equetro, an extended-release formulation, was given an FDA indication for the treatment of acute mania and mixed episodes. Carbamazepine may be used alone or in combination with lithium, valproate, lamotrigine, and antipsychotics (American Psychiatric Association 2002). It is less preferable than lithium or valproate because of the complex pharmacokinetic interactions and lower therapeutic index, which make it more difficult to use in combination with many medications (Schatzberg et al. 2010). Carbamazepine has shown efficacy in patients with mixed episodes and rapid cycling. Studies have reported that in maintenance therapy, carbamazepine, either alone or in combination with lithium or antipsychotics, has efficacy in the prophylaxis of bipolar disorder (Stahl 2008).

Carbamazepine enhances GABA activity, decreases the release of glutamate, and blocks calcium influx. It inhibits the cAMP-signaling pathway and subsequently brings about long-term gene expression (Manji and Lenox 2000). It is also hypothesized to act by blocking voltage-sensitive sodium channels (Stahl 2008). Carbamazepine is metabolized in the liver primarily by CYP3A4 enzymes and excreted by the kidneys. Because carbamazepine is an inducer of CYP3A4, it induces its own metabolism and that of other medications, including valproate, lamotrigine, topiramate, benzodiazepines, antipsychotics, antidepressants, and oral contraceptives, thereby decreasing their efficacy and requiring an upward dosage adjustment. Carbamazepine levels may be increased by medications that inhibit CYP3A4, including fluoxetine (Prozac), fluvoxamine (Luvox), cimetidine (Tagamet), calcium channel blockers, and some antibiotics, thus requiring a downward dose adjustment (American Psychiatric Association 2002; Pedersen and Leahy 2010; Stahl 2011).

Carbamazepine stimulates its own hepatic metabolism; thus, the dose requirement is likely to increase after stabilization. The serum plasma level should be monitored and is ideally maintained between 4 and 12 µg/mL. If given with valproate or lamotrigine, it can decrease valproate and lamotrigine levels (American Psychiatric Association 2002).

After treatment begins and during maintenance, a CBC should be done every 2–4 weeks for the first 2 months and then every 3–6 months. Liver, kidney, and thyroid function should be tested every 6–12 months. Because of the possibility of hyponatremia, sodium levels should be monitored. Individuals of Asian descent should consider screening for the presence of the HLA-B*1502 allele because individuals with this allele are at an increased risk for developing Stevens-Johnson syndrome and should not take the drug (Stahl 2011).

Common side effects of carbamazepine include sedation, dizziness, headache, unsteadiness, nausea, vomiting, diarrhea, blurred vision, and weight gain. Less common are skin rashes, leukopenia, thrombocytopenia, hyponatremia, hypo-osmolality, and liver enzyme elevations. These side effects are usually mild and resolve spontaneously or with a dose reduction.

Life-threatening or dangerous side effects include hepatic failure, renal failure, cardiac conduction disturbances, hematological disorders (e.g., agranulocytosis, aplastic anemia), exfoliative dermatitis (e.g., Stevens-Johnson syndrome), and pancreatitis. Carbamazepine may be fatal in overdose, and deaths have been reported with ingestions of more than 6 g. Signs of toxicity include ataxia, sedation, diplopia, respiratory dysfunction, tachycardia, arrhythmia, hypotension, hyperirritability, nystagmus, ophthalmoplegia, impaired consciousness, stupor, convulsions, and coma. Treatment includes gastric lavage and hemoperfusion (American Psychiatric Association 2002).

Carbamazepine is a Category D pregnancy risk and should not be taken during pregnancy because of the increased risk of congenital anomalies and neural tube defects, especially if taken during the first trimester. Women should not breast-feed while taking carbamazepine (American Psychiatric Association 2002).

Oxcarbazepine

Oxcarbazepine is an anticonvulsant used off-label for the manic phase of bipolar disorder. As an analog of carbamazepine, it is better tolerated and has less sedation, bone marrow toxicity, and CYP3A4 interactions. It is frequently used as an augmenting agent for other anticonvulsants, lithium, and SGAs (Schatzberg et al. 2010) but may be used as a first-line agent for patients unwilling to monitor serum levels or needing a medication that is better tolerated. Oxcarbazepine stabilizes neuronal membranes by blocking and interacting with the open channel conformation of voltage-sensitive sodium channels. It also inhibits the release of glutamate (Stahl 2011).

Common side effects of oxcarbazepine include sedation, dizziness, diplopia, headache, nausea, vomiting, nystagmus, somnolence, ataxia, abnormal gait, tremor, abdominal pain, fatigue, vertigo, and vision abnormalities. Less common are hypotension, asthenia, insomnia, speech disorder, rash, dyspepsia, muscle weakness, and angioedema. Oxcarbazepine is associated with clinically significant hyponatremia, a dangerous and potentially life-threatening adverse event (American Psychiatric Association 2002). Older adults require lower doses and are more susceptible to side effects. Dosing should begin low and be slowly increased (Kennedy 2008). Oxcarbazepine carries a Category C pregnancy risk.

Lamotrigine

Lamotrigine, an anticonvulsant, was the second FDA-approved drug for use in the maintenance treatment of bipolar I disorder to prevent the recurrence of both mania and depression in adults age 18 years or older. Lamotrigine can be used in combination with lithium, valproate, carbamazepine, and SGAs for augmentation purposes.

Lamotrigine acts to reduce the release of glutamate and aspartate through its blockade of voltage-sensitive sodium channels (Stahl 2008). Lamotrigine has a 98% absorption rate following oral administration. It is metabolized in the liver and excreted renally. It is highly bound to melanin-containing tissues (eyes, pigmented skin). Its half-life is 33 hours but may change if taking enzyme-inducing or -inhibiting medication. Lamotrigine takes several weeks to improve bipolar depression (Pedersen and Leahy 2010; Stahl 2011).

Lamotrigine must be titrated very slowly for patients at risk for developing Stevens-Johnson syndrome. To avoid an increased risk of rash, the recommended initial dose and subsequent dose escalations must take into consideration whether the patient is also taking carbamazepine, an enzyme inducer, or valproate, an enzyme inhibitor. Oral contraceptives may decrease plasma levels of lamotrigine. Discontinuation should occur over 2 weeks (Stahl 2011), and if the patient stops the medication for more than 2 days, the entire titration process must be restarted from the beginning. Refer to Table 4–3 for guidelines on titration of lamotrigine.

Lamotrigine has a tolerable side-effect profile except for the rare, life-threatening Stevens-Johnson rash. The risk of this one potentially serious side effect can be minimized by very slow upward titration during the initiation phase of drug therapy. Other serious effects are withdrawal seizures on abrupt withdrawal and rare blood dyscrasias, rare aseptic meningitis, and rare activation of suicidal ideation (Stahl 2011). Less dangerous side effects include dizziness, ataxia, headache, tremor, insomnia, poor coordination, vertigo, blurred vision, diplopia, fatigue, nausea, vomiting, dyspepsia, abdominal pain, constipation, rhinitis, dysarthria, palpitations, anxiety, chills, decreased memory, malaise, and benign rash (10%). Unlike other anticonvulsants, lamotrigine does not produce weight gain or sedation (American Psychiatric Association 2002).

Table 4-3. Titration of lamotrigine

Week(s)	For patients taking valproate	For patients not taking carbamazepine or valproate (mg/day)	For patients taking carbamazepine and not taking valproate (mg/day)
1, 2	25 mg every other day	25	50
3, 4	25 mg/day	50	100
5	50 mg/day	100	200
6	100 mg/day	200	300
7	100 mg/day	200	400

Lamotrigine is a Category C pregnancy risk and should not be taken during pregnancy because of the increased risk of cleft palate or cleft lip with first-trimester exposure. Women should not breast-feed while taking lamotrigine (Stahl 2011).

Gabapentin

Gabapentin may be used off-label as an augmenting agent to lithium, atypical antipsychotics, and other anticonvulsants in the treatment of bipolar disorder. It is not FDA approved for bipolar disorder. Gabapentin may affect the transport of amino acids across neuronal membranes and stabilize them. It binds to voltage-sensitive calcium channels, diminishing excessive neuronal activity and neurotransmitter release. It enhances and is structurally related to GABA while inhibiting the release of glutamate (Stahl 2011).

Antacids may decrease the absorption of gabapentin and reduce the bioavailability. A risk of central nervous system (CNS) depression occurs with other CNS depressants, including alcohol, opioids, antihistamines, and sedative-hypnotics. Gabapentin taken with kava, valerian, or chamomile can increase CNS depression (Pedersen and Leahy 2010; Stahl 2011).

Adverse reactions and side effects include sedation, dizziness, ataxia, fatigue, nystagmus, tremor, confusion, depression, anxiety, malaise, weakness, constipation, weight gain, anorexia, flatulence, paresthesias, and facial edema.

Gabapentin is usually well tolerated. For sedation, a larger dose can be given at night and less during the day. Morphine and hydrocodone increase gabapentin levels and may increase the risk of toxicity.

Gabapentin is a Category C pregnancy risk and should not be taken during pregnancy.

Topiramate

Topiramate is an anticonvulsant that is used off-label as an adjunctive agent to treat bipolar disorder. It is associated with weight loss and is sometimes given as an adjunct to mood stabilizers and antipsychotics that cause weight gain. The mechanism of action of topiramate is unknown, but it seems to enhance GABA function and reduce glutamate function by modulating voltage-sensitive sodium and calcium channels. It may take several weeks to have an effect on mood stabilization.

No significant monitoring is done other than for side effects, the most common of which include sedation, asthenia, dizziness, ataxia, paresthesias, nervousness, nystagmus, tremor, nausea, appetite loss, weight loss, confusion, depression, impaired concentration and memory, psychomotor slowing, speech problems, abnormal vision, diplopia, anxiety, fatigue, malaise, vertigo, weakness, and taste perversion. Topiramate may decrease blood levels and effects of oral contraceptives, risperidone, lithium, or valproate.

Topiramate is a Category C pregnancy risk and should not be taken during pregnancy because of the possible increased risk of congenital malformations (Pedersen and Leahy 2010). Hypospadias occurred in some male infants whose mothers took topiramate during pregnancy.

First-Generation Antipsychotics

Before lithium was approved as the first medication to treat bipolar disorder in 1970, the FGAs were the mainstay medications used to control the symptoms of acute mania. After lithium was introduced, they were still used initially for patients with bipolar mania and psychotic symptoms but usually were discontinued within the first few months after the lithium took full effect. Chlorpromazine, approved in 1974, is the only FGA approved by the FDA for the treatment of acute mania. Other FGAs such as haloperidol, loxapine (Loxitane), thiothixene, and perphenazine are frequently used off-label. The FGAs are still used in combination with lithium and anticonvulsants in psychotic patients with bipolar mania and mixed episodes. Because of the risk of tardive dyskinesia, their long-term use is limited, and they are usually discontinued with mood stabilization (Schatzberg et al. 2010).

The FGAs block dopamine type 2 (D_2) receptors in the striatum, pituitary, and mesolimbic pathways. Because they are not selective, they act as antagonists on α-adrenergic, histamine, and muscarinic acetylcholine receptors (Schatzberg et al. 2010). They are well absorbed following oral or intramuscular administration and are distributed in high concentrations within the CNS.

The FGAs act as antagonists on histamine receptors, causing symptoms of sedation, antiemetic effect, and weight gain; on α-adrenergic receptors, causing dizziness, sedation, hypotension, vertigo, hypersalivation, and sexual dysfunction; and on muscarinic acetylcholine receptors, causing anticholinergic symptoms of sedation, dry mouth, blurred vision, constipation, and urinary retention. Other symptoms include extrapyramidal reactions, akathisia, galactorrhea, amenorrhea, and photosensitivity. Benztropine and trihexyphenidyl have both shown efficacy in reducing dystonia and other extrapyramidal side effects related to the FGAs.

Elderly patients should have a lower dose of chlorpromazine and be monitored closely. Those with dementia-related psychosis are at an increased risk for death and cerebrovascular events; thus, the FDA has issued a black box warning for the antipsychotics as a class of medications.

Chlorpromazine carries a Category C pregnancy risk. According to Stahl (2011), case reports indicate extrapyramidal symptoms, jaundice, hyperreflexia, and hyporeflexia in infants whose mothers took FGAs during pregnancy. They generally should not be used during the first trimester or while breast-feeding and should be used only with caution in the second and third trimesters.

FGAs are a less expensive alternative to the atypical antipsychotics for treating the symptoms of bipolar disorder and should be considered for patients without insurance or the financial means to pay for the more expensive newer agents.

Second-Generation Antipsychotics

In the past decade, the SGAs, all of which are Category C for pregnancy and bear the black box warning for increased risk of death in the elderly with dementia-related psychosis, have played an increasing role in the treatment of bipolar disorder and are now commonly prescribed as monotherapy or in combination with the traditional mood stabilizers for the acute treatment of manic, mixed, and depressive episodes as well as maintenance therapy. The evidence suggests that SGAs are more effective than placebo for the treatment of acute mania and maintenance prophylaxis and more effective when combined with lithium or valproate (Cipriani et al. 2011). Several SGAs are now approved for treating acute mania and maintenance, including risperidone, aripiprazole, quetiapine, ziprasidone, and asenapine. Olanzapine plus fluoxetine in combination and quetiapine are also approved for treating bipolar depression.

The positive aspects of these drugs include their rapid onset of action and their ability to treat both poles in the acute phase and maintenance prophylaxis; the negative aspects include weight gain and metabolic complications. Clozapine and olanzapine offer the most risk of weight gain, whereas ziprasidone and aripiprazole offer the least risk. Weight gain not only can lead to type 2 diabetes and cardiovascular diseases but also is a leading cause of medication nonadherence. Routine monitoring of weight along with regular exercise and healthy diets are critical for patients taking these medications. Please refer to Chapter 12, "Management of Metabolic Side Effects of Psychotropic Medications," for more information on metabolic syndrome and other potential adverse effects related to the FGAs and SGAs.

Olanzapine

Olanzapine is a D_2 receptor antagonist that reduces positive symptoms of psychosis and stabilizes mood symptoms. It also is a serotonin type 2A (5-HT_{2A}) receptor antagonist, causing enhancement of dopamine release, reducing motor side effects, and improving cognitive and mood symptoms. Olanzapine also acts as a histamine type 1 receptor antagonist, α_1-adrenergic receptor antagonist, and muscarinic type 1 receptor antagonist. It is olanzapine's action on these various receptors, as well as its rapid onset of action, that makes it a good choice for treatment-refractory bipolar symptoms.

Improvement of manic symptoms occurs within 1 week with oral administration; the intramuscular formulation reduces agitation in 15–30 minutes. The half-life of olanzapine is 21–54 hours. The protein binding is 93% (Pedersen and Leahy 2010).

As with all antipsychotics, before initiating treatment, patients' weight, body mass index, waist circumference, and blood pressure should be assessed, and a CBC, comprehensive metabolic profile, and lipid profile should be obtained. Olanzapine may increase the effects of antihypertensive agents and antagonize levodopa and other dopaminergic agents. The dose may need to be lowered if given with CYP1A2 inhibitors (e.g., fluvoxamine) and raised if given with CYP1A2 inducers (e.g., carbamazepine, tobacco smoke).

Common side effects of olanzapine include dizziness, sedation, dry mouth, constipation, dyspepsia, weight gain, peripheral edema, joint pain, back pain, chest pain, extremity pain, abnormal gait, ecchymosis, tachycardia, and orthostatic hypotension. Weight gain increases the risk for diabetes mellitus, dyslipidemia, and metabolic syndrome. Life-threatening or dangerous side effects include hyperglycemia with ketoacidosis or hyperosmolar coma or death, neuroleptic malignant syndrome, seizures, and tardive dyskinesia.

Risperidone

Risperidone, a D_2 receptor antagonist, reduces positive symptoms of psychosis and stabilizes mood symptoms. It also is a 5-HT_{2A} receptor antagonist, which enhances dopamine release, reduces motor side effects, and improves cognitive and mood symptoms. The onset of action is approximately 1–2 weeks with oral administration and 3 weeks for the intramuscular dosing. The half-life of risperidone is 20–24 hours, but its metabolites are actively metabolized by CYP2D6 enzymes. Risperidone may increase the effects of antihypertensive agents and antagonize levodopa/dopamine agonists. Coadministration with carbamazepine may decrease plasma levels of risperidone; coadministration with fluoxetine and paroxetine may increase plasma levels of risperidone.

Hyperglycemia with ketoacidosis or hyperosmolar coma or death, neuroleptic malignant syndrome, seizures, and tardive dyskinesia are dangerous and life-threatening side effects associated with risperidone. Extrapyramidal side effects such as dystonia are more common with this agent, as are hyperprolactinemia, lactation, and gynecomastia in both males and females.

Aripiprazole

Aripiprazole is a partial agonist at D_2 receptors, which reduces dopamine when concentrations are high and increases dopamine when concentrations are low. It also is a 5-HT_{2A} receptor antagonist, which enhances dopamine release, reduces motor side effects, and improves cognitive and mood symptoms. It is absorbed 87% following oral administration and 100% with intramuscular administration. The half-life is 75 hours for aripiprazole and 94 hours for its major metabolite dehydroaripiprazole. Aripiprazole is metabolized primarily by the liver enzymes CYP2D6 and CYP3A4. Approximately 18% is excreted unchanged in the feces (Pedersen and Leahy 2010; Stahl 2011).

When switching to aripiprazole from another antipsychotic, patients do best by adding a full dose of aripiprazole to the maintenance dose of the first antipsychotic for at least several days before slowly discontinuing the first antipsychotic (Stahl 2011). Ketoconazole (Nizoral) and other CYP3A4 inhibitors (e.g., fluvoxamine and fluoxetine) may increase plasma levels of aripiprazole; carbamazepine and other inducers of CYP3A4 may decrease plasma levels of aripiprazole. Quinidine and other inhibitors of CYP2D6 (e.g., paroxetine, fluoxetine, and duloxetine [Cymbalta]) may increase plasma levels. Aripiprazole may enhance the effects of antihypertensive drugs and antagonize levodopa and other dopaminergic agents.

Common side effects of aripiprazole include dizziness, insomnia, akathisia, activation, nausea, and vomiting. Weight gain is lower with aripiprazole than with other SGAs but still may occur with some patients. Children may be more at risk for weight gain. Aripiprazole may be safe and effective for behavior disturbances in children and adolescents, especially at lower doses.

Quetiapine

Quetiapine, a D_2 receptor antagonist, reduces positive symptoms of psychosis and stabilizes mood symptoms. It also is a 5-HT_{2A} receptor antagonist, which enhances dopamine release, reduces motor side effects, and improves cognitive and mood symptoms. Actions at 5-HT_{1A} receptors may contribute to efficacy for cognitive and mood symptoms. This SGA also has a high affinity as a histamine antagonist, which lends to its sedating side effects (Stahl 2011).

CYP3A4 inhibitors and CYP2D6 inhibitors may reduce clearance of quetiapine and raise plasma levels, but dosage reduction is not necessary. Quetiapine may increase effects of antihypertensive agents.

Common side effects of quetiapine include sedation, weight gain, dizziness, hypotension, dry mouth, constipation, tachycardia, and an increased risk for diabetes and dyslipidemia. Life-threatening or dangerous side effects include hyperglycemia sometimes associated with ketoacidosis or hyperosmolar coma or death, neuroleptic malignant syndrome, and seizures.

Ziprasidone

Ziprasidone, similar to the other SGAs, blocks D_2 receptors, which stabilizes mood symptoms and reduces positive symptoms of psychosis, and 5-HT_{2A} receptors, which enhances dopamine release, reduces motor side effects, and improves cognitive and mood symptoms. Actions at 5-HT_{2C} and 5-HT_{1A} receptors may contribute to efficacy for cognitive and mood symptoms (Stahl 2011).

The protein binding is almost complete with ziprasidone, which is extensively metabolized by the CYP3A4 enzyme. It also may prolong the QTc interval more than do other SGAs and should be used cautiously in those with a significant family history of cardiac deficits. Symptom improvement may be observed within 1 week of initiation of treatment (Pedersen and Leahy 2010; Stahl 2011).

Ziprasidone should be taken with a meal of about 500 calories. Food can double the bioavailability by increasing absorption and thus increasing plasma drug levels.

This SGA is known to have more activating side effects at low doses and sedating effects at high doses in addition to other common side effects such as dizziness, extrapyramidal symptoms, sedation, dystonia, nausea, dry mouth, asthenia, skin rash, and orthostatic hypotension. Ziprasidone is a Category C pregnancy risk and is secreted in breast milk. Ziprasidone should not be used in patients with a known history of QTc prolongation, recent acute myocardial infarction, uncompensated heart failure, and cardiac impairment in general.

Asenapine

Asenapine has a mechanism of action and side-effect profile similar to those of the SGAs previously discussed in this chapter. The half-life is approximately

13–39 hours. It inhibits CYP2D6 and is a substrate for CYP1A2. Symptoms can improve as early as 1 week after initiation of treatment (Stahl 2011). The dosage form is a sublingual tablet, and patients should be advised not to eat or drink for 10 minutes following administration.

Other Pharmacological Agents

Benzodiazepines also may be used for sedation early in treatment with lithium or an anticonvulsant to help manage the symptoms because lithium and anticonvulsants do not have immediate antimanic effects. Lorazepam and clonazepam provide a more benign alternative to antipsychotic agents for attenuating symptoms such as agitation, insomnia, anxiety, and hyperactivity while waiting for the mood stabilizer to take effect (American Psychiatric Association 2002). Little evidence supports the use of benzodiazepines for long-term management of bipolar disorder. Benzodiazepines are not recommended for elderly patients as first-line treatments; they are more likely to develop cognitive impairment and are more prone to falls if prescribed these medications (American Psychiatric Association 2002).

Calcium channel blockers also have been tried with variable results. They do not figure prominently in the available practice guidelines as first- or second-line interventions. Their mechanism of action is inactivation of calcium channels to block calcium influx, which leads to inhibition of neural signal transmission and neurotransmitter synthesis and release (Currier and Goodnick 1998). Several small double-blind trials have found that verapamil (Calan, Isoptin) and other calcium channel blockers (e.g., diltiazem [Cardizem], nifedipine [Adalat, Procardia], nimodipine [Nimotop]) have antimanic efficacy. For maintenance treatment, there appears to be some evidence for the role of verapamil (Giannini et al. 1987).

Omega-3 fatty acids eicosapentaenoic acid (EPA) and docosahexaenoic acid (DHA) have been proposed as individual or adjunctive treatments for bipolar disorder. EPA is an essential fatty acid that can be metabolized to DHA and is a normal component of a diet that contains fish. Both EPA and DHA are found in large quantities in the brain, especially in cell membranes. The mechanisms underlying omega-3 activity that may be beneficial in mood stabilization involve inhibition of cell-signaling pathways causing enhanced cell membrane fluidity, anti-inflammation via select cytokine inhibition, and phosphoinositide–protein kinase C antagonism.

Animal studies have reported that higher fish consumption predicts a lower occurrence of bipolar disorder. A meta-analysis was completed on RCTs of 4 weeks or longer that used omega-3 as augmentation for patients with bipolar mania and bipolar depression diagnoses and receiving conventional mood stabilizers. The findings provide strong evidence that supplementation of mood stabilizers with omega-3 significantly reduced depressive symptoms in patients with bipolar depression but showed no significance for use in improving bipolar mania. From the analysis, it appears that EPA or higher EPA-to-DHA ratio preparations are potentially more effective. The researchers recommended that patients with bipolar depression be encouraged to add increased dietary omega-3 to their diet or add a daily supplement of 1,000–1,500 mg of mixed EPA and DHA (higher EPA-to-DHA ratio) (Sarris et al. 2011).

Treatment of Special Populations

Children and Adolescents

Children and adolescents with bipolar disorder experience a great deal of impairment in social, emotional, and academic functioning. The course and symptom profile of children and adolescents are somewhat different from those of adults. Children are more apt to show hyperactivity and irritability that may be accompanied by episodes of violent, explosive outbursts over trivial matters. The American Psychiatric Association (2002) practice guideline notes that the mood swings in children are less defined, and discrete lengthy episodes and euphoric moods are absent. Adolescents, in contrast, frequently have euphoric moods, but otherwise, the symptom profile is similar to that of children. They both have more mixed episodes, rapid cycling, psychosis, and comorbid disorders (e.g., disruptive behavior disorders, attention-deficit/ hyperactivity disorder, anxiety disorders) that have overlapping symptoms as compared with adults.

The evidence for effective psychopharmacological agents remains limited for children and adolescents. The same agents used to treat bipolar disorder in adults are used for this population, even though many of them have not been FDA approved. Lithium and a few SGAs have been approved by the FDA for use in children and adolescents, but no medications are currently approved for treatment in children younger than 10 years. Several older open-label trials in which lithium was used to treat bipolar mania in children found successful response rates ranging from 23% to 55% (Liu et al. 2011). Older open-label studies in which anticonvulsants (e.g., carbamazepine, valproate, lamotrigine, oxcarbazepine, topiramate) were used to treat bipolar mania have been conducted with mild and moderate support (Washburn et al. 2011). No anticonvulsant is FDA approved to treat bipolar disorder in children and adolescents, but anticonvulsants are nonetheless used off-label with success. One open-label study that used omega-3 fatty acids showed a 35% efficacy rate (Liu et al. 2011).

More placebo-controlled, double-blind studies have examined the use of SGAs for the treatment of bipolar disorder in children and adolescents, with results showing a high level of efficacy ranging from 53% to 66% greater than placebo. In a few comparative studies, the results suggested that the SGAs have superior efficacy as compared with lithium and anticonvulsants for treating bipolar disorder in children and adolescents. However, SGAs are associated with somnolence, greater weight gain, dyslipidemias, glycemic dyscontrol, and the risk for tardive dyskinesia. The FDA has approved several SGAs for treating bipolar disorder in children and adolescents, including risperidone, aripiprazole, and quetiapine for 10- to 17-year-olds and olanzapine for 13- to 17-year-olds. In general, these medications are started at a low dose and titrated up slowly.

In clinical practice, bipolar children and adolescents are usually taking combination medications that require frequent adjustments to address recurring symptoms and side effects (Washburn et al. 2011). Little evidence-based research on combination therapy in this population is available. A study cited in Hamrin and Iennaco (2010) noted that children and adolescents with bipolar disorder were typically given 3.4 psychiatric medications and had an average of 6.3 trials. When treating bipolar disorder in children and adolescents, the psychiatric APRN needs to carefully weigh all the variables involved in the decision-making process.

Older Adults

Although the prevalence rates of bipolar disorder for the older adult are low, ranging from 0.2% to 0.4%, inpatient psychiatric admissions are approximately 10%. Most older adult inpatients have the first episode of bipolar disorder before age 30, but 10%–15% have an onset after age 50. Older adults also differ in the course of the disorder, having longer and more frequent episodes of illness (American Psychiatric Association 2002). Differential diagnoses are more challenging with older adults because comorbid medical and psychiatric disorders are more prevalent (Sajatovic et al. 2006). It has been estimated that 70% of older adults who present with a first episode of mania in later life have a neurological problem (Sorrell 2011). Compared with younger populations, older bipolar adults are at highest risk for suicide (Sherrod et al. 2010).

Older patients generally require lower doses of medications. Concomitant medications and medical conditions may alter the pharmacokinetics of psychiatric medication. Older adults are at an increased risk for developing adverse reactions and toxicity. Medication management requires frequent monitoring, including laboratory testing. Adherence is a problem with this population because of self-administration limitations, doubts about the necessity of the medication, and a desire to discontinue the medication (Hoblyn 2004).

Caution should be taken when prescribing antipsychotic medication for older adults. In 2005, the FDA issued an advisory that atypical antipsychotic medications increase mortality among elderly patients with dementia, and a black box warning was required. This advisory did not apply to conventional antipsychotic medication; however, when conventional antipsychotic medications were found to be associated with a significantly higher risk of death than were atypical antipsychotics (Wang et al. 2005), the FDA, in 2007, issued a black box warning on the conventional antipsychotics as well. The greatest increases in risk occur soon after therapy is initiated and with higher dosages of antipsychotic medications (Wang et al. 2005).

Medically Compromised Patients

Medically compromised patients have a higher risk of exacerbating the course or severity of bipolar disorder as well as complicating its treatment. They also have a poorer prognosis. Conditions requiring the use of diuretics, angiotensin-converting enzyme inhibitors, nonsteroidal anti-inflammatory drugs, cyclooxygenase-2 inhibitors, or salt-restricted diets all affect lithium excretion. Conditions associated with abnormal thyroid, cardiac, renal, or hepatic function may further restrict the choice or dosage of medication. Conditions that require the use of steroids (e.g., asthma, inflammatory bowel disease) may exacerbate the course of bipolar disorder. Drug-drug interactions with pre-scribed medications and herbal and over-the-counter products are a serious problem with the medically compromised patient.

Comorbid psychiatric conditions also pose complicated diagnostic pic-tures and are associated with fewer and slower remissions, higher rates of sui-cide, and poorer outcome. Substance abuse presents a difficult prescribing problem because alcohol-related dehydration may raise lithium levels to tox-icity and may alter plasma levels of valproate and carbamazepine because of hepatic dysfunction. Patients with attention-deficit/hyperactivity disorder should not be prescribed stimulants until the bipolar disorder is stabilized, or the stimulant will exacerbate mood swings.

Pregnant or Breast-Feeding Patients

Pregnant women frequently have exacerbations of bipolar disorder. Because many medications for bipolar disorder are associated with a high risk of birth defects, prescribing for pregnant women presents a challenge. Women of child-bearing age should be encouraged to use contraceptives when taking certain medications such as lithium or valproate. Carbamazepine, oxcarbazepine, and topiramate increase the metabolism of oral contraceptives, so alternative types of birth control should be selected (American Psychiatric Association 2002).

First-trimester exposure to lithium is associated with Ebstein's anomaly (1–2 per 1,000), which produces cardiac anomalies ranging from displace-ment of the tricuspid valve into the ventricle to atrial septal defects. First-trimester exposure to valproate and carbamazepine is associated with neural tube defects (1%–5%), craniofacial abnormalities, limb malformations, and cardiac defects. A recent systematic review examined the effects of exposure to lithium, valproate, carbamazepine, and lamotrigine during pregnancy and found that all four of these mood stabilizers, but especially valproate and var-ious combinations of these medications, were associated with a high risk of child malformations, perinatal complications, and long-term neurodevel-opmental problems (Galbally et al. 2010). Women who choose to continue taking lithium, valproate, or carbamazepine during pregnancy should be screened for neural tube defects and cardiac abnormalities before the twenti-eth week of gestation. If the woman is taking lithium, care must be taken at delivery because the swift fluid changes increase lithium levels, and doses may need to be lowered (American Psychiatric Association 2002).

There is no evidence of birth abnormalities with the use of FGAs, and these medications are recommended in place of lithium and anticonvulsants (Stahl 2008). The high-potency FGAs (e.g., haloperidol, perphenazine [Trilafon], and thiothixene [Navane]) are preferred because they have fewer hypotensive, anticholinergic, and antihistaminergic effects; however, neonates may develop extrapyramidal side effects when these drugs are used near delivery. Little information is available regarding the teratogenic risks of the SGAs, so they should be taken cautiously; however, they are preferred by most practitioners.

Some early studies concluded that benzodiazepines with a long half-life such as diazepam (Valium) and chlordiazepoxide (Librium) could result in malformations with first-trimester exposure; however, later studies showed no significant indications, and, thus, the risk is considered very small. The recommended benzodiazepine to use, if necessary, is lorazepam. However, if benzodiazepines are used near delivery, the neonate could develop withdrawal symptoms (American Psychiatric Association 2002).

The postpartum period is associated with a very high risk for first onset and recurrence of bipolar disorder. All medications used to treat bipolar disorder are secreted in breast milk; thus, risks and benefits need to be evaluated. The use of lithium or lamotrigine in nursing women is not recommended, and valproate, lamotrigine, carbamazepine, or SGAs should be used cautiously (American Psychiatric Association 2002).

Gender Issues in Bipolar Disorders

Women have more mixed and depressive episodes, suicide attempts, and rapid cycling than do men, whereas men have more manic episodes than do women. Comorbid anxiety disorders and eating disorders are more frequent in women, whereas substance use disorders are more prevalent in men. Thyroid dysfunction is more prevalent in women, and women may be more susceptible to the thyroid effects of lithium. Women also report more atypical symptoms, especially increased appetite and weight gain. During the premenstrual phase, symptoms of bipolar disorder may worsen for women. Treatment with antipsychotics causes higher elevation of serum prolactin levels in women, resulting in more galactorrhea, sexual dysfunction, and menstrual disorders. Polycystic ovarian syndrome with amenorrhea, hyperandrogenism, weight gain, and insulin resistance occurs more frequently in women taking valproate (American Psychiatric Association 2002).

Summary

When prescribing psychopharmacological agents for bipolar disorder, many factors, including efficacy, side effects, and patient variables, need to be considered. Lithium, anticonvulsants, and SGAs alone or in combination are clearly effective for treating bipolar disorder. The advantages of the SGAs are rapid onset of action. quick and easy titration, relative safety in overdose, and established efficacy in treating both manic and depressive symptoms. Their limitations are cost and the number of serious side effects. including weight gain, metabolic syndrome, sedation, and akathisia, which may limit adherence and present long-term health problems. The advantages of the mood stabilizers are lower cost and a long history of research supporting their effectiveness. The limitations are slower onset of action, more difficult titration, and side effects such as tremor, rash, gastrointestinal distress, and impaired memory, which also may limit adherence. In addition, some of them have a narrow therapeutic window that necessitates frequent serum monitoring.

Psychiatric APRNs must know the pharmacodynamics and pharmacokinetics of each medication as well as the safety profile, efficacy, and cost. These criteria along with the patient's comorbid conditions, symptoms, and preferences will allow for the construction of a personalized psychopharmacological treatment protocol for each patient.

Clinical Pearls

- In general, combination therapy (e.g., lithium, anticonvulsants, antipsychotics) is well tolerated. Subtle variations exist among the agents used in the treatment of the various forms of bipolar disorder.
- Lithium is an excellent choice for bipolar mania and may be underused because it is an older agent and lacks promotional marketing by pharmaceutical companies. Lithium is an excellent choice for patients who have suicidal ideation.

- Valproate is a first-line treatment for mixed states and rapid cycling and is a good choice to treat aggression, agitation, and impulsivity in many other types of psychiatric disorders. A significant advantage of valproate is the ability to rapidly administer loading doses that may produce a rapid antimanic response (3 days) with minimal side effects.

- Oxcarbazepine has a lower risk of leukopenia, aplastic anemia, agranulocytosis, elevated liver enzymes, or Stevens-Johnson syndrome than does carbamazepine; oxcarbazepine seems to have the same therapeutic action as carbamazepine but with fewer side effects. Oxcarbazepine may be a good choice for patients who would be noncompliant with serum testing or those who are more prone to side effects.

- Lamotrigine is effective in preventing both manic and depressive relapses and is well tolerated with little weight gain or sedation. Titration of lamotrigine is "low and slow" because of the potential risk of Stevens-Johnson syndrome.

- Gabapentin may be useful for patients with chronic neuropathic pain and fibromyalgia.

- Topiramate may be helpful for bipolar patients with weight gain, especially those with psychotropic drug-induced weight gain. With longer-term use, however, topiramate may contribute to mental confusion and memory impairment.

- Chlorpromazine, an FGA, is much less expensive than the SGAs. Chlorpromazine is very good if sedation is needed during a manic episode.

- Olanzapine, an SGA, is very good if rapid onset of antipsychotic action is needed without drug titration and for use in treatment-refractory bipolar disorder, especially at higher doses.

- Risperidone is well accepted for the treatment of behavior disorders in children and adolescents (but this group may have more weight gain and sedation) and for the treatment of agitation and aggression in elderly patients with dementia.

- Aripiprazole is very good for patients concerned about weight gain or for those already overweight, those with diabetes or dyslipidemia, those requiring rapid onset of action without dosage titration, and those who wish to avoid sedation.

* Quetiapine's antagonism of the histamine receptor may induce sleep in the patient experiencing mania.

References

Altshuler LL, Bartzokis G, Grieder T, et al: Amygdala enlargement in bipolar disorders and hippocampal reduction in schizophrenia: an MRI study demonstrating neuroanatomic specificity. Arch Gen Psychiatry 55:663–664, 1998

American Psychiatric Association: Diagnostic and Statistical Manual of Mental Disorders, 4th Edition, Text Revision. Washington, DC, American Psychiatric Association, 2000

American Psychiatric Association: Practice Guideline for the Treatment of Patients With Bipolar Disorder, 2nd Edition. April 2002. Available at: http://psychiatryonline.org/content.aspx?bookid=28&sectionid=1669577. Accessed February 28, 2013.

Berns GS, Nemeroff CB: The neurobiology of bipolar disorder. Am J Med Genet 123C:76–84, 2003

Bogart GT, Chavez B: Safety and efficacy of quetiapine in bipolar depression. Ann Pharmacother 43:1848–1856, 2009

Calabrese JR, Bowden CL, Sachs G, et al: A placebo-controlled 18-month trial of lamotrigine and lithium maintenance treatment in recently depressed patients with bipolar disorder. J Clin Psychiatry 64:1013–1024, 2003

Cipriani A, Barbui C, Salanti G, et al: Comparative efficacy and acceptability of antimanic drugs in acute mania: a multiple-treatments meta-analysis. Lancet 378:1306–1315, 2011

Currier MB, Goodnick PJ: Calcium antagonists and newer anticonvulsants, in Mania: Clinical and Research Perspectives. Edited by Goodnick PJ. Washington, DC, American Psychiatric Press, 1998, pp 337–362

Dubovsky SL, Davies R, Dubovsky AM: Mood disorders, in The American Psychiatric Publishing Textbook of Clinical Psychiatry, 4th Edition. Edited by Hales RE, Yudofsky SC. Washington, DC, American Psychiatric Publishing, 2003, pp 439–452

Frank E, Kupfer DJ, Thase ME, et al: Two-year outcomes for interpersonal and social rhythm therapy in individuals with bipolar I disorder. Arch Gen Psychiatry 62:996–1004, 2005

Galbally M, Roberts M, Buist A: Mood stabilizers in pregnancy: a systematic review. Aust NZ J Psychiatry 44:967–977, 2010

Geddes JR, Calabrese JR, Goodwin GM: Lamotrigine for treatment of bipolar depression: independent meta-analysis and meta-regression of individual patient data from five randomized trials. Br J Psychiatry 194:4–9, 2009

Ghaemi SN, Bauer M, Cassidy F, et al: Diagnostic guidelines for bipolar disorder: a summary of the International Society for Bipolar Disorders Diagnostic Guidelines Task Force Report. Bipolar Disord 10 (1 pt 2):117–128, 2008

Giannini AJ, Tarasqewski R, Loiselle RH: Verapamil and lithium in the maintenance therapy of manic patients. J Clin Pharmacol 27:980–982, 1987

Goodwin FK, Jamison KR: Manic-Depressive Illness: Bipolar Disorders and Recurrent Depression, 2nd Edition. New York, Oxford University Press, 2007

Goodwin GM, Consensus Group of the British Association for Psychopharmacology: Evidence-based guidelines for treating bipolar disorder: revised second edition— recommendations from the British Association for Psychopharmacology. J Psychopharmacol 23:346–388, 2009

Hamrin V, Iennaco JD: Psychopharmacology of pediatric bipolar disorder. Expert Rev Neurother 10:1053–1088, 2010

Hirschfeld RMA: Bipolar depression: the real challenge. Eur Neuropsychopharmacol 14 (suppl 2):S83–S88, 2004

Hirschfeld RMA: Guideline Watch: Practice Guideline for the Treatment of Patients With Bipolar Disorder, 2nd Edition. Arlington, VA, American Psychiatric Association, 2005

Hirschfeld RMA, Lewis L, Vornik LA: Perceptions and impact of bipolar disorder: how far have we really come? Results of the National Depressive and Manic-Depressive Association 2000 survey of individuals with bipolar disorder. J Clin Psychiatry 64:161–174, 2003

Hoblyn J: Bipolar disorder in later life: older adults presenting with new onset manic symptoms usually have underlying medical or neurologic disorder. Geriatrics 59:41–44, 2004

Kasper S, Calabrese JR, Johnson G, et al: International Consensus Group on the Evidence-Based Pharmacological Treatment of Bipolar I and II Depression. J Clin Psychiatry 69:1632–1646, 2008

Keck PE Jr, Nelson EB, McElroy SL: Advances in the pharmacologic treatment of bipolar depression. Biol Psychiatry 53:671–679, 2003b

Kennedy GL: Bipolar disorder in late life: mania. Prim Psychiatry 15:28–33, 2008

Krüger S, Young T, Bräunig P: Pharmacotherapy of manic-depressive mixed states [in German]. Psychiatr Prax 33 (suppl 1):S32–S39, 2006

Lenox RH, Hahn CG: Overview of the mechanism of action of lithium in the brain: fifty-year update. J Clin Psychiatry 61 (suppl 9):5–15, 2000

Liu HY, Potter MP, Woodworth KY, et al: Pharmacologic treatments for pediatric bipolar disorder: a review and meta-analysis. J Am Acad Child Adolesc Psychiatry 50:749–762, 2011

Macritchie K, Geddes J, Scott J, et al: Valproate for acute mood episodes in bipolar disorder. Cochrane Database of Systematic Reviews 2003, Issue 1. Art. No.: CD004052. DOI: 10.1002/14651858.CD004052

Manji HK, Lenox RH: The nature of bipolar disorder. J Clin Psychiatry 61 (suppl 13):42–57, 2000

Martinowich K, Schloesser RJ, Manji HK: Bipolar disorder: from genes to behavior pathways. J Clin Invest 119:726–736, 2009

McIntyre RS, Yoon J: Efficacy of antimanic treatments in mixed states. Bipolar Disord 14:22–36, 2012

Miklowitz DJ, Otto MW, Frank E, et al: Psychosocial treatments for bipolar depression: a 1-year randomized trial from the Systematic Treatment Enhancement Program (STEP). Arch Gen Psychiatry 64:419–426, 2007

National Institute of Mental Health: Mental Disorders in America: The Numbers Count. Bethesda, MD, National Institutes of Health, 2008

Nivoli AMA, Murru A, Goikolea JM, et al: New treatment guidelines for acute bipolar mania: a critical review. J Affect Disord 140:125–141, 2012

Pedersen DD, Leahy LG: Pocket Psych Drugs: Point-of-Care Clinical Guide. Philadelphia, PA, FA Davis, 2010

Ruggero CJ, Zimmerman M, Chelminski I, et al: Borderline personality disorder and the misdiagnosis of bipolar disorder. J Psychiatr Res 44:405–408, 2010

Sachs GS, Nierenberg AA, Calabrese JR, et al: Effectiveness of adjunctive antidepressant treatment for bipolar depression. N Engl J Med 356:1711–1722, 2007

Sadock BJ, Sadock VA: Kaplan and Sadock's Synopsis of Psychiatry: Behavioral Sciences/Clinical Psychiatry, 10th Edition. Philadelphia, PA, Lippincott Williams & Wilkins, 2007

Sajatovic M, Blow FC, Ignacio RV: Psychiatric comorbidity in older adults with bipolar disorder. Int J Geriatr Psychiatry 21:582–587, 2006

Sanger TM, Tohen M, Vieta E, et al: Olanzapine in the acute treatment of bipolar I disorder with a history of rapid cycling. J Affect Disord 73:155–161, 2003

Sarris J, Mischoulon D, Schweitzer I: Omega-3 for bipolar disorder: meta-analyses of use in mania and bipolar depression. J Clin Psychiatry 73:81–86, 2011

Schatzberg AF, Cole JO, DeBattista C: Manual of Clinical Psychopharmacology, 7th Edition. Arlington, VA, American Psychiatric Association, 2010

Sherrod T, Quinlan-Colwell A, Lattimore TB, et al: Older adults with bipolar disorder: guidelines for primary care providers. J Gerontol Nurs 36:20–27, 2010

Smith LA, Cornelius V, Warnock A, et al: Acute bipolar mania: a systematic review and meta-analysis of co-therapy vs. monotherapy. Acta Psychiatr Scand 115:12–20, 2006

Sorrell JM: Caring for older adults with bipolar disorder. J Psychosoc Nurs Ment Health Serv 49:21–25, 2011

Stahl SM: Stahl's Essential Psychopharmacology: Neuroscientific Basis and Practical Applications, 3rd Edition. New York, Cambridge University Press, 2008

Stahl SM: The Prescriber's Guide: Stahl's Essential Psychopharmacology, 4th Edition. New York, Cambridge University Press, 2011

Strakowski SM, Fleck DE, Maj M: Broadening the diagnosis of bipolar disorder: benefits vs. risks. World Psychiatry 10:181–186, 2011

Suppes T, Dennehy EB, Gibbons EW: The longitudinal course of bipolar disease. J Clin Psychiatry 61 (suppl 9):23–30, 2000

Tondo L, Baldessarini RJ, Hennen J, et al: Lithium treatment and risk of suicidal behavior in bipolar disorder patients. J Clin Psychiatry 59:405–414, 1998

Tondo L, Hennen J, Baldessarini RJ: Rapid-cycling bipolar disorder: effects of long-term treatments. Acta Psychiatr Scand 108:4–14, 2003

Van der Loos MLM, Mulder P, Hartong EG, et al: Long term outcome of bipolar depressed patients receiving lamotrigine as add-on to lithium with the possibility of the addition of paroxetine in nonresponders: a randomized, placebo-controlled trial with a novel design, Bipolar Disord 13:111–117, 2011

Wang PS, Schneeweiss S, Avorn J, et al: Risk of death in elderly users of conventional vs. atypical antipsychotic medications. N Engl J Med 353:2335–2340, 2005

Washburn JJ, West AE, Heil JA: Treatment of pediatric bipolar disorder: a review. Minerva Psichiatr 52:21–35, 2011

5

Psychotic Disorders

Serena M. Natal, M.S.N., A.P.R.N.,
P.M.H.-F.N.P., B.C.

Taresa Pittman, B.S.N., R.N.

Shannon Richmond, M.S.N., A.P.R.N.,
P.M.H.-F.N.P., B.C.

Linden Spital, M.S.N., A.P.R.N., P.M.H.-
F.N.P., B.C.

Megan Walsh, M.S.N., A.P.R.N.,
P.M.H.-F.N.P., B.C.

Schizophrenia cannot be understood without understanding despair.
—R.D. Laing, Scottish psychiatrist (1927–1989)

129

Overview of Schizophrenia Spectrum and Other Psychotic Disorders

Psychosis has a myriad of definitions, with no one definition globally accepted. In this chapter, *psychosis* is defined as a group of symptoms commonly seen in psychiatric disorders. Psychosis is not in and of itself a disorder; instead, it is a mixture of symptoms that can occur in the presence of other DSM-IV-TR (American Psychiatric Association 2000) psychiatric disorders. Psychosis is a state of diminished affective response and impaired ability to recognize reality, communicate, and socialize (Stahl 2010).

The importance of psychosis and psychotic disorders (Table 5–1) can be directly correlated to their ranking on the World Health Organization's disabling diseases list. According to this listing, active psychosis is the third most debilitating disease around the world, and its presence may decrease the patient's life by nearly 10 years (World Health Organization 2001). If nonorganic causes are not considered, statistically, the most prominent types of psychosis are affective (49.4%), schizophrenic (26.8%), schizoaffective (16.9%), and other unspecified psychoses (2.8%) (Marneros and Pillmann 2004). Lifetime prevalence of nonaffective psychosis or schizophrenia is estimated to be between 1% and 2% (Kendler et al. 1996; Saha et al. 2005). This can increase to 10% if a first-degree relative has the disorder and up to 50% if both parents have the disorder (Siegel and Ralph 2011; Tsuang et al. 2001). Some studies have found even higher risk percentages in monozygotic twins. These numbers and percentages have been consistent across various multicountry studies.

Schizoaffective disorder has a prevalence rate ranging from 0.2%–1.1% in the general public to 9% among psychiatrically hospitalized adults (Fuji and Ahmed 2007). Schizoaffective disorder is generally considered less common than schizophrenia and has fewer statistical data available regarding worldwide prevalence. Schizophreniform disorder and brief psychotic disorder are arguably the least researched psychotic disorders in terms of prevalence. It is suggested that the disorders combined have a 2% lifetime prevalence with a higher percentage in adult psychiatric inpatients (5%–10%) (Fuji and Ahmed 2007).

Delusional disorders were extensively studied during the middle of the twentieth century. However, the diagnostic criteria used during these studies were not the same as those in DSM-IV-TR; therefore, the results may cur-

Table 5–1.   Psychotic disorders at a glance

Disorder	Features
Schizophrenia	Commonly begins before age 30. Generally chronic, and premorbid level of functioning not achieved.
Delusional disorder	Delusions are not bizarre and involve situations that could conceivably occur in real life. Disorder is usually chronic, and delusions cause functional impairment.
Brief psychotic disorder	Psychotic symptom(s) occur for less than a month but for at least 1 day with a return to baseline.
Schizophreniform disorder	Psychotic symptoms last at least 1 month but less than 6 months. Mood symptoms brief in comparison to psychotic symptoms.
Schizoaffective disorder	Must include mania or depression in addition to psychotic symptoms. Mood symptoms significant part of illness (e.g., 25% of psychotic period) but shorter in duration than psychosis.

rently have little significance (Fuji and Ahmed 2007). Delusional disorders are thought to be less prevalent than schizophrenia.

Symptoms of psychosis are commonly categorized as positive, negative, cognitive, and mood. The positive symptoms include perceptual disturbances, such as hallucinations and delusions; disordered speech and behavior; and thought dysregulation. In distinguishing hallucinations and delusions, it is important to note that hallucinations are faulty perceptions that may involve any of the five senses. Additionally, delusions can be defined as fixed false beliefs that the patient holds to be true despite attempts made to persuade otherwise. They can be categorized as persecutory, grandiose, religious, somatic, reference, thought withdrawal, or thought insertion. Negative symptoms are commonly manifested as avolition, amotivation, anhedonia, and deficits in affect regulation, depth of thought, and breadth of speech (also known as alogia). Hallmark cognitive symptoms include compromised attention, memory, and executive and social functioning. Disruptions in mood can range from euphoric to depressive. Less intuitively, mood alterations also may include suicidal and homicidal ideation.

In addition to the categorical symptoms, motor disturbances may be associated with any type of psychosis. Psychomotor agitation or retardation, odd positioning, and various catatonic states are all potential motor disturbance symptoms. (Nasrallah 2011; Sadock and Sadock 2007; Schilling et al. 2006; Stahl 2010).

Table 5–2.   DSM-IV-TR diagnostic criteria for schizophrenia

A.   *Characteristic symptoms:*   Two (or more) of the following, each present for a significant portion of time during a 1-month period (or less if successfully treated):

   (1)   delusions

   (2)   hallucinations

   (3)   disorganized speech (e.g., frequent derailment or incoherence)

   (4)   grossly disorganized or catatonic behavior

   (5)   negative symptoms, i.e., affective flattening, alogia, or avolition

   Note: Only one criterion A symptom is required if delusions are bizarre or hallucinations consist of a voice keeping up a running commentary on the person's behavior or thoughts, or two or more voices conversing with each other.

B.   *Social/occupational dysfunction:*   For a significant portion of the time since the onset of the disturbance, one or more major areas of functioning such as work, interpersonal relations, or self-care are markedly below the level achieved prior to the onset (or when the onset is in childhood or adolescence, failure to achieve expected level of interpersonal, academic, or occupational achievement).

C.   *Duration:*   Continuous signs of the disturbance persist for at least 6 months. This 6-month period must include at least 1 month of symptoms (or less if successfully treated) that meet criterion A (i.e., active-phase symptoms) and may include periods of prodromal or residual symptoms. During these prodromal or residual periods, the signs of the disturbance may be manifested by only negative symptoms or two or more symptoms listed in criterion A present in an attenuated form (e.g., odd beliefs, unusual perceptual experiences).

D.   *Schizoaffective and mood disorder exclusion:*   Schizoaffective disorder and mood disorder with psychotic features have been ruled out because either (1) no major depressive, manic, or mixed episodes have occurred concurrently with the active-phase symptoms; or (2) if mood episodes have occurred during active-phase symptoms, their total duration has been brief relative to the duration of the active and residual periods.

E.   *Substance/general medical condition exclusion:*   The disturbance is not due to the direct physiological effects of a substance (e.g., a drug of abuse, a medication) or a general medical condition.

Table 5–2. DSM-IV-TR diagnostic criteria for schizophrenia *(continued)*

F. *Relationship to a pervasive developmental disorder:* If there is a history of autistic disorder or another pervasive developmental disorder, the additional diagnosis of schizophrenia is made only if prominent delusions or hallucinations are also present for at least a month (or less if successfully treated).

Classification of longitudinal course (can be applied only after at least 1 year has elapsed since the initial onset of active-phase symptoms):

Episodic With Interepisode Residual Symptoms (episodes are defined by the reemergence of prominent psychotic symptoms); *also specify if:* With Prominent Negative Symptoms

Episodic With No Interepisode Residual Symptoms

Continuous (prominent psychotic symptoms are present throughout the period of observation); *also specify if:* With Prominent Negative Symptoms

Single Episode In Partial Remission; *also specify if:* With Prominent Negative Symptoms

Single Episode In Full Remission

Other or Unspecified Pattern

Certain disorders, as defined by DSM-IV-TR criteria, are characterized by the existence of psychosis, including schizophrenia (Table 5–2), schizophreniform disorder (Table 5–3), schizoaffective disorder (Table 5–4), delusional disorder (Table 5–5), brief psychotic disorder (Table 5–6), shared psychotic disorder, substance-induced psychosis, and psychotic disorder due to a general medical condition (Table 5–7). Other disorders, such as depression, mania, cognitive disorders, and Alzheimer's dementia, can occur with or without the presence of psychosis.

Etiology of Psychotic Disorders

It has been suggested that traumatic exposure in pregnancy or early childhood development can interact with genetic vulnerabilities, potentially disposing a patient to the onset of a psychotic disorder. Currently, no factors have been ruled out as definitive causes; however, several risks have been identified that

Table 5–3.   DSM-IV-TR diagnostic criteria for 295.40 schizophreniform disorder

A.   Criteria A, D, and E of schizophrenia are met.

B.   An episode of the disorder (including prodromal, active, and residual phases) lasts at least 1 month but less than 6 months. (When the diagnosis must be made without waiting for recovery, it should be qualified as "Provisional.")

Specify if:

Without Good Prognostic Features

With Good Prognostic Features: as evidenced by two (or more) of the following:

(1)   onset of prominent psychotic symptoms within 4 weeks of the first noticeable change in usual behavior or functioning

(2)   confusion or perplexity at the height of the psychotic episode

(3)   good premorbid social and occupational functioning

(4)   absence of blunted or flat affect

Table 5–4.   DSM-IV-TR diagnostic criteria for 295.70 schizoaffective disorder

A.   An uninterrupted period of illness during which, at some time, there is either a major depressive episode, a manic episode, or a mixed episode concurrent with symptoms that meet criterion A for schizophrenia.

   Note: The major depressive episode must include criterion A1: depressed mood.

B.   During the same period of illness, there have been delusions or hallucinations for at least 2 weeks in the absence of prominent mood symptoms.

C.   Symptoms that meet criteria for a mood episode are present for a substantial portion of the total duration of the active and residual periods of the illness.

D.   The disturbance is not due to the direct physiological effects of a substance (e.g., a drug of abuse, a medication) or a general medical condition.

Specify type:

Bipolar Type: if the disturbance includes a manic or a mixed episode (or a manic or a mixed episode and major depressive episodes)

Depressive Type: if the disturbance only includes major depressive episodes

Table 5–5. DSM-IV-TR diagnostic criteria for 297.1 delusional disorder

A. Nonbizarre delusions (i.e., involving situations that occur in real life, such as being followed, poisoned, infected, loved at a distance, or deceived by spouse or lover, or having a disease) of at least 1 month's duration.

B. Criterion A for schizophrenia has never been met. **Note:** Tactile and olfactory hallucinations may be present in delusional disorder if they are related to the delusional theme.

C. Apart from the impact of the delusion(s) or its ramifications, functioning is not markedly impaired and behavior is not obviously odd or bizarre.

D. If mood episodes have occurred concurrently with delusions, their total duration has been brief relative to the duration of the delusional periods.

E. The disturbance is not due to the direct physiological effects of a substance (e.g., a drug of abuse, a medication) or a general medical condition.

Specify type (the following types are assigned based on the predominant delusional theme):

Erotomanic Type: delusions that another person, usually of higher status, is in love with the individual

Grandiose Type: delusions of inflated worth, power, knowledge, identity, or special relationship to a deity or famous person

Jealous Type: delusions that the individual's sexual partner is unfaithful

Persecutory Type: delusions that the person (or someone to whom the person is close) is being malevolently treated in some way

Somatic Type: delusions that the person has some physical defect or general medical condition

Mixed Type: delusions characteristic of more than one of the above types but no one theme predominates

Unspecified Type

have a much higher connection in patients with psychotic disorder. Some of these potential risks are not well elucidated, such as socioeconomic status, education level, and season of birth, whereas others have more empirical evidence to support them. Genetic factors, such as chromosomal mutations and genetic

Table 5–6.   DSM-IV-TR diagnostic criteria for 298.8 brief psychotic disorder

A.   Presence of one (or more) of the following symptoms:

(1)   delusions

(2)   hallucinations

(3)   disorganized speech (e.g., frequent derailment or incoherence)

(4)   grossly disorganized or catatonic behavior

Note: Do not include a symptom if it is a culturally sanctioned response pattern.

B.   Duration of an episode of the disturbance is at least 1 day but less than 1 month, with eventual full return to premorbid level of functioning.

C.   The disturbance is not better accounted for by a mood disorder with psychotic features, schizoaffective disorder, or schizophrenia and is not due to the direct physiological effects of a substance (e.g., a drug of abuse, a medication) or a general medical condition.

Specify if:

With Marked Stressor(s) (brief reactive psychosis):   if symptoms occur shortly after and apparently in response to events that, singly or together, would be markedly stressful to almost anyone in similar circumstances in the person's culture

Without Marked Stressor(s):   if psychotic symptoms do *not* occur shortly after, or are not apparently in response to events that, singly or together, would be markedly stressful to almost anyone in similar circumstances in the person's culture

With Postpartum Onset: if onset within 4 weeks postpartum

---

polymorphisms, are believed to present significant risk factors, as supported by studies that show increased risk of schizophrenia in family members of schizophrenic patients. However, to date, no specifically identified gene predisposes individuals to the schizophrenic spectrum. Obstetrical complications, including abnormal fetal growth and development, hypoxia, and maternal stress or illness, also have been connected with the eventual development of disorders on the schizophrenic spectrum. These early developmental problems may affect the neurogenesis and neuronal migration within the growing fetal brain

Table 5–7. DSM-IV-TR diagnostic criteria for psychotic disorder due to a general medical condition

A.   Prominent hallucinations or delusions.

B.   There is evidence from the history, physical examination, or laboratory findings that the disturbance is the direct physiological consequence of a general medical condition.

C.   The disturbance is not better accounted for by another mental disorder.

D.   The disturbance does not occur exclusively during the course of a delirium.

Code based on predominant symptom:

.81   **With Delusions:**   if delusions are the predominant symptom

.82   **With Hallucinations:**   if hallucinations are the predominant symptom

Coding note: Include the name of the general medical condition on Axis I, e.g., 293.81 psychotic disorder due to malignant lung neoplasm, with delusions; also code the general medical condition on Axis III.

Coding note: If delusions are part of vascular dementia, indicate the delusions by coding the appropriate subtype, e.g., 290.42 vascular dementia, with delusions.

and lead to neural vulnerabilities, priming the brain for mental illness. Another potential precipitating factor in the development of psychosis is the use of illicit substances, such as phencyclidine (PCP), lysergic acid diethylamide (LSD), and marijuana (Marneros and Pillmann 2004). Finally, in keeping with the biopsychosocial model of mental illness, social risk factors for psychotic disorders have been linked with urban environments, minority ethnicity and especially the migration of Afro-Caribbean and East African native populations, and prior exposure to social adversity and traumatic life events (Dean and Murray 2005; Marneros and Akiskal 2007; Marneros and Pillmann 2004).

Pathophysiology of Schizophrenia

Currently, there is no single neurobiological disruption or mechanism that has been found to be responsible for causing schizophrenia and other psychotic disorders. Most of the research and investigation into the neurobiology of psychotic disorders have focused on the specific disorder of schizophrenia. Therefore, most of the information provided in this section focuses on hypotheses that have resulted from research on this particular disorder. We provide a brief snapshot of what is currently known about the neurobiology of schizophrenia as a basis for the subsequent discussion of psychopharmacology. However, many of the hypotheses reflect symptomatology applicable to a wide variety of psychotic disorders.

For many years, the hypotheses surrounding the causes of positive psychotic symptoms were derived from the effects and mechanisms of action of the conventional antipsychotics. Additional effects of nonmedicinal or highly abused substances such as cocaine, amphetamines, and hallucinogenic drugs producing psychotic symptoms also supported these hypotheses (Nasrallah 2011; Sadock and Sadock 2007; Stahl 2008; Tsai and Coyle 2002). The information gathered from these observations was pertinent only to the positive symptoms of psychotic disorders and neglected to address what neurobiological mechanisms were responsible for negative, mood, and cognitive symptoms (Nasrallah 2011; Sadock and Sadock 2007; Stahl 2008; Tsai and Coyle 2002). This realization sparked interest in a search for various neurobiological mechanisms to explain the symptoms of schizophrenia and psychosis. Several hypotheses in the literature now address neurotransmitter, neurocircuitry/ brain areas, neurodevelopmental, and structural aspects of these disorders.

One of the longest-held hypotheses about the neurobiology of schizophrenia is the dopamine hypothesis. Because the positive symptoms of this disorder appeared when people ingested amphetamines and cocaine, substances that increase amounts of dopamine, it was believed that an excess of dopamine in the mesolimbic pathway of the brain was responsible for causing schizophrenia (Nasrallah 2011; Sadock and Sadock 2007; Stahl 2008; Tsai and Coyle 2002). The pharmacological options available to treat psychosis were traditionally dopamine (D_2) receptor antagonists, which decrease available dopamine (Citrome 2011; Nasrallah 2011; Sadock and Sadock 2007; Stahl 2008; Tsai and Coyle 2002).

Research into the role dopamine plays in the negative, cognitive, and mood symptoms of schizophrenia also has been conducted, especially in regard to the various dopaminergic pathways. The four major dopaminergic pathways in the brain are mesolimbic, mesocortical, nigrostriatal, and tuberoinfundibular (Stahl 2008; Vallone et al. 2000). The first three dopaminergic pathways are of particular importance in the symptomatology of schizophrenia. The mesolimbic pathway originates in the ventral tegmental area and terminates in the nucleus accumbens. The mesocortical pathway also arises in the ventral tegmental area but extends to the prefrontal cortex. The nigrostriatal pathway derives from the substantia nigra and terminates in the striatum. When one considers the symptoms of schizophrenia and compares them with the functions of the dopaminergic pathways, the various pieces of the disorder fit together. The mesolimbic pathway plays a role in the regulation of pleasure, motivation, and reward and has been associated with the positive symptoms of schizophrenia (Stahl 2008; Vallone et al. 2000). The mesocortical pathway functions in regulating cognition and is understandably associated with the negative, cognitive, and mood symptoms of schizophrenia (Stahl 2008). This pathway also seems to play a role in learning and memory (Vallone et al. 2000). The nigrostriatal pathway functions in the regulation of motor movements and is correlated with motor disturbances within the disorder, as well as the side effects of antipsychotic medications (Stahl 2008; Vallone et al. 2000). The tuberoinfundibular pathway is involved in the regulation of prolactin (Vallone et al. 2000).

Currently, the thought is that decreased dopamine in the mesocortical pathway leading to the prefrontal cortex is responsible for the three remaining symptom categories (Citrome 2011; Nasrallah 2011; Stahl 2008). Mesocortical dopaminergic hypoactivity may precede the onset of schizophrenia and may be associated with behavioral risk of schizophrenia. Once illness emerges, mesolimbic hyperactivity has been associated with positive symptoms of psychosis (Stahl 2008).

Dopamine and D_2 receptors are not the only neurotransmitter and receptors that are implicated in the pathophysiology of schizophrenia. Recent research supports the role of N-methyl-D-aspartate (NMDA) receptors and the excitatory neurotransmitter glutamate in schizophrenia. NMDA receptors are one of three types of voltage-gated receptors associated with glutamate in the brain. Other receptors implicated in schizophrenia include α-amino-3-hydroxy-5-methyl-4-isoxazolepropionic acid (AMPA) and kainate, which are not discussed in this section (Bunney and Bunney 2000; Citrome 2011; Stahl 2008; Tsai and Coyle 2002). In schizophrenia, a hypofunction of the NMDA receptors is believed to occur. The hypofunctioning of NMDA receptors has far-reaching neurobiological effects. Typically, NMDA receptors will inhibit dopamine activity in the mesolimbic pathway. When their function is decreased, the amount of dopamine activity is increased, which is known to cause positive symptoms. The effects of PCP and ketamine, an anesthetic, support the role of NMDA receptors in schizophrenia. These two substances antagonize NMDA receptors and mimic not only positive but also negative and cognitive symptoms of schizophrenia (Nasrallah 2011; Stahl 2008; Tsai and Coyle 2002). Use of this hypothesis to guide treatment is problematic because increasing the function of NMDA receptors has the potential to cause excitotoxicity and neuronal death (Stahl 2008; Tsai and Coyle 2002).

Areas in the prefrontal cortex and accompanying connectivity with temporal-limbic brain areas have been implicated in the neurobiology of schizophrenia. The dorsolateral and ventromedial prefrontal cortices, as well as the orbitofrontal cortex and the nucleus accumbens, are all involved (Bunney and Bunney 2000; Citrome 2011; Stahl 2008). The function of each area parallels related symptoms. For example, the dorsolateral prefrontal cortex has been associated with the cognitive dysfunction of schizophrenia (Stahl 2008), whereas temporal areas have been implicated in positive symptoms such as hallucinations. Various neuroimaging studies support the phenomenon termed *hypofrontality* in schizophrenia. Hypofrontality refers to the decrease in frontal lobe activity observed in schizophrenic patients while performing cognitive tasks (Bunney and Bunney 2000; Sadock and Sadock 2007; Stahl 2008).

Finally, various structural changes have been observed in the brains of those with schizophrenia, compared with those without the disorder. Typically, the structural changes include a decreased volume of brain matter—specifically, a decrease in neuronal volume and size—in the prefrontal cortex and temporal areas (Bunney and Bunney 2000; Gur et al. 2000; Sadock and Sadock 2007; Tsai and Coyle 2002). Decreased cortical brain matter and enlargement of cerebral ventricles also have been observed in those with schizophrenia (Sadock and Sadock 2007). Research findings are inconclusive as to whether volume changes are causative or progressive effects of the disorder. Volume changes also may be a result of treatment strategies for schizophrenia. A recent longitudinal study by Ho and colleagues (2011) found an association between decreased brain volume and treatment with antipsychotic medications.

In summary, the neurobiology of schizophrenia and psychotic disorders is extremely complex and remains poorly understood. Neurological function and activity continue to remain a mystery. Further neurobiological research may unify the aforementioned hypotheses. The unique presentations of schizophrenia and other psychotic disorders highlight the importance of individualized psychopharmacological treatment. Therefore, a thorough and holistically oriented assessment should be completed with each patient before treatment.

Antipsychotic Medications

In addition to their U.S. Food and Drug Administration (FDA)–approved indication for schizophrenia, antipsychotics are commonly prescribed off-label for other psychiatric disorders (Table 5–8).

Prescribing Considerations

The class of antipsychotic medication is divided into conventional agents, also known as first-generation antipsychotics (FGAs), and atypical agents, also known as second-generation antipsychotics (SGAs). FGAs are defined by their D_2 receptor antagonistic activity in the mesolimbic dopamine pathway. The blockade of D_2 receptors in the mesolimbic pathway diminishes positive symptoms of psychosis. Oral administration of FGAs leads to wide distribution of the drug, affecting every D_2 receptor throughout the brain. In contrast, SGAs antagonize both the serotonin receptor and the dopamine receptor (Stahl 2008).

Choice of medication treatment is based on history of response and weighing potential side effects associated with specific antipsychotics and their classes. In general, because of their efficacy and tolerability profile, SGAs are considered the first-line choice of medication treatment, but FGAs remain widely used because of their efficacy. Over the past decade, algorithms have been established for treatment of psychosis and schizophrenia, such as those from the Texas Medication Algorithm Project (e.g., Miller et al. 1999)—based on expert consensus—and from the Clinical Antipsychotic Trials of Intervention Effectiveness (e.g., Lieberman et al. 2005), a large-scale National Institute of Mental Health–funded clinical trial. However, the clinician must

Table 5–8. Off-label uses for commonly prescribed antipsychotics

Drug	Anxiety disorders	Bipolar disorder	Dementia	Delirium	Agitation
Chlorpromazine (Thorazine)		X			X
Haloperidol (Haldol)				X	
Loxapine (Loxitane)		X			
Perphenazine (Trilafon)		X		X	
Pimozide (Orap)	X				
Thiothixene (Navane)		X			
Aripiprazole (Abilify)	X	X		X	
Olanzapine (Zyprexa)	X	X			
Quetiapine (Seroquel)	X		X	X	X
Risperidone (Risperdal)	X		X	X	

consider that for a variety of reasons, clinical trials and their participants may not reflect efficacy in the field, especially in the individual patient with psychosis.

Pharmacokinetics and Pharmacodynamics

Most antipsychotic agents are metabolized through the same cytochrome P450 (CYP) enzymes—namely, CYP2D6, CYP3A4, CYP2C9, and CYP1A2. All antipsychotics are subject to various drug interactions because of their extensive CYP metabolism. Antipsychotics are generally absorbed through the gut wall into the liver where they are partially converted to a biotransformed product in the bloodstream while another portion of the drug remains unaltered (Stahl 2008).

Specific pharmacokinetics of antipsychotics include their lipophilic nature and highly protein- and tissue-bound compounds that attain large volumes of distribution (Table 5–9). Their oral absorption is variable, and first-pass metabolism occurs via the liver. This contributes to minimal or fluctuating oral bioavailability. Once the antipsychotic dose has been stabilized, most conventional agents can be dosed once or twice daily because of their extended half-lives (Jibson 2011).

Many psychotropic medications are metabolized through the CYP isoenzyme system pathway. The enzymes involved in this system catalyze oxidative metabolism in various organs such as the liver and small intestine to break down drugs. Numerous subsystems are categorized as substrates, inducers, or inhibitors. Drugs metabolized by CYP enzymes are classified as substrates (e.g., haloperidol [Haldol] and olanzapine [Zyprexa]). CYP enzyme inducers increase metabolism and decrease the effects of the drug (e.g., carbamazepine [Tegretol]). CYP enzyme inhibitors decrease metabolism and increase the effects of the drug (e.g., escitalopram [Lexapro] and chlorpromazine [Thorazine]). The inducing and inhibiting effects can contribute to inefficacy, toxicity, drug interactions, and adverse reactions. Knowledge of this system is of particular importance when multiple medications are prescribed (psychotropic and nonpsychotropic). An example of a CYP system interaction can be seen with the concomitant use of aripiprazole (Abilify; an SGA) and fluoxetine (Prozac; an antidepressant). Aripiprazole is metabolized by CYP2D6 and CYP3A6. Fluoxetine is a CYP2D6 inhibitor and may increase the levels

Table 5–9. Pharmacokinetics of antipsychotic medications

Drug	Time to peak (hours)	Half-life (hours)	Metabolism
Chlorpromazine (Thorazine)	2–4 po	30	Hepatic metabolism via CYP2D6 transformation and active metabolites. Low oral bioavailability relative to intramuscular injection due to first-pass metabolism.
Fluphenazine	Rapid	33	Hepatic metabolism via CYP2D6 and other transformations.
Haloperidol (Haldol)	2–6 po; 0.5 im	20	Hepatic metabolism via CYP3A4 and CYP2D6 transformations.
Loxapine (Loxitane)	1.5–3 po	12	Extensively metabolized by most of the CYP system enzymes.
Perphenazine (Trilafon)	1–3 po	9–12	Hepatic metabolism via CYP2D6 and CYP3A4 transformations and active metabolites.
Pimozide (Orap)	6–8 po	55	Hepatic metabolism via CYP3A4 and other transformations.
Thiothixene (Navane)	1–3 po	33	Hepatic metabolism via CYP1A2 and other transformations.
Thioridazine	1 po	21–25	Hepatic metabolism via CYP2D6 transformations and active metabolites (mesoridazine, sulforidazine).

Table 5–9. Pharmacokinetics of antipsychotic medications *(continued)*

Drug	Time to peak (hours)	Half-life (hours)	Metabolism
Trifluoperazine	1.5–6.0 po	22	Hepatic metabolism via CYP1A2 and other transformations.
Aripiprazole (Abilify)	3–5 po; 1–3 im	75–94	Hepatic metabolism via CYP2D6 and CYP3A4 transformations and an active metabolite (dehydro-aripiprazole). Half-life prolonged in CYP2D6 slow metabolizers.
Asenapine (Saphris)	0.5–1.5 po	24	Hepatic metabolism via CYP1A2 transformation and glucuronidation.
Clozapine (Clozaril)	2.5 po	12	Hepatic metabolism via CYP1A2 transformation and active metabolite (norclozapine).
Iloperidone (Fanapt)	2–4 po	18–26	Hepatic metabolism via CYP2D6 and CYP3A4 transformations and active metabolites. Prolonged half-life up to 37 hours in CYP2D6 slow metabolizers.
Olanzapine (Zyprexa)	5–8 po; 0.25–0.75 im	30–38	Hepatic metabolism via CYP1A2 transformation and direct glucuronidation.
Paliperidone (Invega)	24 po	23 po	Minimal hepatic metabolism; excreted primarily unchanged in urine, necessitating dose reduction in renal insufficiency.

Table 5–9.　Pharmacokinetics of antipsychotic
medications *(continued)*

Drug	Time to peak (hours)	Half-life (hours)	Metabolism
Quetiapine (Seroquel)	1.5 IR po; 6 ER po	6–12	Hepatic metabolism via CYP3A4 transformation and active hydroxy metabolite.
Risperidone (Risperdal)	1.5 po	20	Hepatic metabolism via CYP2D6 and CYP3A4 transformations and active hydroxy metabolite. Prolonged half-life in CYP2D6 slow metabolizers.
Ziprasidone (Geodon)	6–8 po; <1 im	7 po; 2–5 im	Hepatic metabolism via CYP3A4 and other transformations.

Note.　CYP = cytochrome P450; ER = extended release; im = intramuscular; IR = immediate release; po = by mouth.

Source.　Adapted from Jibson 2011.

of aripiprazole. Prescribing with this in mind would warrant a decreased dose of aripiprazole for someone taking fluoxetine and monitoring for efficacy. If prescribing a recommended dose, one would keep in mind that the potential for side effects would be increased.

Side Effects

Antipsychotic medications, both first and second generation, affect the dopamine pathways of the brain. Dopamine, as mentioned previously, is a neurotransmitter that is closely connected to brain areas that regulate pleasure/reward, mood, and movement. Because of its wide-reaching effects, dopamine has been implicated in most side effects that can be associated with psychopharmacological treatments.

Extrapyramidal Symptoms

One of the most common side effects with FGAs is extrapyramidal symptoms (EPS), or disturbances of movement. Although movement disorders can be caused by all antipsychotic agents, many fewer occur with second-generation medications (Caroff et al. 2011). Symptoms of parkinsonism, dystonia, tardive dyskinesia, and akathisia are all associated with antipsychotic treatment. Parkinsonian symptoms include not only tremors and slowed initiation of spontaneous movement but also diminished reflexes and muscle rigidity, exemplified by lead pipe or cogwheel movements (Reveley and Deakin 2000). Dystonia is a form of muscle rigidity that is episodic and unrelenting for the period of the episode (Caroff et al. 2011). Contractions of the muscles within the head and neck are most common and can lead to contortions, contractions, and abnormal postures. Oculogyric crisis, in which the patient's eye muscles contract and cause the eyes to sustain an either upward or lateral gaze, is a form of dystonia (Reveley and Deakin 2000). Tardive dyskinesia is different from dystonia in that it is a repetitive movement, not a sustained contraction. Tardive dyskinesia is abnormal, involuntary movements and is most often noticed in facial features (i.e., lip smacking, jaw moving, protruding of the tongue) (Stoklosa and Ongur 2011). Akathisia is also a motor side effect but is more associated with a patient's subjective feeling of restlessness or inability to sit still (Reveley and Deakin 2000). Because of these feelings, the patient is constantly in motion, exhibiting foot tapping, frequent shifting of weight, and similar activities.

Neuroleptic malignant syndrome is an extreme form of EPS and is a very rare side effect of antipsychotic agents. Most closely associated with atypical antipsychotics at higher doses, this syndrome can be life-threatening. Symptoms include general muscle rigidity and catatonic states, hyperthermia, autonomic dysregulation, and altered consciousness (Caroff et al. 2011). Generally, this condition can reverse itself with the withdrawal of the dopamine antagonist. On rare occasions, neuroleptic malignant syndrome can progress to hypermetabolic crisis, and some patients can have prolonged residual symptoms that need interventions such as benzodiazepines, dopamine agonists, or electroconvulsive therapy to resolve (Caroff et al. 2011).

Metabolic Disturbances

Metabolic disturbances are more frequently seen with SGAs because of their combination of serotonin and histamine antagonism. The combined blockade of these receptors can lead to increased appetite and weight gain (Stahl 2011). Weight gain itself increases risk for cardiometabolic disorders because obesity can cause insulin resistance, which will encourage an increased production of insulin, leading to hyperinsulinemia and destruction of beta cells in the liver (Stahl 2011). However, factors inherent to SGAs are also thought to cause dyslipidemia and insulin resistance unlinked to weight gain (Argo et al. 2011). Either way, an increase in fasting triglycerides and insulin resistance in the patient has significant potential to progress to diabetes and thus increase the risk of cardiovascular disease and possibly premature death (Stahl 2011).

Prolactin Elevation

Within the tuberoinfundibular pathway of dopamine, the release of the prolactin hormone is regulated. Prolactin is a hormone present in all mammals that encourages the production of milk and stimulates lactation. All antipsychotics work to decrease dopamine within the mesolimbic tract, through either antagonism or receptor blockade, to decrease positive symptoms (Stahl 2011). Dopamine acts in the tuberoinfundibular pathway to inhibit the release of prolactin; consequently, the decrease of dopamine in this pathway causes an increase in the level of prolactin (Madhusoodanan et al. 2010). Prolactin elevation can thus cause lactation, acne, and amenorrhea, all of which can cause subjective levels of distress within the patient.

Exacerbation of Negative Symptoms

Medication-induced negativism, or idiopathic negative symptoms, can be caused by antipsychotic treatments. Because of the previously mentioned need to decrease dopamine in the mesolimbic tract to treat positive symptoms of psychosis, antipsychotics encourage hypoactive dopamine production (Nasrallah 2011). This may be caused by either dopamine antagonism or a secondary dopamine decrease resulting from inhibition by serotonin receptors (Stahl 2011). Unfortunately, in the mesocortical tract, hypoactive dopamine receptors can produce a dampening of cognition and affective flattening (Nasrallah 2011). As a result, the patient taking antipsychotics can potentially experience a worsening of negative symptoms despite resolution of positive symptomatology. This phenomenon is more closely associated with FGAs.

Sedation and Anticholinergic Side Effects

Sedation, along with weight gain and EPS, is one of the most common side effects of antipsychotic medications. Dopamine, muscarinic-cholinergic, histamine, and α_1-adrenergic blockade can all cause sedation (Stahl 2011). This may be a desired effect in acute or aggressive presentations, but long-term treatment with a sedating agent may lead to patient nonadherence (Stahl 2011). Anticholinergic effects also may complicate patient adherence. Anticholinergic side effects are generally thought of as dry mouth, blurred vision, urinary retention, and constipation but also may include dizziness, drowsiness, and complications in cognition (Nasrallah 2011). These are more frequently seen with FGAs because of their strong dopamine blockade.

Treatment of Special Populations

The antipsychotic medications have been used for decades, but caution is generally the rule of thumb with various populations, including women who are pregnant or breast-feeding, elderly patients, medically compromised patients, and children and adolescents.

Pregnant or Breast-Feeding Patients

For the most part, both FGAs and SGAs are FDA Category C for pregnancy and are contraindicated in breast-feeding mothers. The exception to this categorization is clozapine, which is not generally thought to be a first-line agent but is Category B for pregnancy. Psychiatric advanced practice registered nurses (APRNs) must use their best clinical judgment to evaluate the risks and benefits for both the patient and her unborn infant when psychiatric symptoms arise before or during pregnancy. Chlorpromazine and haloperidol both have been used to alleviate the symptoms of psychosis and stabilize the symptoms of schizophrenia during pregnancy. Similarly, caution must be exercised when treating the woman who is nursing her infant because active metabolites of the antipsychotics may be released through breast milk. Remember, when treating women during this phase of life, the APRN is now treating two individuals with distinctly unique metabolisms.

Elderly Patients

When the psychiatric APRN is evaluating and prescribing antipsychotics for an elderly patient, he or she must be aware of the FDA-issued black box warning for potential increased risk of mortality in elderly patients with dementia (see also Table 1–4 in Chapter 1, "Introduction to Clinical Psychopharmacology for Nurses"). Additionally, the elderly have a greater potential for drug-drug interactions because of the high incidence of polypharmacy and multiple medical complications, which may contraindicate the prescribing of the antipsychotics. Finally, with advancing age, the individual's metabolism may slow, nutritional intake may be sparse, and sleep patterns may be disrupted, all of which would be further compromised by the potential adverse effects of the antipsychotic medications.

Medically Compromised Patients

Given the potential increased risk for patients to gain weight and develop metabolic syndrome related to the use of the antipsychotics, judicious monitoring must be part of every psychiatric APRN's repertoire. Guidelines for the management of side effects and metabolic syndrome are addressed in greater detail in Chapter 12, "Management of Metabolic Side Effects of Psychotropic Medications." Because patients with chronic psychiatric illness experience a marked increase in morbidity and mortality compared with the general population and may, in fact, have their life expectancy shortened by decades, it is critical to monitor and address any potential medical complications as soon as they arise.

Children and Adolescents

When prescribing antipsychotics to children and adolescents, off-label use must be both discussed and documented with the child and his or her parents or guardian. The following SGAs have FDA approval for children and adolescents:

- Risperidone (Risperdal): irritability related to the autistic spectrum disorders (ages 5–16), schizophrenia (age 13 or older), and bipolar disorder, manic or mixed (age 10 or older)

- Quetiapine (Seroquel): schizophrenia (age 13 or older) and bipolar disorder, manic (age 10 or older)
- Olanzapine: schizophrenia (age 13 or older) and bipolar disorder, manic or mixed (age 13 or older)
- Aripiprazole (Abilify): schizophrenia (age 13 or older); bipolar disorder, manic or mixed (age 10 or older); and irritability related to the autistic spectrum disorders (age 6 or older)

The following FGAs have FDA approval for children and adolescents:

- Chlorpromazine: severe behavior disorders (ages 6 months to 12 years)
- Haloperidol: severe behavior disorders and agitation (age 3 or older), Tourette syndrome (age 3 or older), and psychosis (age 3 or older)
- Pimozide (Orap): Tourette syndrome, severe (age 12 or older)

Given that children often metabolize drugs more quickly than do adults, the psychiatric APRN will need to monitor closely for efficacy and potential side effects. Because children do not enjoy taking medications, the clinician must monitor for "cheeking" and check in with the parent or guardian to ensure adherence. Finally, although some of these agents are indicated and approved for behavior disorders and symptoms, the antipsychotics are not a substitute for behavior modification interventions and family therapy.

Summary

As the knowledge base on schizophrenia and other psychotic disorders continues to broaden with ongoing research, holistic treatment options will continue to evolve. With an increased understanding of the neurobiology that underlies psychosis and other clinical symptoms, pharmacological treatments will be more accurately tailored to demonstrated symptom categories and associated motor disturbances, thus becoming more efficacious. To achieve the best possible clinical outcomes, medication selection and dosing must be grounded in careful consideration of pharmacokinetic and side-effect profiles and targeted toward facilitating patient adherence to treatment.

Clinical Pearls

- Many patients with schizophrenia are loners and may be uncomfortable when other people violate their personal space. The clinician should respect the patient's personal space and not intrude on that space unless invited.

- Nursing staff must always treat patients as human beings with dignity and respect, regardless of whether they are homeless or disheveled. They should make eye contact with those patients who can tolerate that and speak in a matter-of-fact manner but with empathy. A small act of kindness, such as offering a shower, clean clothes, and a meal, is one of the fastest and easiest ways to develop a therapeutic relationship. Occasionally, offering coffee, soda, or a cigarette may prove beneficial when all other interventions have been exhausted.

- Always be safety conscious. Do not attempt to approach an aggressive client alone. It is best to have other staff members and/or security in close proximity to you when addressing a hostile patient—using, if necessary, a "show of force." Continue to offer choices to the patient, maintain his or her dignity, and use physical interventions only after all other interventions have been thoroughly explored.

- When a patient is suspicious or mistrustful about medications (which often occurs with paranoid delusions or hallucinations), medication teaching often becomes more complex. We always want to provide medication education to our patients, but if a patient is paranoid about medications, it may be helpful to state the specific symptom that the medication will target (e.g., "This is your medication, Zyprexa [olanzapine], and it will help with your thinking"). It may be less beneficial to discuss every potential side effect or negative outcome associated with the medication.

- The vast majority of schizophrenic patients are not violent toward others. Most command hallucinations tell patients that they are in danger or will be harmed. Paranoid patients may become assaultive if they perceive a person as a threat, which is usually due to their dysfunctional beliefs and paranoia. Look for cues of increasing agitation—such as pacing, cursing, yelling, or responding to internal stimuli loudly—

and intervene early. It may be necessary to decrease stimuli, provide time out in the patient's room or the quiet room, and offer medications as needed. Stress to patients the need for them to maintain control, and explain to them that medication may help them relax and feel better.

References

American Psychiatric Association: Diagnostic and Statistical Manual of Mental Disorders, 4th Edition, Text Revision. Washington, DC, American Psychiatric Association, 2000

Argo T, Carnahan R, Barnett M, et al: Diabetes prevalence estimates in schizophrenia and risk factor assessment. Ann Clin Psychiatry 23:117–124, 2011

Bunney WE, Bunney BG: Evidence for a compromised dorsolateral prefrontal cortical parallel circuit in schizophrenia. Brain Res Rev 3:138–146, 2000

Caroff S, Hurford I, Lybrand J, et al: Movement disorders induced by antipsychotic drugs: implications of the CATIE schizophrenia trial. Neurol Clin 29:127–148, 2011

Citrome L: Neurochemical models of schizophrenia: transcending dopamine. Curr Psychiat 10 (suppl 9):S10–S14, 2011

Dean K, Murray RM: Environmental risk factors for psychosis. Dialogues Clin Neurosci 7:69–80, 2005

Fuji D, Ahmed I: The Spectrum of Psychotic Disorders. New York, Cambridge University Press, 2007

Gur RE, Turetsky BI, Cowell PE, et al: Temporolimbic volume reductions in schizophrenia. Arch Gen Psychiatry 57:769–775, 2000

Ho B, Andreasen NC, Ziebell S, et al: Long-term antipsychotic treatment and brain volumes: a longitudinal study of first-episode schizophrenia. Arch Gen Psychiatry 68:128–137, 2011

Jibson MD: First-generation antipsychotic medications: pharmacology, administration, and comparative side effects. June 3, 2011. Available at: http://www.uptodate.com/contents/first-generation-antipsychotic-medications-pharmacology-administration-and-comparative-side-effects. Accessed February 24, 2012.

Kendler KS, Gallagher TJ, Abelson JM, et al: Lifetime prevalence, demographic risk factors, and diagnostic validity of nonaffective psychosis as assessed in a US community sample: the National Comorbidity Survey. Arch Gen Psychiatry 53:1022–1031, 1996

Lieberman JA, Stroup TS, McEvoy JP, Et al: Effectiveness of antipsychotic drugs in patients with chronic schizophrenia. N Engl J Med 353:1209–1223, 2005

Madhusoodanan S, Parida S, Jimene C: Hyperprolactinemia associated with psychotropics: a review. Hum Psychopharmacol Clin Exp 25:281–297, 2010

Marneros A, Akiskal H: The Overlap of Affective and Schizophrenic Spectra. New York, Cambridge University Press, 2007

Marneros A, Pillmann F: Acute and Transient Psychoses. Cambridge, UK, Cambridge University Press, 2004

Miller AL, Chiles JA, Chiles JK, et al: The Texas Medication Algorithm Project (TMAP) schizophrenia algorithms. J Clin Psychiatry 60:649–657, 1999

Nasrallah H: The primary and secondary symptoms of schizophrenia: current and future management. Curr Psychiatr 10 (suppl 9):S5–S9, 2011

Reveley M, Deakin J: The Psychopharmacology of Schizophrenia. London, Arnold Publishers, 2000

Sadock BJ, Sadock VA: Kaplan and Sadock's Synopsis of Psychiatry: Behavioral Sciences/Clinical Psychiatry, 10th Edition. Philadelphia, PA, Lippincott Williams & Wilkins, 2007

Saha S, Chant D, Welham J, et al: A systematic review of the prevalence of schizophrenia. PLoS Med 2(5): e141, 2005

Schilling J, Nieginski E, Moreau D, et al: Straight A's in Psychiatric and Mental Health Nursing: A Review Series. Ambler, PA, Lippincott Williams & Wilkins, 2006

Siegel S, Ralph L: Demystifying Schizophrenia for the General Practitioner. Sudbury, MA, Jones & Bartlett, 2011

Stahl SM: Stahl's Essential Psychopharmacology: Neuroscientific Basis and Practical Applications, 3rd Edition. New York, Cambridge University Press, 2008

Stahl SM: The Prescriber's Guide: Stahl's Essential Psychopharmacology, 4th Edition. New York, Cambridge University Press, 2011

Stoklosa J, Ongur D: Rational antipsychotic choice: weighing the risk of tardive dyskinesia and metabolic syndrome. Harv Rev Psychiatry 19:271–276, 2011

Tsai G, Coyle JT: Glutamatergic mechanisms in schizophrenia. Annu Rev Pharmacol Toxicol 42:165–179, 2002

Tsuang MT, Stone WS, Faraone SV: Genes, environment and schizophrenia. Br J Psychiatry 178:s18–s24, 2001

Vallone D, Picetti R, Borrelli E: Structure and function of dopamine receptors. Neurosci Biobehav Rev 24:125–132, 2000

World Health Organization: The World Health Report 2001—Mental Health: New Understanding, New Hope. Geneva, Switzerland, World Health Organization, 2001

6

Attention-Deficit/Hyperactivity and Autistic Spectrum Disorders

Patti A. Varley, M.N., A.P.R.N., P.M.H.-
C.N.S., B.C.

Laura G. Leahy, M.S.N., P.M.H.-
A.P.R.N.

I prefer to distinguish ADD as attention abundance disorder. Everything is just so interesting... remarkably at the same time.

—Frank Coppola, M.A., ADHD Coach

Autism: Where the "randomness of life" collides and clashes with an individual's need for the sameness.

—Eileen Miller, *The Girl Who Spoke with Pictures: Autism Through Art*

In this chapter, we explore two neurodevelopmental disorders that significantly impact children and adolescents. Attention-deficit/hyperactivity disorder (ADHD), once thought to affect only children and adolescents, has in recent years been found to also impair the functioning of adults. The ADHD symptoms of inattention, restlessness, and reduced concentration are woven throughout the affective, psychotic, and other mental disorders. The impact and treatment of those symptoms will be addressed in this chapter.

Similarly, the autistic spectrum disorders have seen much media attention in recent years, and their symptoms, impact on functioning, and treatment options will be addressed in this chapter.

Attention-Deficit/Hyperactivity Disorder

Over the past four decades, attention-deficit/hyperactivity disorder (ADHD) has been a diagnosis fraught with much controversy. Prior to 1980, when the diagnosis attention-deficit disorder was included in DSM-III (American Psychiatric Association 1980), other names had been used to describe this constellation of symptoms. Such names included hyperkinetic reaction of childhood, hyperkinetic syndrome, hyperactive child syndrome, minimal brain damage, minimal brain dysfunction, minimal cerebral dysfunction, and minor cerebral dysfunction. The disorder was once thought to be either simply a behavior disorder or a result of trauma to the brain. Some even believed that the disorder was caused by a lack of discipline. Today we know that the symptoms related to ADHD are neurodevelopmental in origin. Despite the controversies, the core features of the disorder—reduced attention span, distractibility, difficulty focusing, and hyperactivity—have remained throughout.

ADHD contributes much disruption to the patient's educational, occupational, family, and social life. It continues across the life span (Table 6–1); the symptoms do not disappear once the individual reaches adolescence, as was previously thought. Adults can continue to show symptoms of disorganization, difficulty sustaining attention, failure to complete tasks, and forgetfulness, although the symptoms of hyperactivity may be diminished.

Figure 6–1 illustrates the various levels of impairment related to ADHD across the life span (Melmed 2011).

The National Institute of Mental Health (2009) has been conducting the Multimodal Treatment of Attention Deficit Hyperactivity Disorder (MTA)

Table 6–1. Symptoms of attention-deficit/hyperactivity disorder across the life span

Childhood	Adolescence	Adulthood
Hyperactivity, "on the go"	Easily distracted, inattentiveness	Inattentiveness
Low frustration tolerance	Easily bored	Poor organization; poor time and money management
Aggression	Impatience	Frequently missed deadlines, appointments, or events
Easily distracted	Emotional immaturity compared with peers	Poor ability to track bills or checkbook
Difficulty developing routines	Frequently changes activities	Psychomotor restlessness
Impulsivity	Lack of focus while driving	Emotional reactivity

Source.   Adapted from Wasserstein 2005.

study since the early 1990s. This ongoing study of ADHD involving multiple settings, long-term follow-up, long-term interventions, differential interventions, and head-to-head medication trials has solidified the evidence base for this disorder. In fact, by 1998, the American Medical Association called ADHD "one of the best-researched disorders in medicine and the overall data on its validity are far more compelling than for many medical conditions" (Goldman et al. 1998, p. 6).

Psychiatric advanced practice registered nurses (APRNs) who treat symptoms of ADHD in children, adolescents, and adults understand that caution must be used to thoroughly evaluate the patient because the symptoms of ADHD (Table 6–2) cross the spectrum of all the other psychiatric disorders. Improper diagnosis and treatment choices may result in poorer patient outcomes or exacerbation of other mental illnesses.

Useful screening instruments such as the Vanderbilt ADHD Diagnostic Parent Rating Scale (VADPRS; Wolraich et al. 2003) and Teacher Rating Scale (VADTRS; Wolraich et al. 1998) and the Adult ADHD Self-Report Scale—Version 1.1 (Adult ASRS-v1.1; Kessler et al. 2005) are available to guide the clinician's evaluation. Copies of these assessment scales are provided in Appendix 4, "Psychiatric Rating Scales").

Potential Areas of Impairment

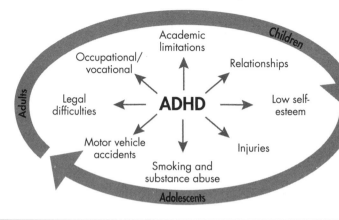

Figure 6–1.   Potential areas of impairment related to attention-deficit/hyperactivity disorder (ADHD) across the life span.

Source.   Adapted from Melmed 2011.

Autistic Spectrum Disorders

Autistic spectrum disorders have received much attention in the media in recent years. Paralleling ADHD, the autistic spectrum disorders have experienced a 10-fold increase in prevalence over the past 40 years (AutismSpeaks 2012). It is now estimated that 1 in every 88 children in the United States will be affected by autism, with the prevalence increasing annually. The autistic spectrum disorders are now ranked as the fastest-growing serious developmental disability in the United States, with annual costs of $126 billion (AutismSpeaks 2012). This class of disorders includes autistic disorder (Table 6–3), Asperger's disorder (Table 6–4), pervasive developmental disorder not otherwise specified (NOS), Rett's disorder, childhood disintegrative disorder, and child psychosis NOS.

Although many national and international research initiatives have explored autism and its associated spectrum of disorders, no definitive medical tests or treatments are indicated for these disorders. Individuals with autistic spectrum or developmental disorders commonly present for treatment of symptoms that disrupt their abilities of daily functioning, personal and social relationships, and attainment of education or occupational functioning. Such symptoms might variably include irritability, anxiety, agitation and aggression, obsessive thoughts and compulsive behaviors, perseveration, inattention and cognitive dysfunction, and, less commonly, psychotic symptoms. Although other psychiatric disorders can occur comorbidly with the autistic spectrum disorders, the aforementioned symptoms also may solely be a part of the developmental disability. Treatment entails a thorough evaluation of the symptoms to formulate a management plan that incorporates a combination of therapeutic, behavioral, and psychopharmacological interventions. For the purposes of this chapter, the focus will remain on the psychotropic medications used in the treatment of the mood and behavioral symptoms associated with autism.

Biological Underpinnings of Neurodevelopmental Disorders

Attention-Deficit/Hyperactivity Disorder

Over the years, a plethora of research has explored the etiology and neurobiological underpinnings of ADHD. In the early 1970s, Satterfield et al. (1974) suggested that children with ADHD symptoms have low levels of arousal accompanied by low levels of inhibition in the central nervous system (CNS). The anterior cingulate cortex, located in the prefrontal cortex, controls goal-directed behaviors, emotional reactivity, error processing, and attention. Problems with executive functioning (e.g., working memory, attention, and organizational skills) are related to the dorsolateral prefrontal cortex, which is responsible for problem solving, self-monitoring, planning, and cognitive flexibility. The symptoms of impulsivity, disorganization, and distractibility are associated with the orbitofrontal cortex, whereas symptoms of hyperactivity are associated with the motor cortex (Stahl 2007).

Table 6–2.   DSM-IV-TR diagnostic criteria for attention-deficit/
hyperactivity disorder

A.   Either (1) or (2):

    (1)   six (or more) of the following symptoms of **inattention** have persisted for at least 6 months to a degree that is maladaptive and inconsistent with developmental level:

    Inattention

        (a)   often fails to give close attention to details or makes careless mistakes in schoolwork, work, or other activities

        (b)   often has difficulty sustaining attention in tasks or play activities

        (c)   often does not seem to listen when spoken to directly

        (d)   often does not follow through on instructions and fails to finish schoolwork, chores, or duties in the workplace (not due to oppositional behavior or failure to understand instructions)

        (e)   often has difficulty organizing tasks and activities

        (f)   often avoids, dislikes, or is reluctant to engage in tasks that require sustained mental effort (such as schoolwork or homework)

        (g)   often loses things necessary for tasks or activities (e.g., toys, school assignments, pencils, books, or tools)

        (h)   is often easily distracted by extraneous stimuli

        (i)   is often forgetful in daily activities

    (2)   six (or more) of the following symptoms of **hyperactivity-impulsivity** have persisted for at least 6 months to a degree that is maladaptive and inconsistent with developmental level:

    Hyperactivity

        (a)   often fidgets with hands or feet or squirms in seat

        (b)   often leaves seat in classroom or in other situations in which remaining seated is expected

        (c)   often runs about or climbs excessively in situations in which it is inappropriate (in adolescents or adults, may be limited to subjective feelings of restlessness)

        (d)   often has difficulty playing or engaging in leisure activities quietly

        (e)   is often "on the go" or often acts as if "driven by a motor"

        (f)   often talks excessively

Table 6–2. DSM-IV-TR diagnostic criteria for attention-deficit/ hyperactivity disorder *(continued)*

Impulsivity

(g)   often blurts out answers before questions have been completed

(h)   often has difficulty awaiting turn

(i)   often interrupts or intrudes on others (e.g., butts into conversations or games)

B.   Some hyperactive-impulsive or inattentive symptoms that caused impairment were present before age 7 years.

C.   Some impairment from the symptoms is present in two or more settings (e.g., at school [or work] and at home).

D.   There must be clear evidence of clinically significant impairment in social, academic, or occupational functioning.

E.   The symptoms do not occur exclusively during the course of a pervasive developmental disorder, schizophrenia, or other psychotic disorder and are not better accounted for by another mental disorder (e.g., mood disorder, anxiety disorder, dissociative disorder, or a personality disorder).

Code based on type:

314.01   **Attention-Deficit/Hyperactivity Disorder, Combined Type:** if both criteria A1 and A2 are met for the past 6 months

314.00   **Attention-Deficit/Hyperactivity Disorder, Predominantly Inattentive Type:**   if criterion A1 is met but criterion A2 is not met for the past 6 months

314.01   **Attention-Deficit/Hyperactivity Disorder, Predominantly Hyperactive-Impulsive Type:**   if criterion A2 is met but criterion A1 is not met for the past 6 months

Coding note: For individuals (especially adolescents and adults) who currently have symptoms that no longer meet full criteria, "In Partial Remission" should be specified.

Table 6–3.   DSM-IV-TR diagnostic criteria for 299.00 autistic disorder

A.   A total of six (or more) items from (1), (2), and (3), with at least two from (1), and one each from (2) and (3):

    (1)   qualitative impairment in social interaction, as manifested by at least two of the following:

        (a)   marked impairment in the use of multiple nonverbal behaviors such as eye-to-eye gaze, facial expression, body postures, and gestures to regulate social interaction

        (b)   failure to develop peer relationships appropriate to developmental level

        (c)   a lack of spontaneous seeking to share enjoyment, interests, or achievements with other people (e.g., by a lack of showing, bringing, or pointing out objects of interest)

        (d)   lack of social or emotional reciprocity

    (2)   qualitative impairments in communication as manifested by at least one of the following:

        (a)   delay in, or total lack of, the development of spoken language (not accompanied by an attempt to compensate through alternative modes of communication such as gesture or mime)

        (b)   in individuals with adequate speech, marked impairment in the ability to initiate or sustain a conversation with others

        (c)   stereotyped and repetitive use of language or idiosyncratic language

        (d)   lack of varied, spontaneous make-believe play or social imitative play appropriate to developmental level

    (3)   restricted repetitive and stereotyped patterns of behavior, interests, and activities, as manifested by at least one of the following:

        (a)   encompassing preoccupation with one or more stereotyped and restricted patterns of interest that is abnormal either in intensity or focus

        (b)   apparently inflexible adherence to specific, nonfunctional routines or rituals

        (c)   stereotyped and repetitive motor mannerisms (e.g., hand or finger flapping or twisting, or complex whole-body movements)

        (d)   persistent preoccupation with parts of objects

B.   Delays or abnormal functioning in at least one of the following areas, with onset prior to age 3 years: (1) social interaction, (2) language as used in social communication, or (3) symbolic or imaginative play.

C.   The disturbance is not better accounted for by Rett's disorder or childhood disintegrative disorder.

Table 6–4.   DSM-IV-TR diagnostic criteria for 299.80 Asperger's disorder

A.   Qualitative impairment in social interaction, as manifested by at least two of the following:

   (1)   marked impairment in the use of multiple nonverbal behaviors such as eye-to-eye gaze, facial expression, body postures, and gestures to regulate social interaction

   (2)   failure to develop peer relationships appropriate to developmental level

   (3)   a lack of spontaneous seeking to share enjoyment, interests, or achievements with other people (e.g., by a lack of showing, bringing, or pointing out objects of interest to other people)

   (4)   lack of social or emotional reciprocity

B.   Restricted repetitive and stereotyped patterns of behavior, interests, and activities, as manifested by at least one of the following:

   (1)   encompassing preoccupation with one or more stereotyped and restricted patterns of interest that is abnormal either in intensity or focus

   (2)   apparently inflexible adherence to specific, nonfunctional routines or rituals

   (3)   stereotyped and repetitive motor mannerisms (e.g., hand or finger flapping or twisting, or complex whole-body movements)

   (4)   persistent preoccupation with parts of objects

C.   The disturbance causes clinically significant impairment in social, occupational, or other important areas of functioning.

D.   There is no clinically significant general delay in language (e.g., single words used by age 2 years, communicative phrases used by age 3 years).

E.   There is no clinically significant delay in cognitive development or in the development of age-appropriate self-help skills, adaptive behavior (other than in social interaction), and curiosity about the environment in childhood.

F.   Criteria are not met for another specific pervasive developmental disorder or schizophrenia.

Differences in neurotransmitters are seen among the three subtypes of ADHD, which contribute to the varying manifestation of symptoms in children and adults with the disorder. Those with primarily the inattentive type of ADHD have changes in their norepinephrine transporter gene, which affects levels of norepinephrine in the brain. Patients with primarily the hyperactive-impulsive type of ADHD have changes in the dopamine transporter gene, which regulates dopamine (Stannard Gromisch 2010; Wasserstein 2005). Studies from Vanderbilt University (Snyder 2009) have noted that patients with the combined type of ADHD have alterations in their choline transporter gene, thus implicating acetylcholine as the modulating neurotransmitter. The imbalance among these neurotransmitters contributes to the often debilitating symptoms across the life span.

Autistic Spectrum Disorders

According to the DSM-IV-TR diagnostic criteria (American Psychiatric Association 2000), the autistic spectrum disorders being discussed in this chapter are based on delays in development that extend beyond the normal and anticipated time frame. The etiology of these disorders remains unclear; however, some medications (e.g., thalidomide [Thalomid], valproic acid [Depakene, Depakote], misoprostol [Cytotec]) taken by a woman during pregnancy have been implicated as risk factors.

Autism is characterized as a polygenetic neurodevelopmental disorder with multiorgan system involvement, although it predominantly involves CNS dysfunction (Minshew and Williams 2007). As nurses are aware, disturbances in the brain produce a constellation of cognitive and neurological deficits. These deficits are clearly seen in the developmental disorders. Magnetic resonance imaging (MRI) shows approximately a 10% increase in the brain size of the toddler with autism as compared with the average 3- to 4-year-old (Redcay and Courchesne 2005). Marc and Olson (2009) suggested that cytokines play a role in autism on the basis of the alteration in the permeability of the blood-brain barrier and subsequent inflammation. This also may be the reason for increased brain size in individuals with autism. Functional MRI studies have shown that skill deficits often found in those with autism and the developmental disorders are accompanied by a reduction in neural activity in the brain regions that normally govern the specific functional domain (Pelphrey et al. 2005).

Elevated urinary serotonin levels have been found in those with the autistic spectrum disorders and are thought to manifest as behavioral symptoms (Castellani et al. 2009). Similarly, elevated levels of plasma glutamate have been excitotoxic and may lead to neurodegeneration and cognitive dysfunction seen clinically in those with developmental disorders (Ha et al. 2009). Although autism and the developmental disorders remain a mystery in terms of their neurotransmission and associated neuropathways, a flurry of research over the past few years continues to offer plausible explanations for the various symptoms of these disorders.

Medications Used to Treat Symptoms Associated With Autism

The psychotropic medications used to treat the symptoms associated with autism are borrowed from the various classes of psychiatric drugs: psychostimulants (see "Medications Used to Treat Symptoms of Attention-Deficit/Hyperactivity Disorder" below), antidepressants (see Chapter 3, "Depressive Disorders"), mood stabilizers (see Chapter 4, "Bipolar Disorders"), and antipsychotics (see Chapter 5, "Psychotic Disorders"). Table 6–5 offers information on the U.S. Food and Drug Administration (FDA)–approved and off-label psychotropics used in the treatment of autistic spectrum disorders.

Medications Used to Treat Symptoms of Attention-Deficit/Hyperactivity Disorder

Table 6–6 lists the FDA-approved medications used to treat the symptoms of ADHD. The purpose of the psychostimulant and other medications used in the treatment of ADHD is to increase dopamine and norepinephrine in the prefrontal cortex. Essentially, both the methylphenidate class and the mixed amphetamine salts class of psychostimulants block the transporter proteins, whereas only the amphetamine salts increase the release of both neurotransmitters from the presynaptic vesicles.

Table 6–5.   Medications commonly prescribed to treat symptoms associated with autism

Drug	FDA approval (adults unless otherwise noted)	Off-label uses (symptoms)
Dextroamphetamine/ amphetamine (Adderall, Adderall XR)	ADHD	Impulsivity, hyperactivity, inattention
Methylphenidate (Ritalin, Concerta, Metadate ER)	ADHD	Impulsivity, hyperactivity, inattention
Atomoxetine (Strattera)	ADHD	Inattention, decreased concentration, anxiety
Bupropion (Wellbutrin SR and XL)	Depression	Inattention, decreased concentration, depression
Fluoxetine (Prozac)	Depression (7 years and older), OCD (7 years and older), anxiety, PMDD	Repetitive behaviors, anxiety, depression
Sertraline (Zoloft)	OCD (6 years and older), anxiety, depression, PTSD, PMDD	Repetitive behaviors, anxiety, depression
Fluvoxamine (Luvox)	OCD (8 years and older)	Repetitive behaviors, ritualistic behaviors
Clomipramine (Anafranil)	OCD (10 years and older)	Ritualistic behaviors, repetitive behaviors
Risperidone (Risperdal)	Irritability associated with autistic spectrum disorders (5 years and older)	Irritability, tantrums, aggression, self-injury
Aripiprazole (Abilify)	Irritability associated with autistic spectrum disorders (6 years and older)	Irritability, tantrums, aggression, self-injury
Haloperidol (Haldol)	Severe behavior disorders (3 years and older)	Aggression, tantrums
Chlorpromazine (Thorazine)	Severe behavior disorders (6 months and older)	Aggression, tantrums
Buspirone (BuSpar)	Anxiety	Anxiety, self-injury, aggression

Note.   ADHD=attention-deficit/hyperactivity disorder; FDA=U.S. Food and Drug Administration; OCD=obsessive-compulsive disorder; PMDD=premenstrual dysphoric disorder; PTSD= posttraumatic stress disorder.

Table 6–6. U.S. Food and Drug Administration (FDA)–approved medications used in the treatment of attention-deficit/hyperactivity disorder (ADHD)

Drug	Mechanism of action	Black box warnings	Drug properties and guidelines	Typical daily dose: child/adolescent	Typical daily dose: adult
Methylphenidate (Ritalin, Methylin)	Blocks reuptake and increases NE and DA	Drug dependence	No CYP metabolism; half-life: 2–3 hours	6 years and older: 2.5–5 mg po bid; increase by 5–10 mg weekly; maximum: 60 mg	5–15 mg po bid–tid; increase by 10 mg weekly; maximum: 60 mg
Methylphenidate extended release (Methylin ER, Metadate CD and ER, Ritalin LA and SR)	Blocks reuptake and increases NE and DA	Drug dependence	No CYP metabolism; half-life: 3–4 hours	10 mg po qam; increase by 5–10 mg weekly; maximum: 60 mg	20 mg po qam; increase by 10 mg weekly; maximum: 60 mg
Methylphenidate transdermal (Daytrana Patch)	Blocks reuptake and increases NE and DA	Drug dependence	No CYP metabolism; effect may last 5 hours after patch removed; remove patch before 15 hours	6 years and older: 10 mg/9 hours daily applied to hip (alternate daily); increase to next dose weekly; maximum: 30 mg/9 hours daily	Same as for children

Table 6–6.   U.S. Food and Drug Administration (FDA)–approved medications used in the treatment of attention-deficit/hyperactivity disorder (ADHD) *(continued)*

Drug	Mechanism of action	Black box warnings	Drug properties and guidelines	Typical daily dose: child/adolescent	Typical daily dose: adult
Methylphenidate extended release OROS (Concerta)	Blocks reuptake and increases NE and DA	Drug dependence	No CYP metabolism; avoid use in patients with gastrointestinal issues; hard polymer shell excreted in stool	6–12 years: 18 mg po qam; increase by 18 mg weekly; maximum: 54 mg 13 years and older: 18 mg po qam; maximum: 72 mg	18–65 years: 18 mg po qam; increase by 18 mg weekly; maximum: 72 mg; 5 mg methylphenidate is equivalent to 6 mg Concerta
Dexmethylphenidate (Focalin)	Blocks reuptake and increases NE and DA; stimulates sympathomimetic CNS activity	Drug dependence	No CYP metabolism	6 years and older: 2.5 mg po bid; increase by 5–10 mg weekly; maximum: 20 mg; convert at 50% of total daily dose	2.5 mg po bid; increase by 5–10 mg weekly; maximum: 20 mg

Table 6–6. U.S. Food and Drug Administration (FDA)–approved medications used in the treatment of attention-deficit/hyperactivity disorder (ADHD) (*continued*)

Drug	Mechanism of action	Black box warnings	Drug properties and guidelines	Typical daily dose: child/adolescent	Typical daily dose: adult
Dexmethylphenidate XR (Focalin XR)	Blocks reuptake and increases NE and DA; stimulates sympathomimetic CNS activity	Drug dependence	No CYP metabolism	6 years and older: 5 mg po qam; increase by 5 mg weekly; maximum: 30 mg	10 mg po qam; increase by 10 mg weekly; maximum: 40 mg; convert from IR at same total daily dose
Dextroamphetamine (Dexedrine, Dexedrine Spansules ER)	Blocks reuptake and increases NE and DA; stimulates NE and DA release from presynaptic vesicle	Abuse potential; dependency	CYP metabolism unknown; half-life: 10–12 hours; pH-dependent excretion; avoid grapefruit juice	3–5 years (IR only): 2.5 mg po qam; maximum: 40 mg 6 years and older (IR/ER): 5 mg po qam–tid IR; 5 mg po qam ER; maximum: 40 mg	10 mg po qam; maximum: 60 mg; divide dose qd–tid

Table 6–6.   U.S. Food and Drug Administration (FDA)–approved medications used in the treatment of attention-deficit/hyperactivity disorder (ADHD) *(continued)*

Drug	Mechanism of action	Black box warnings	Drug properties and guidelines	Typical daily dose: child/adolescent	Typical daily dose: adult
Dextroamphetamine/ amphetamine (Adderall)	Blocks reuptake and increases NE and DA; stimulates NE and DA release from presynaptic vesicle	Drug dependence	pH-dependent excretion; avoid grapefruit juice; half-life: 9–14 hours	3–5 years: 2.5 mg po qam; increase by 2.5 mg weekly; maximum: 40 mg 6 years and older: 5 mg po qam; increase by 5 mg weekly; maximum: 40 mg; divide dose qd–tid	5 mg po bid; increase by 5 mg weekly; maximum: 40 mg; divide dose qd–tid

Table 6–6. U.S. Food and Drug Administration (FDA)–approved medications used in the treatment of attention-deficit/hyperactivity disorder (ADHD) *(continued)*

Drug	Mechanism of action	Black box warnings	Drug properties and guidelines	Typical daily dose: child/adolescent	Typical daily dose: adult
Dextroamphetamine/ amphetamine extended release (Adderall XR)	Blocks reuptake and increases NE and DA; stimulates NE and DA release from presynaptic vesicle	Drug dependence	pH-dependent excretion; avoid grapefruit juice	6–12 years: 10 mg po qam; increase by 5–10 mg weekly; maximum: 30 mg 13–17 years: 10–20 mg po qam; increase by 10 mg weekly; maximum: 40 mg; convert from IR at same total daily dose	20 mg po qam; increase by 10 mg weekly; maximum: 60 mg; convert from IR at same total daily dose
Lisdexamfetamine (Vyvanse)	Stimulates sympathomimetic CNS activity	Abuse potential	CYP2D6 inhibitor	6–17 years: 10 mg po qam; increase by 10 mg weekly; maximum: 70 mg	30 mg po qam; increase by 10–20 mg weekly; maximum: 70 mg

Table 6–6. U.S. Food and Drug Administration (FDA)–approved medications used in the treatment of attention-deficit/hyperactivity disorder (ADHD) *(continued)*

Drug	Mechanism of action	Black box warnings	Drug properties and guidelines	Typical daily dose: child/adolescent	Typical daily dose: adult
Atomoxetine (Strattera)	Selectively inhibits NE reuptake at presynaptic neuron	Suicidality	CYP2C19 and CYP2D6 substrates; half-life: 5–22 hours (poor CYP2D6 metabolizers); monitor hepatic function	6 years and older and ≤70 kg: 0.5 mg/kg po qpm × 3 days then increase by 1.2 mg/kg; maximum: 1.4 mg/kg 6 years and older and >70 kg: 40 mg po qpm × 3 days, then increase by 60 mg daily; may increase to 100 mg daily over 2–4 weeks; maximum: 100 mg	40 mg po daily × 3 days then increase by 80 mg po daily; maximum: 100 mg; may divide dose

Table 6–6. U.S. Food and Drug Administration (FDA)–approved medications used in the treatment of attention-deficit/hyperactivity disorder (ADHD) (*continued*)

Drug	Mechanism of action	Black box warnings	Drug properties and guidelines	Typical daily dose: child/adolescent	Typical daily dose: adult
Clonidine (Catapres, Kapvay ER)	Stimulates α_2-adrenergic receptors in prefrontal cortex	None	CYP metabolism unknown; half-life: 12–16 hours; monitor for hypotension; dose must be tapered on discontinuation—*do not* stop abruptly	6–17 years (Kapvay ER only): 0.1 mg po qhs; increase by 0.1 mg weekly; maximum: 0.4 mg	Currently not FDA approved for adult ADHD
Guanfacine (Tenex, Intuniv ER)	Stimulates α_2-adrenergic receptors in prefrontal cortex	None	CYP3A4/5 substrate; half-life: 18 hours; monitor for hypotension; dose must be tapered on discontinuation—*do not* stop abruptly	6–17 years (Intuniv ER only): 1 mg po; increase by 1 mg weekly; maximum: 4 mg	Currently not FDA approved for adult ADHD

Note. bid=twice a day; CD=controlled dispense; CNS=central nervous system; CYP=cytochrome P450; DA=dopamine; ER=extended release; IR=immediate release; LA=long acting; NE=norepinephrine; po=by mouth; qam=every morning; qd=once a day; qhs=every night; qpm=every day after noon; tid=three times a day; SR=sustained release; XR=extended release.

Psychostimulant Medications

For the most part, the psychostimulant medications, both the methylphenidate formulations and the amphetamine or mixed amphetamine formulations, target the neurotransmitters norepinephrine and dopamine in the prefrontal cortex. They act to block the reuptake of these neurochemicals in the presynaptic neuron, thus enhancing their action in the synapse. Additionally, dextroamphetamine and the mixed amphetamines act as agonists, not only blocking the reuptake of norepinephrine and dopamine but also stimulating their release from the presynaptic neuron.

There are exceptions to the pharmacodynamics of the psychostimulant medications. Lisdexamfetamine (Vyvanse), a prodrug, stimulates sympathomimetic activity in the CNS. Atomoxetine (Strattera), a nonstimulant indicated for ADHD, selectively inhibits only norepinephrine at the presynaptic neuron and improves concentration and attention while simultaneously reducing anxiety. Clonidine (Catapres) and guanfacine (Intuniv) stimulate the α_2-adrenergic receptors in the prefrontal cortex, providing a calming effect and decreasing impulsivity.

It is recommended that grapefruit juice be avoided with dextroamphetamine (Dexedrine) and the mixed amphetamine salts, which are dependent on pH for excretion. With regard to pharmacokinetics, the psychostimulants have minimal to no action on the cytochrome P450 (CYP) system in the liver and, therefore, do not contribute to many drug-drug interactions. The exceptions are atomoxetine, which is a substrate of CYP2D6 and CYP2C19, and guanfacine, which is a substrate of CYP3A4 and CYP3A5.

Other Medications

Two additional psychotropic medications—bupropion XL (Wellbutrin XL) and modafinil (Provigil)—have been used off-label in the treatment of ADHD. Bupropion is a dopamine and norepinephrine reuptake inhibitor like the psychostimulants but is not a controlled substance. Bupropion may be an appropriate choice if ADHD symptoms occur with comorbid depression. It also has been helpful for adults, who may be sensitive to the "stimulation" of the methylphenidate and amphetamine products. Bupropion requires daily dosing to be effective, and its onset of action may not be apparent for 2–6 weeks. Bupropion is metabolized by CYP2B6, and the metabolite (hydroxybupropion) is an inhibitor of CYP2D6. Bupropion also may lower the seizure threshold.

Although the mechanism of action of modafinil is currently unknown, this agent is hypothesized to stimulate the release of histamine, which improves attention, wakefulness, mental clarity, and concentration. The FDA denied modafinil's application for an ADHD indication in 2006, citing a risk of approximately 1 in 1,000 for the development of Stevens-Johnson syndrome, a rare necrotizing fasciitis (International Medical News Group 2006). Modafinil and its single isomer armodafinil (Nuvigil) are metabolized by CYP enzymes. Modafinil is a 3A4 partial substrate and inducer and a 2C19 inhibitor; thus, caution should be exercised when other medications are added to a regimen with modafinil.

Dosing Considerations

Attention-Deficit/Hyperactivity Disorder

Dosing guidelines for the medications approved for the treatment of ADHD can be found in Table 6–6. At times, the shorter-acting formulations may be used to facilitate time of onset along with the longer-acting, controlled-release formulations. The shorter-acting agents also may be used to decrease the effect of "rebound" hyperactivity when the longer-acting agents wear off.

Autistic Spectrum Disorders

The most commonly prescribed medications used to treat behavioral, self-injurious, and repetitive and other symptoms associated with the autistic spectrum disorders can be found in Table 6–5. Dosing in this population should begin at a very low subtherapeutic dose and be titrated very slowly because those with developmental disorders may respond in unpredictable ways.

Treatment Monitoring

Attention-Deficit/Hyperactivity Disorder

The methylphenidate and the amphetamine formulations of the psychostimulants have similar nuisance side effects, which are not medically dangerous.

The patient may experience decreased appetite, headaches, stomach upset, and insomnia. These side effects often dissipate within a week or so. Taking the medication with food typically helps to reduce these adverse events. The rebound effect is likely the worst side effect. This phenomenon occurs when the medication begins to wear off, and the original symptoms—hyperactivity and impulsivity—return in excess. Augmenting with a low-dose, short-acting psychostimulant can be helpful.

Cardiovascular side effects may occur as an adverse event related to the psychostimulants. The American Heart Association recommends obtaining an electrocardiogram before beginning treatment with a psychostimulant, but the American Academy of Pediatrics does not (Simon and Zieve 2012). It is important for the prescribing APRN to complete a thorough cardiac history of both the patient and the family before prescribing psychostimulants and to monitor blood pressure and heart rate.

Because the psychostimulants are Schedule II controlled substances, it is wise to monitor for potential abuse. These psychotropic medications do have a black box warning for potential abuse and dependence. Additionally, there have been reported incidences of diversion with these medications. The patient and family should store the supply in a safe, locked space where they cannot fall into the wrong hands. Parents and guardians also should monitor to ensure that the child or adolescent has swallowed the medication because incidences of "sharing" have been reported in school systems.

Autistic Spectrum Disorders

Monitoring the medications used in the treatment of autism and the developmental disorders is very important because individual side effects may be unusual. Additionally, these disorders are treated with the psychotropic medications commonly used to treat other psychiatric disorders. (Further information on treatment monitoring of the antidepressants, mood stabilizers, and antipsychotics can be found in Chapter 3, "Depressive Disorders," Chapter 4, "Bipolar Disorders," and Chapter 5, "Psychotic Disorders," respectively.) However, note that the prescribing nurse should expect the unexpected when treating developmental disorders. Those rare side effects that are typically not observed in clinical practice may appear. Additionally, individuals along this spectrum may require what normally would be considered subtherapeutic doses or supratherapeutic doses of the medication. Because one cannot gauge the response to either efficacy or side effects, patience is needed by all involved to obtain the optimal results.

Treatment of Special Populations

Autistic Spectrum Disorders in Specific Patient Groups

Because no specific class of psychotropic medications is targeted toward treatment of individuals with autism and developmental disorders, the focus of this section is on the use of psychostimulants in specific patient populations.

Attention-Deficit/Hyperactivity Disorder in Specific Patient Groups

The psychostimulants are the first-line treatment for all forms of ADHD in children, adolescents, and adults. A few unique considerations are involved in psychostimulant treatment of individuals with autism, those who are elderly, those who are medically compromised, and those who are pregnant or breast-feeding an infant.

Individuals With Autism and ADHD-Like Symptoms

In a comprehensive review of studies, Cortese et al. (2012) concluded that the psychostimulants may be effective in reducing the ADHD-like symptoms associated with autistic spectrum disorders. The side effects are consistent with those observed in the general population, although slightly higher levels of irritability and emotional outbursts were reported.

Given the complexity of symptoms in autism and the developmental disorders, the APRN should continue to use his or her best clinical judgment to make treatment decisions and recommendations.

Elderly or Medically Compromised Patients With Depression, Fatigue, or Apathy

Although the psychostimulants are used primarily in the treatment of ADHD, they have found another niche in the treatment of depression, fatigue, and apathy in elderly patients (Franzen et al. 2012). Given the high degree of polypharmacy in this population, nurses need to be mindful of the potential side effects, drug-drug interactions, and medical safety issues, particularly appetite reduction, insomnia, and potential cardiac risks, to which the elderly are already prone. The stimulants have been successful in the treatment of apathy in older adults who have lost interest and motivation in life (Padala et al. 2010). Again, safety must be a priority because the stimulants may further disrupt sleep, appetite, and cardiac status.

In general, the psychostimulants are not a first-line treatment for depression; however, they have been used to augment antidepressant therapies, especially when the continuing symptom is fatigue. They also have been used to treat depression in medically compromised patients requiring immediate improvement (Franzen et al. 2012). This situation may present in a patient who has been diagnosed with cancer, HIV, or stroke. The stimulants offered rapid onset of action, were well tolerated, and worked effectively in a very brief study of elderly depressed patients with medical comorbidities (Wallace et al. 1995).

Although the stimulants may be effective in the treatment of depression, fatigue, and apathy in older adults, this population may be more prone to adverse events such as anxiety, delirium, palpitations, hallucinations, and headache. Weighing the risks and benefits is critical, as it is with all patient populations.

Pregnant or Breast-Feeding Women With ADHD

Although most of the medications used in the treatment of ADHD are pregnancy risk Category C, as are most of the psychotropics, women generally are not advised to continue taking psychostimulants during pregnancy or lactation. Because the stimulants may decrease the woman's appetite, the growing fetus may not receive important nutrients for healthy development.

Summary

Medications Used to Treat Attention-Deficit/ Hyperactivity Disorder

The psychostimulant medications have shown efficacy in the treatment of all three types of ADHD for almost 50 years. APRNs who treat and prescribe for children, adolescents, adults, and the elderly should be aware that the symptoms of ADHD are seen in many other psychiatric disorders. With this in mind, the APRN should conduct a thorough evaluation and, whenever possible, obtain collateral information from family, educators, employers, or friends to ensure the treatment of the correct diagnosis. The psychostimulant medications are currently the first-line treatment for ADHD in children, adolescents, and adults.

Many of the myths once held to be true regarding the psychostimulants have been disproved. We are now aware that after 24 months of study, children prescribed these medications are within 1 inch and 2 pounds of the height and weight, respectively, of their same-age unmedicated peers (MTA Cooperative Group 2004). Most patients with ADHD will respond to the psychostimulant medications, although other psychotropic agents also have shown efficacy in improving symptoms and quality of life for the patient with ADHD. Finally, dependence and further substance abuse are rare when individuals with ADHD receive treatment; in fact, the psychostimulants may be protective by reducing the risk of the impulsive individual seeking alternative substances with which to self-medicate symptoms.

Medications Used to Treat Symptoms Associated With Autistic Spectrum Disorders

Medications used in the treatment of the autistic spectrum disorders are typically prescribed off-label. The psychotropics are used to treat the symptoms of aggression, self-injurious behaviors, severe tantrums, irritability, anxiety, repetitive and ritualistic behaviors, obsessive thoughts, and compulsive behaviors. The APRN treating this population should be alert to the possibility that individuals with autism or developmental disorders may not respond in the same way to medication therapies as do nonautistic individuals. Because this field is ever-evolving, the APRN is advised to maintain a current list of references on the use of psychotropic medications to reduce the symptoms associated with autism and the developmental disorders.

Clinical Pearls

- The dose of the psychostimulants should be optimized before considering switching to another medication.
- The symptoms of ADHD may mimic those of other disorders such as learning disorders, depression, anxiety, dementia, and even menopause.

- The clinician should attempt to avoid prescribing medications during the school day if at all possible to improve compliance and convenience.

- When combining medications, nurses should know what each agent does and what side effects and symptoms it controls. When a second agent is added, nurses can determine which drug is responsible for the side effects or symptom control and which one to adjust.

- Treatment should continue as long as it is efficacious, it causes no side effects, and evidence indicates that the disorder detrimentally affects the individual's life.

- For patients with autistic disorders, psychotropic medications are used to treat the mood and behavioral symptoms that affect their life.

- Patients with autism may experience atypical side effects or respond to the medication in an unpredictable manner.

References

American Psychiatric Association: Diagnostic and Statistical Manual of Mental Disorders, 3rd Edition. Washington, DC, American Psychiatric Association, 1980

American Psychiatric Association: Diagnostic and Statistical Manual of Mental Disorders, 4th Edition, Text Revision. Washington, DC, American Psychiatric Association, 2000

AutismSpeaks: What is autism? 2012. Available at: http://www.autismspeaks.org/what-autism. Accessed March 15, 2012.

Castellani ML, Conti CM, Kempuraj DJ, et al: Autism and immunity: revisited study. Int J Immunopathol Pharmacol 22:15–19, 2009

Cortese S, Castelnau P, Morcillo C, et al: Psychostimulants for ADHD-like symptoms in individuals with autism spectrum disorders. Expert Rev Neurother 12(4):461–473, 2012

Franzen JW, Padala PR, Wetzel MW, et al: Psychostimulants for older adults. Curr Psychiatry 11:23–32, 2012

Goldman LS, Genel M, Bezman RJ, et al: Diagnosis and treatment of attention-deficit/hyperactivity disorders in children and adolescents. JAMA 279:1100–1107, 1998

Ha J, Lee C-S, Maeng J-S, et al: Chronic glutamate toxicity in mouse cortical neuron culture. Brain Res 1273:138–143, 2009

International Medical News Group: FDA cites Stevens-Johnson in modafinil's ADHD rejection. 2006. Available at: http://www.thefreelibrary.com/FDA+cites+Stevens+Johnson+in+modafinil's+ADHD+rejection.-a0152011010. Accessed February 22, 2012.

Kessler RC, Adler L, Ames M, et al: The World Health Organization Adult ADHD Self-Report Scale (ASRS): a short screening scale for use in the general population. Psychol Med 35:245–256, 2005

Marc D, Olson K: Neuroimmunology of autism spectrum disorder. NeuroScience, Inc., April 2009. Available at: https://www.neurorelief.com/uploads/content_files/Neuroimmunology%20of%20Autism%20White%20paper.pdf. Accessed January 8, 2013.

Melmed R: ADHD: interesting cases in diagnosis and management. Presented at: 20th annual conference on The Young Child With Special Needs, Las Vegas, NV, March 2–5, 2011. Content available for purchase from Contemporary Forums at: http://www.onlinecelibrary.com/youngchildspecialneeds/?select=session&sessionID=232. Accessed February 10, 2013.

Minshew NJ, Williams DL: The new neurobiology of autism. Arch Neurol 64:945–950, 2007

MTA Cooperative Group: National Institute of Mental Health Multimodal Treatment Study of ADHD follow-up: changes in effectiveness and growth after the end of treatment. Pediatrics 113:762–769, 2004

National Institute of Mental Health: The multimodal treatment of attention deficit hyperactivity disorder study (MTA): questions and answers. Revised November 2009. Available at: http://www.nimh.nih.gov/trials/practical/mta/the-multimodal-treatment-of-attention-deficit-hyperactivity-disorder-study-mta-questions-and-answers.shtml. Accessed January 8, 2013.

Padala PR, Burke WJ, Shostrom VK, et al: Methylphenidate for apathy and functional status in dementia of the Alzheimer type. Am J Geriatr Psychiatry 18:371–374, 2010

Pelphrey KA, Morris JP, McCarthy G: Neural basis of eye gaze processing deficits in autism. Brain 128 (pt 5):1038–1048, 2005

Redcay E, Courchesne E: When is a brain enlarged in autism? A meta-analysis of all brain size reports. Biol Psychiatry 58:1–9, 2005

Satterfield JH, Cantwell DP, Satterfield BT: Pathophysiology of the hyperactive child syndrome. Arch Gen Psychiatry 31:839–844, 1974

Simon H, Zieve D (eds): Attention deficit hyperactivity disorder (ADHD) (in-depth report): medications. February 27, 2012. Available at: http://health.nytimes.com/health/guides/disease/attention-deficit-hyperactivity-disorder-adhd/medications.html. Accessed January 8, 2013.

Snyder B: Genetics may explain three types of ADHD. Reported: Vanderbilt University Medical Center's Weekly Newspaper, December 11, 2009. Available at: http://www.mc.vanderbilt.edu/reporter/index.html?ID=7947. Accessed January 8, 2013.

Stannard Gromisch E: Neurotransmitters involved in ADHD. 2010. Available at: http://psychcentral.com/lib/2010/neurotransmitters-involved-in-adhd. Accessed January 8, 2013.

Wallace A, Kofoed LL, West AN: Double-blind, placebo controlled trial of methylphenidate in older, depressed, medically ill patients. Am J Psychiatry 152:929–931, 1995

Wasserstein J: Diagnostic issues for adolescents and adults with ADHD. J Clin Psychol 61:535–547, 2005

Wolraich ML, Feurer I, Hannah JN, et al: Obtaining systematic teacher reports of disruptive behavior disorders utilizing DSM-IV. J Abnorm Child Psychol 26:141–152, 1998

Wolraich ML, Lambert W, Doffing MA, et al: Psychometric properties of the Vanderbilt ADHD diagnostic parent rating scale in a referred population. J Pediatr Psychol 28:559–567, 2003

7

Substance Use Disorders

Laura G. Leahy, M.S.N., P.M.H.-A.P.R.N.

It is far more important to know what person the disease has
than what disease the person has.

—Hippocrates

Over the past few years, the United States has experienced a growing trend of individuals who are abusing psychotherapeutic medications for nonmedical purposes. Medications such as the opioid pain relievers (e.g., oxycodone [OxyContin, Percocet]), sedative-hypnotics (benzodiazepines [e.g, Xanax (alprazolam)] and barbiturates [e.g., phenobarbital]), and psychostimulants (e.g., Adderall [mixed amphetamine salts]) are among those most frequently abused. Because many of these drugs are available in the home medicine cabinet and via the Internet and mail-order companies, it has become easier to obtain them while maintaining anonymity. Additionally, the misperception that prescription medications are safer than illegal drugs has contributed to the rise in abuse of prescription medications (National Institute on Drug Abuse 2011).

Substance use disorders affect millions of individuals in the United States on an annual basis. Alcohol abuse alone affects more than 17 million people and was the cause of approximately 85,000 deaths in 2010, 22,000 of which were due to alcohol-related diseases (Alcohol Abuse Treatments 2012). In 2008, opioid drug overdoses in the United States accounted for 36,450 deaths. Opioid pain relievers were involved in 14,800 deaths (73.8%) of the 20,044 prescription drug overdoses (Centers for Disease Control and Prevention 2011). According to the National Institute on Drug Abuse (2010), "nicotine is one of the most heavily used addictive drugs, and through the use of tobacco products, is the leading preventable cause of disease, disability and death in the United States." Ninety percent of lung cancer cases can be attributed to cigarette smoking, and the effects of secondhand smoke result in about 38,000 deaths per year (National Institute on Drug Abuse 2010). Nurses witness firsthand the effect of substance abuse on an individual's physical health, emotional well-being, and overall quality of life.

For decades, the idea that those with substance abuse and dependence might be self-medicating has been a useful tool for both practitioners and patients. In the 1970s and 1980s, Khantzian et al. (1974; Khantzian 1985) explored self-medicating to define a psychoanalytic basis for substance abuse, whereas Duncan (1974) used it to define a behavioral basis. Over the years, this model of self-medication has benefited the practitioner-patient relationship by allowing patients to communicate more freely with less shame and guilt regarding their substance abuse issues and allowing clinicians to include this information in their assessments (Coletsos and Bursztajn 2011). Advanced practice registered nurses (APRNs) frequently question patients about the role and benefit such substance abuse serves in their lives and how the substances help them in daily life. This line of questioning insinuates that the APRN believes that the substance may be aiding the patient in relieving certain mood, thought, or behavioral symptoms and allowing the patient to cope with daily life stressors.

Since the "decade of the brain" in the 1990s, practitioners involved in treating substance use disorders have grown to believe that, like the psychiatric disorders, substance use disorders are diseases of the brain. This concept actually has been verified through the identification of the multiple genetic markers (refer to Appendix 3, "Psychopharmacogenetic Variations: Implications for Practice," for more information on genetic markers in psychiatry) that predispose an individual to substance abuse and addiction (Kendler 2005). Many genes contribute to the risk for substance addiction (Comings et al. 2001; Uhl et al. 2002).

Addictive disorders are thought to be associated with variants of genes that code for three enzymes that act on dopamine: dopamine β-hydroxylase (DBH), catechol O-methyltransferase (COMT), and monoamine oxidase (MAO). Alcoholic individuals have elevated frequencies of the gene that encodes DBH, and cocaine abusers with low-activity DBH have increased sensitivity to cocaine-induced euphoria (Köhnke et al. 2006; Weinshenker et al. 2002). The Val allele of the COMT gene is associated with alcoholism, methamphetamine use, heroin addiction, and polysubstance abuse (Kreek et al. 2005).

The substance use disorders certainly are among the most frequent co-occurring disorders in patients with mental illness, and they disrupt not only many aspects of the individual's family, occupational, and social life but also their physical health and well-being. Substance abusers are vulnerable to elevated blood pressure, hepatotoxicity, cirrhosis, and blood cell damage, in addition to various psychiatric comorbidities (Mokdad et al. 2004).

The underlying vulnerability that these disorders share is termed *the addictive process*. According to Goodman (2009), the addictive process is believed to involve impairments in motivation/reward systems, affect regulation, and behavioral inhibition. "The addictive process is not what makes cocaine, ice cream, or sex pleasurable for people in general; rather, it is what makes the drive for cocaine or ice cream or sex so much more inexorable for those who have an addictive disorder" (Goodman 2009, p. 1). Goodman (2009) further postulates that the development of a substance abuse disorder is shaped by the addictive process, which leads to the behaviors of consequence and the selection of the preferred substance of abuse. Bearing in mind the addictive process, we are challenged to work with our patients in identifying the elements of impairment and incorporating strategies to address more healthy ways of coping, the physiological manifestations, and the social implications of substance abuse and dependence.

Overview of Substance Use Disorders

Because nurses are faced with individuals who abuse and find themselves dependent on various substances, it is beneficial to understand the neurophysiological underpinnings of addiction to collaborate with patients in developing the most appropriate course of treatment. Because the number of potential substances of abuse is unlimited, I will limit my discussion to three categories of substances: alcohol, opioids/opiates, and nicotine.

In the remainder of this chapter, I guide the reader through the neurobiology of substance abuse and dependence (DSM-IV-TR [American Psychiatric Association 2000] diagnostic criteria for these disorders are presented in Tables 7–1 and 7–2). I identify the various pathways leading to such dangerous and potentially life-threatening behaviors. The pharmacological properties of agents used to treat substance abuse disorders are described to help the APRN make informed treatment decisions for the patient with substance abuse and/or dependence. I also discuss safety concerns and treatment of special populations.

Neurobiology of Substance Abuse and Dependence

The major neuropathway influencing the cycle of substance abuse and dependence involves the flow of dopamine through the limbic system. The limbic system controls the dopamine "motivation/reward" circuit, which is activated by drugs of abuse. The system floods with dopamine and creates a highly powerful, pleasurable sensation that endures longer than the natural rewards experienced through engaging in activities such as eating or sexual intercourse. Some drugs of abuse can release 2–10 times more dopamine than is released with natural rewards (Comings et al. 1997). Long-term use of these substances causes neuroadaptation; thus, life's natural pleasures are no longer able to create positive sensations, and more of the drug of abuse is required to potentiate the same effect. This process contributes to individuals developing tolerance to the substance of abuse and ultimately physiological and/or psychological addiction.

Table 7–1.   DSM-IV-TR diagnostic criteria for substance dependence

A maladaptive pattern of substance use, leading to clinically significant impairment or distress, as manifested by three (or more) of the following, occurring at any time in the same 12-month period:

(1) tolerance, as defined by either of the following:

    (a) a need for markedly increased amounts of the substance to achieve intoxication or desired effect

    (b) markedly diminished effect with continued use of the same amount of the substance

(2) withdrawal, as manifested by either of the following:

    (a) the characteristic withdrawal syndrome for the substance (refer to criteria A and B of the criteria sets for withdrawal from the specific substances)

    (b) the same (or a closely related) substance is taken to relieve or avoid withdrawal symptoms

(3) the substance is often taken in larger amounts or over a longer period than was intended

(4) there is a persistent desire or unsuccessful efforts to cut down or control substance use

(5) a great deal of time is spent in activities necessary to obtain the substance (e.g., visiting multiple doctors or driving long distances), use the substance (e.g., chain-smoking), or recover from its effects

(6) important social, occupational, or recreational activities are given up or reduced because of substance use

(7) the substance use is continued despite knowledge of having a persistent or recurrent physical or psychological problem that is likely to have been caused or exacerbated by the substance (e.g., current cocaine use despite recognition of cocaine-induced depression, or continued drinking despite recognition that an ulcer was made worse by alcohol consumption)

Specify if:

With Physiological Dependence: evidence of tolerance or withdrawal (i.e., either item 1 or 2 is present)

Without Physiological Dependence: no evidence of tolerance or withdrawal (i.e., neither item 1 nor 2 is present)

Course specifiers (see DSM-IV-TR text for definitions):

Early Full Remission	Early Partial Remission
Sustained Full Remission	Sustained Partial Remission
On Agonist Therapy	In a Controlled Environment

Table 7–2. DSM-IV-TR diagnostic criteria for substance abuse

A. A maladaptive pattern of substance use leading to clinically significant impairment or distress, as manifested by one (or more) of the following, occurring within a 12-month period:

   (1) recurrent substance use resulting in a failure to fulfill major role obligations at work, school, or home (e.g., repeated absences or poor work performance related to substance use; substance-related absences, suspensions, or expulsions from school; neglect of children or household)

   (2) recurrent substance use in situations in which it is physically hazardous (e.g., driving an automobile or operating a machine when impaired by substance use)

   (3) recurrent substance-related legal problems (e.g., arrests for substance-related disorderly conduct)

   (4) continued substance use despite having persistent or recurrent social or interpersonal problems caused or exacerbated by the effects of the substance (e.g., arguments with spouse about consequences of intoxication, physical fights)

B. The symptoms have never met the criteria for substance dependence for this class of substance.

The nucleus accumbens (NA), along with the ventral tegmental area (VTA) of the brain, is the "gatekeeper" of addiction. (Refer to Figures A1–1 and A1–2 in the appendix to Chapter 1, "Introduction to Clinical Psychopharmacology for Nurses," for depictions of the brain and its neuropathways.) Motivation and reward are modulated by dopamine following a pathway originating in the VTA, passing through the NA, and extending outward to the prefrontal cortex (PFC). This pathway contributes to increased risk of alcohol use, cigarette smoking, and use of other illicit drugs (Comings et al. 1997). According to Stahl (2008), the idea of willpower relates to the hypoactivation of dopamine on the receptors extending from the VTA to the NA and to the hyperactivation of dopamine in the PFC, which essentially allows the "executive functioning" level of the brain to respond by "just saying No."

Temptation in addiction, according to Stahl (2008), involves activation of the amygdala in anticipating the drug. This activation, via dopamine, leads to hyperactivation in the VTA, which sends the reward signal to the NA. Simultaneously, the ventromedial PFC is hypoactivated by dopamine, inducing drug cravings and impairing cognition. Essentially, the executive functioning level of the brain is failing to identify and ward off the potential danger and consequences as a result of the powerful action of dopamine in the NA. This circuit begins to loop, and the cravings increase, leading to compulsive use and ultimately addiction and dependence.

When individuals compulsively use substances to increase reward and pleasure, the PFC becomes grossly hypoactivated—as in attention-deficit/hyperactivity disorder—which causes the amygdala to hyperactivate, yielding drug-induced cravings and impulsive behaviors. Stahl (2008) postulated that this circuit follows the pathway through the VTA, which is also hyperactivated, creating reward sensitivities in the NA and activating drug-seeking behaviors. The PFC has lost its executive regulatory abilities, and addiction ensues.

Dopamine is not the only neurochemical implicated in substance abuse and dependence. γ-Aminobutyric acid (GABA), an inhibitory neurotransmitter; glutamate, an excitatory neurotransmitter; serotonin; and epinephrine are also involved in substance abuse. During *intoxication* (Table 7–3), increasing dopamine leads to mood elevation, increasing serotonin contributes to euphoria and sedation, increasing epinephrine leads to hypertension, and increased GABA leads to ataxia, sedation, and disinhibition (National Institute on Drug Abuse 2007). Our bodies are, with long-term substance use, capable of neuroadaptation as a result of decreased GABA inhibition and increased glutamate excitability. However, when the substance is abruptly withdrawn, GABA rapidly decreases, contributing to anxiety, insomnia, and seizures; epinephrine further increases, causing hypertension and tachycardia; serotonin decreases, contributing to insomnia and mood disorders; and dopamine ultimately decreases, leading to dysphoria (National Institute on Drug Abuse 2007). This process is more commonly referred to as *withdrawal* (Table 7–4). With this mental illustration, one can see the correlation between substance abuse and other psychiatric illnesses and their associated symptoms and neurotransmitters.

Table 7–3. DSM-IV-TR diagnostic criteria for substance intoxication

A. The development of a reversible substance-specific syndrome due to recent ingestion of (or exposure to) a substance. **Note:** Different substances may produce similar or identical syndromes.

B. Clinically significant maladaptive behavioral or psychological changes that are due to the effect of the substance on the central nervous system (e.g., belligerence, mood lability, cognitive impairment, impaired judgment, impaired social or occupational functioning) and develop during or shortly after use of the substance.

C. The symptoms are not due to a general medical condition and are not better accounted for by another mental disorder.

Table 7–4. DSM-IV-TR diagnostic criteria for substance withdrawal

A. The development of a substance-specific syndrome due to the cessation of (or reduction in) substance use that has been heavy and prolonged.

B. The substance-specific syndrome causes clinically significant distress or impairment in social, occupational, or other important areas of functioning.

C. The symptoms are not due to a general medical condition and are not better accounted for by another mental disorder.

Pharmacological Properties of Agents Used to Treat Substance Use Disorders

The pharmacodynamics, mechanisms of action, pharmacokinetics, and metabolism of the psychopharmacological agents prescribed for alcohol, opiate, and nicotine abuse and dependence are outlined in Tables 7–5, 7–6, and 7–7, respectively.

These tables also include side effects, precautions, and adult dosing guidelines for the agents used in the treatment of substance use disorders.

Table 7–5. Medications used in the treatment of alcohol and opioid/opiate abuse and dependence

	Naltrexone (Depade, ReVia)	Extended-release injectable naltrexone (Vivitrol)	Acamprosate (Campral)	Disulfiram (Antabuse)	Topiramate (Topamax)
FDA-approved indications	Opioid addiction; alcohol dependence	Opioid dependence; alcohol dependence	Alcohol dependence	Alcohol dependence	Off-label for alcohol dependence
Mechanism of action	Blocks opioid receptors, resulting in reduced craving and reduced reward in response to drinking	Same as oral naltrexone; 30-day duration	Affects glutamate and GABA neurotransmitter systems	Inhibits metabolism of alcohol, causing a buildup of acetaldehyde	Increases GABA neurotransmission and reduces glutamate neurotransmission
Common side effects	Nausea, vomiting, decreased appetite, headache, dizziness, fatigue, anxiety	Same as oral naltrexone plus joint pain, muscle aches/cramps	Diarrhea, somnolence, insomnia, depression	Metallic aftertaste, dermatitis, transient mild drowsiness, hypotension, ataxia	Paresthesias, taste perversion, anorexia, weight loss, somnolence, cognitive dysfunction

Table 7–5. Medications used in the treatment of alcohol and opioid/opiate abuse and dependence *(continued)*

	Naltrexone (Depade, ReVia)	Extended-release injectable naltrexone (Vivitrol)	Acamprosate (Campral)	Disulfiram (Antabuse)	Topiramate (Topamax)
Precautions	Hepatic disease; renal impairment; pregnancy Category C Advise patient to carry a wallet card to alert medical personnel in the event of an emergency.[a]	Same as oral naltrexone plus hemophilia or other bleeding problems	Moderate renal impairment (dose adjustment may be required); suicidality; pregnancy Category C	Hepatic cirrhosis or insufficiency; epilepsy; cerebrovascular disease or cerebral damage; psychoses; diabetes mellitus; hypothyroidism; renal impairment; pregnancy Category C	Narrow-angle glaucoma; kidney stones; renal or hepatic impairment; severe underweight; use of CNS depressants; pregnancy Category C
Serious adverse reactions	Will precipitate severe withdrawal if patient is dependent on opioids; hepatotoxicity (although does not appear to be hepatotoxic at recommended doses)	Same as oral naltrexone plus injection-site reactions that may be severe; instruct patient to closely monitor site and seek care immediately if reaction is worsening	Rare events include suicidal ideation and behavior	Disulfiram-alcohol reaction, hepatotoxicity, optic neuritis, peripheral neuropathy, psychotic reactions	Metabolic acidosis, acute myopia and secondary narrow-angle glaucoma, oligohydrosis, hyperthermia

Table 7–5. Medications used in the treatment of alcohol and opioid/opiate abuse and dependence *(continued)*

	Naltrexone (Depade, ReVia)	Extended-release injectable naltrexone (Vivitrol)	Acamprosate (Campral)	Disulfiram (Antabuse)	Topiramate (Topamax)
Potential drug interactions	Opioid medications (blocks action)	Same as oral naltrexone	No clinically relevant interactions known	Anticoagulants, tricyclic antidepressants, caffeine	Other anticonvulsants, hydrochlorothiazide, metformin, pioglitazone, lithium, amitriptyline
CYP metabolism	No CYP metabolism	No CYP metabolism	No CYP metabolism	CYP2E1 and 2C9 inhibitors; CYP3A4 and 3A5 substrates	CYP2C19 inhibitor; CYP3A4 inducer

Table 7–5. Medications used in the treatment of alcohol and opioid/opiate abuse and dependence *(continued)*

	Naltrexone (Depade, ReVia)	Extended-release injectable naltrexone (Vivitrol)	Acamprosate (Campral)	Disulfiram (Antabuse)	Topiramate (Topamax)
Typical adult dosing	Oral dose: 50 mg/day Before prescribing, patient must be opioid free for a minimum of 7–10 days	Intramuscular injection dose: 380 mg/month Before injection, patient must be opioid free for a minimum of 7–10 days	Oral dose: 666 mg tid (two 333-mg tablets) With renal impairment: 333-mg tablet tid Before prescribing, evaluate renal function and establish abstinence	Oral dose: 250 mg/day (range: 125–500 mg) Warn patient 1) not to take disulfiram within 12 hours of alcohol and 2) to avoid alcohol in diet, over-the-counter medications (e.g., cough syrups), and toiletries	Oral dose: 25 mg at bedtime, increase dose by 25–50 mg/day weekly, divided into morning and evening doses Target dosage: 200 mg/day Before prescribing, evaluate renal function and obtain serum electrolytes and bicarbonate
Laboratory follow-up	Monitor liver function	Monitor liver function		Monitor liver function	

Note. CNS=central nervous system; CYP=cytochrome P450; FDA=U.S. Food and Drug Administration; GABA=γ-aminobutyric acid; tid=three times a day.

[a]For wallet card information, see www.niaaa.nih.gov/guide.

Source. Adapted from Leahy 2012).

Table 7–6. Medications used in the treatment of opioid/opiate abuse and dependence

	Methadone (Dolophine, Methadose)	Buprenorphine (Subutex)	Buprenorphine-Naloxone (Suboxone)
FDA-approved indications	Opioid dependence; severe pain	Opioid dependence; severe pain	Opioid dependence (induction and maintenance treatment)
Mechanism of action	Opioid agonist; 5-HT and NE reuptake inhibitor; NMDA antagonist	Partial agonist at μ receptor; κ receptor antagonist	Partial agonist at μ opioid receptor and antagonist at multiple receptors
Precautions	Monitor for QTc prolongation, avoid grapefruit juice; multiple FDA black box warnings: incomplete cross-tolerance, respiratory depression, cardiac conduction effects, opioid addiction treatment	Initial prescription: supply 1 day only; strictly regulated; APRNs not able to write prescriptions; relapse to opioid use may be life-threatening; pregnancy Category C	Same as buprenorphine; monitor hepatic functions; may require dose adjustments because of opioid toxicity; pregnancy Category C
Serious adverse events	Serotonin syndrome, respiratory depression, QT prolongation	Respiratory depression/arrest, bronchospasm, seizures, hepatotoxicity	Same as buprenorphine
Common side effects	Sedation, headache, hypotension, dizziness, sweating, constipation	Nausea, headache, sedation, vertigo, constipation, hypotension, sweating	Nausea, headache, insomnia, severe constipation (may cause nonadherence)
Potential drug interactions	MAOIs, phenothiazines, TCAs, BZDs, SSRIs, SNRIs	SSRIs, antifungals, antibiotics, BZDs	Same as buprenorphine

Table 7-6.   Medications used in the treatment of opioid/opiate abuse and dependence (*continued*)

	Methadone (Dolophine, Methadose)	Buprenorphine (Subutex)	Buprenorphine-Naloxone (Suboxone)
CYP metabolism	CYP3A4 and 2D6	CYP3A4	CYP3A4
Typical adult dosing	One 15- to 30-mg dose, then 5–10 mg, q 2–4 hours as needed; stabilize dose for 10–14 days, then decrease dose by 10%; detoxification and maintenance only in FDA-approved program	2–4 mg monitored over 2 hours if withdrawal symptoms repeat; 2- to 4-mg dose on day 1; maximum: 8 mg/24 hours; maintenance: 16–24 mg/day	Same as buprenorphine; ratios of 2 mg buprenorphine to 0.5 mg naloxone; day 1: maximum 8 mg/2 mg; maintenance: 16 mg/4 mg to 24 mg/6 mg daily

Note.   APRN = advanced practice registered nurse; BZD = benzodiazepine; CYP = cytochrome P450; FDA = U.S. Food and Drug Administration; 5-HT = serotonin; MAOI = monoamine oxidase inhibitor; NE = norepinephrine; NMDA = *N*-methyl-D-aspartate; SNRI = serotonin-norepinephrine reuptake inhibitor; SSRI = selective serotonin reuptake inhibitor; TCA = tricyclic antidepressant.

Table 7–7. Medications used in the treatment of nicotine dependence

	Nicotine gum/lozenge	Nicotine inhaler	Nicotine nasal spray	Nicotine transdermal patch	Bupropion (Zyban, Wellbutrin)	Varenicline (Chantix)
FDA approval	Over-the-counter smoking cessation	Over-the-counter smoking cessation	Over-the-counter smoking cessation	Over-the-counter smoking cessation	Prescription smoking cessation	Prescription smoking cessation
Mechanism of action	Rapid absorption through oral mucosa	Same as nicotine gum and lozenge	Rapid absorption through nasal mucosa	Absorbed through the skin; most appropriate for those who smoke >10 cigarettes/day	Inhibits neuronal dopamine reuptake and blocks norepinephrine reuptake in the brain	Binds to and blocks nicotine receptors signaling release of dopamine in the brain
Precautions	Pregnancy Category D; *cigarettes*; peptic ulcers; CAD; angina; hypertension; diabetes mellitus; renal and hepatic dysfunction	Same as nicotine gum and lozenge	Same as nicotine gum and lozenge	Same as nicotine gum and lozenge	Pregnancy Category B; renal/hepatic insufficiency; dosages >450 mg/day can lower the seizure threshold	Pregnancy Category C; mania; psychosis; aggression; depression; anxiety; homicidal and suicidal ideation

Table 7–7.   Medications used in the treatment of nicotine dependence (*continued*)

	Nicotine gum/lozenge	Nicotine inhaler	Nicotine nasal spray	Nicotine transdermal patch	Bupropion (Zyban, Wellbutrin)	Varenicline (Chantix)
Potential drug interactions	Decrease effects of diuretics; decrease cardiac output; decrease absorption of glutethimide; increase cortisol and catecholamines	Same as nicotine gum and lozenge	Same as nicotine gum and lozenge	Same as nicotine gum and lozenge	Carbamazepine, cimetidine, phenytoin, and phenobarbital may decrease effects; toxicity increases with levodopa and MAOIs	Decrease in renal clearance with cimetidine; increased incidence of adverse events with nicotine replacement therapy
CYP metabolism	Metabolized primarily through kidney and lungs	Metabolized primarily through kidney and lungs	Metabolized primarily through kidney and lungs	Metabolized primarily through kidney and lungs	CYP2B6 substrate; CYP2D6 inhibitor	No known CYP metabolism
Common side effects	Tingling sensation, peppery taste, numbness of cheek/gum	Rhinitis, throat and mouth irritation	Coughing, worsening of asthma, burning or irritation of nasal passages	Skin irritation, insomnia (if persistent, remove patch at bedtime)	Headache, nausea, anxiety, insomnia, potential increase in suicidal thinking, worsening of depression, agitation	Nausea, GI upset, constipation, insomnia, headache, abnormal dreams

Table 7–7.   Medications used in the treatment of nicotine dependence (*continued*)

	Nicotine gum/lozenge	Nicotine inhaler	Nicotine nasal spray	Nicotine transdermal patch	Bupropion (Zyban, Wellbutrin)	Varenicline (Chantix)
Usual adult dosing	Gum: chew 1 piece every 1–2 hours while awake for 6 weeks, then decrease to 1 piece every 2–4 hours for 2 weeks, then decrease to 1 piece every 4–8 hours for 2 weeks; lozenge: dissolve 1 every 1–2 hours while awake for 6 weeks, then decrease to 1 every 2–4 hours for 2 weeks, then decrease to 1 every 4–8 hours for 2 weeks	Most effective with continuous puffing over 20 minutes using 6–16 cartridges daily; gradually decrease dose over 6–12 weeks	1–2 sprays/hour intranasally, not to exceed 10 sprays/hour or 40 sprays in 24 hours; each spray = 0.5 mg nicotine	Apply highest-dose (21 or 14 mg, depending on prior consumption) patch daily for 6 weeks, then decrease to middle-dose patch for 2 weeks, then decrease to lowest-dose patch for 2 weeks	150 mg/day for 3 days, then increase to 300 mg/day in the morning	Days 1–3: 0.5 mg once daily; days 4–7: 0.5 mg twice daily; day 8–end of treatment, 1 mg twice daily. Treatment is 12 weeks; if abstinent at 12 weeks, an additional 12-week course is recommended to maintain abstinence

Note.   CAD = coronary artery disease; CYP = cytochrome P450; FDA = U.S. Food and Drug Administration; GI = gastrointestinal; MAOI = monoamine oxidase inhibitor.

Pharmacokinetics of Alcohol and Alcoholism Treatment

Most nurses have had the unfortunate opportunity to observe a patient "under the influence" at the higher levels of the blood alcohol threshold. Nurses are called to intervene when the patient who was walking and talking on entering the facility requires intubation after falling into the throes of seizures within moments. Table 7–8 provides an overview of the potential physical and mental symptoms an individual may experience while under the influence of varying levels of alcohol. This may serve as a guideline when evaluating patients in an outpatient setting without the ability to draw a serum alcohol level.

Nurses are aware that alcohol is highly metabolized by the liver by the enzyme alcohol dehydrogenase. Therefore, the potential for interactions between alcohol and other medications, both prescription and over the counter, is increased. In fact, acetaminophen and associated products such as cough and cold preparations and the "-cet" prescription medications (e.g., Percocet, Lorcet, Fioricet) are also highly metabolized in the liver. This pharmacokinetic action can inadvertently lead to hepatotoxicity and potentially death in overdose.

Following large consumptions of alcohol, the enzyme alcohol dehydrogenase is involved in the conversion of alcohol to acetylaldehyde. By interacting with fatty acids, small amounts of alcohol are removed and form fatty acid ethyl esters, which have been shown to contribute to damage in the liver and pancreas (Vonlaufen et al. 2007). Thus, it is imperative for the nurse to obtain a complete history of the patient's current prescription, over-the-counter, and supplemental medications to be able to monitor for competing metabolism and potential interactions. Table 7–5 offers additional information about drug-drug interactions and precautions to be exercised with the alcohol-abusing patient.

Naltrexone (ReVia) is not known to be metabolized by the cytochrome P450 (CYP) system in the liver (Porter et al. 2000), whereas disulfiram (Antabuse) inhibits the hepatic enzymes CYP2E1 and CYP2C9 and is a substrate of the CYP3A4 and CYP3A5 enzymes. The inhibition of these enzymes may increase serum levels of tricyclic antidepressants (TCAs), given their reduced ability to clear the liver. Caffeine levels also may be increased as a result of the same metabolic process when coadministered with disulfiram. Thus, we must caution patients of not only the drug's potential side effects but also the effect of coadministration of disulfiram with other substances and pharmaceutical agents.

Table 7-8. Blood alcohol level (BAL): symptoms and effects

BAL	Symptoms and effects
0.02–0.03	Slight euphoria, loss of shyness Depressant effects are not apparent Mildly relaxed and maybe a bit light-headed
0.04–0.06	Euphoria, feeling of well-being, relaxation, and lowered inhibitions and caution Sensation of warmth Exaggerated behaviors Intensified emotions Minor impairment in reasoning and memory
0.07–0.09	Slight impairment of balance, speech, vision, reaction time, and hearing Reduced judgment and self-control Impaired caution, reason, and memory Belief that they are functioning better than they really are Euphoria 0.08 is legally impaired; it is ILLEGAL to drive at this level
0.10–0.125	Speech may be slurred Loss of good judgment Significantly impaired motor coordination Euphoria Impaired balance, vision, reaction time, and hearing
0.13–0.15	Gross motor impairment and lack of physical control Blurred vision Ataxia/loss of balance Severely impaired judgment and perception Reduced euphoria Anxiety and restlessness begin to appear Dysphoria
0.16–0.19	Dysphoria predominates Nausea may occur Drinker has the appearance of a "sloppy drunk"

Table 7–8.   Blood alcohol level (BAL): symptoms and effects *(continued)*

BAL	Symptoms and effects
0.20	Feeling dazed, confused, and disoriented If injured, may not feel pain Impaired gag reflex May need help to stand or walk Nausea and vomiting "Blackouts"
0.25	Severely impaired mental, physical, and sensory functions Increased risk of asphyxiation from choking or vomit Increased risk of serious injury by falls or other unintentional accidents
0.30	Stupor Little comprehension of where they are May "pass out" suddenly and be difficult to awaken
0.35	Level of surgical anesthesia Coma is possible
0.40	Onset of coma Possible death due to respiratory arrest

Source.   Adapted from Education Specialty Publishing 2011.

Pharmacokinetics of Opiates and Addiction Treatment

Methadone as an opioid agonist inhibits norepinephrine and serotonin reuptake and antagonizes *N*-methyl-D-aspartate (NMDA) receptors, decreasing neuronal excitability and enhancing neural plasticity. It is most similar to the drugs with the greatest abuse potential because they are also full agonists on the μ opioid receptors. Those substances (e.g., heroin, morphine, methadone, oxycodone, hydromorphone [Dilaudid]) with the highest abuse potential are typically categorized as controlled substances on Schedule I (illegal and experimental drugs) or Schedule II (drugs with extremely high potential for abuse) (Center for Substance Abuse Treatment 2004). Refer to Table 1–3 in Chapter 1, "Introduction to Clinical Psychopharmacology for Nurses," for more information on the U.S. Drug Enforcement Administration schedules of controlled substances.

Methadone is extensively metabolized by the CYP system in the liver. In particular, methadone has a high affinity for the liver enzymes CYP3A4 and CYP2D6 (Center for Substance Abuse Treatment 2004), which are also involved in the metabolism of many other commonly prescribed medications. The prescribing APRN needs to exercise caution and evaluate the potential for drug-drug interactions when prescribing methadone to patients abusing opiates. Examples of potential drug-drug interactions and precautions are shown in Table 7–6. Methadone levels may be increased in the patient who is coadministered medications that are CYP3A4 inhibitors. Common psychotropic medications that are considered CYP3A4 inhibitors include fluoxetine (Prozac), sertraline (Zoloft), TCAs, and, to a lesser degree, bupropion (Wellbutrin, Zyban), mirtazapine (Remeron), paroxetine (Paxil), and venlafaxine (Effexor) (McCance-Katz et al. 2010). Thus, either the dose of methadone may need to be increased or the dose of the other agent may need to be decreased. Similarly, buprenorphine (Subutex) and the combination drug buprenorphine-naloxone (Suboxone) also interact with drugs considered to be CYP3A4 inhibitors.

Pharmacokinetics of Nicotine and Smoking-Cessation Treatment

The nicotine replacement therapies are primarily metabolized by the kidneys and lungs. Refer to Table 7–7 for further information on potential drug-drug interactions. Varenicline (Chantix) is not known to be metabolized by the CYP system; thus, the risk of drug-drug interactions is low. Bupropion, a dopamine-norepinephrine reuptake inhibitor, however, is a CYP2B6 substrate and a CYP2D6 inhibitor. Thus, psychopharmacological agents such as carbamazepine (Tegretol), phenytoin (Dilantin), and phenobarbital may decrease the effects of bupropion; toxicity may result from coadministration with levodopa and the MAO inhibitor antidepressants.

Safety Concerns

Detoxification and Withdrawal

For the most part, patients with substance abuse and dependence should undergo detoxification before initiating medications for sobriety and abstinence maintenance. Figures 7–1 and 7–2 offer suggested medical detoxification measures to safely withdraw the patient from alcohol or benzodiazepines (sedative-hypnotics) and opiates, respectively, while maintaining an optimal level of health.

Alcohol/Benzodiazepine (Sedative-Hypnotic) Withdrawal Protocol

Withdrawal diagnosis: Alcohol ❏ Benzodiazepine ❏ Sedative-Hypnotic ❏

Date/time and amount of last ingestion of substance of abuse:_____

Vital signs:

❏ Monitor patient every 4 hours using CIWA-Ar until score is less than 10 for 24 hours while awake (include BP, pulse, respiratory rate, temperature)

❏ STAT page practitioner if patient experiences any of the following: respiratory distress, change in mental status, oral temperature > 101.5°F, urine output < 250 cc/shift, heart rate < 50 or > 120, systolic blood pressure ≥ 180 or ≤ 110, or diastolic blood pressure ≥ 100

Medications: Use CIWA-Ar to determine doses.

CIWA-Ar score	Dose
≤9	None
10–19	Ativan (lorazepam) 2 mg po or im or iv
20–29	Lorazepam 3 mg po or im or iv
≥30	Lorazepam 4 mg po or im or iv

Note. Do not exceed 4 mg in any 4-hour period without practitioner order.

Other medications:

❏ Thiamine 100 mg/day po   ❏ Folic acid 1 mg/day po

❏ Multivitamin with iron po daily

❏ Maalox or Mylanta 30 cc po every 6 hours as needed for abdominal discomfort

❏ Ibuprofen 400 mg po every 4 hours as needed for muscle aches/pains or headache

Diet:

Clear liquids ❏   Regular ❏   Dietary/nutrition consult ❏

Other (specify) _____

Activity:

Bed rest with bathroom privileges ❏   Up and out of bed ad lib ❏

Other (specify) _____

Figure 7–1.   Alcohol/benzodiazepine (sedative-hypnotic) withdrawal protocol.

Alcohol/Benzodiazepine (Sedative-Hypnotic) Withdrawal Protocol *(continued)*

Diagnostic Studies (if not previously completed):

CBC with differential ❏   Comprehensive metabolic panel ❏

Liver function studies ❏   Amylase and lipase ❏

βHCG (females of reproductive age) ❏

Signature of practitioner:_____ Date/time: _____

Figure 7–1. Alcohol/benzodiazepine (sedative-hypnotic) withdrawal protocol *(continued)*.

Note. BP=blood pressure; CBC=complete blood count; CIWA-Ar=Clinical Institute Withdrawal Assessment for Alcohol, Revised; HCG=human chorionic gonadotropin; im=intramuscular; iv=intravenous; po=by mouth.

With alcohol and benzodiazepine withdrawal, the greatest risk is detoxification that is too rapid. Rapid detoxification may precipitate seizures or potentially death. The rationale for "round the clock" dosing of benzodiazepines for withdrawal symptoms is to avoid seizures during the early peak days of withdrawal. Lorazepam (Ativan) is widely used for this purpose because of its shorter duration of action, lower risk of excess sedation, and safer use in elderly or medically compromised patients. Symptom-triggered therapy with a structured assessment scale such as the Clinical Institute Withdrawal Assessment for Alcohol, Revised (CIWA-Ar; Sullivan et al. 1989) has been shown to reduce the amount of medication used and the duration of treatment. (A copy of the CIWA-Ar is provided in Appendix 4, "Psychiatric Rating Scales.")

In terms of opiate withdrawal, many addicted individuals undergo detoxification "cold turkey" without any medical assistance. Withdrawal from opiates may not be life-threatening, as it is with alcohol or benzodiazepine withdrawal, but the process can be very uncomfortable, leading the individual to abandon his or her efforts and return to the desired substance of abuse. The medical withdrawal protocol for opiate abusers shown in Figure 7–2 will provide a more comfortable experience for the individual so that he or she can move forward in the goal of recovery.

Opiate Withdrawal Protocol

Withdrawal diagnosis: Heroin ❑   Prescription opioid ❑

Date/time and amount of last ingestion of substance of abuse:_____

Vital signs:

❑ Monitor patient every 4 hours (include BP, pulse, respiratory rate, temperature)

❑ STAT page practitioner if patient experiences any of the following: respiratory distress, change in mental status, oral temperature > 101.5°F, urine output < 250 cc/shift, heart rate < 50 or > 120, systolic blood pressure ≥ 180 or ≤ 110, or diastolic blood pressure ≥ 100

Medications: Monitor BP before and 20 minutes after each clonidine dose.

Day 1	Clonidine 0.1–0.2 mg every 4 hours not to exceed 1 mg in 24 hours
Days 2–4	Clonidine 0.1–0.2 mg every 4 hours not to exceed 1.2 mg in 24 hours
Day 5 to discontinuation	Reduce dose by half every 24 hours not to exceed reduction of > 0.4 mg/day

Other medications:

❑ Vistaril (hydroxyzine) 25–50 mg every 4 hours as needed for anxiety, nausea, or insomnia

❑ Ibuprofen 400 mg po every 4 hours as needed for muscle aches/pains or headache

❑ Bentyl (dicyclomine) 20 mg po every 6 hours as needed for abdominal cramping

❑ Lomotil (diphenoxylate/atropine) 2 tablets every 6 hours as needed for diarrhea

❑ Multivitamin po daily

Diet:

Clear liquids; encourage adequate fluid intake ❑

Regular ❑   Dietary/nutrition consult ❑

Activity:

Bed rest with bathroom privileges ❑   Up and out of bed ad lib ❑

Figure 7–2.   Opiate withdrawal protocol.

Opiate Withdrawal Protocol *(continued)*

Diagnostic Studies (if not previously completed):

CBC with differential ❑   Comprehensive metabolic panel ❑

Liver function studies ❑   βHCG (females of reproductive age) ❑

Signature of practitioner:_____ Date/time: _____

Figure 7–2. Opiate withdrawal protocol *(continued)*.

Note. BP=blood pressure; CBC=complete blood count; HCG=human chorionic gonadotropin; po=by mouth.

Side Effects and Precautions

Serious adverse events and common side effects of agents used to treat substance use disorders are listed in Tables 7–5, 7–6, and 7–7. There are a few additional safety considerations for the APRN prescribing these agents to persons with substance abuse and dependence disorders. This list of side effects and precautions is by no means exhaustive, and the nurse should consult additional sources if he or she has any question about the safety or efficacy of a specific agent.

The greatest issue of safety when treating any of the substance abuse disorders is the potential that the patient will continue to abuse the substance while taking the pharmacological treatment agent. This is illustrated most prominently when a person with alcohol abuse consumes alcohol while taking disulfiram, which causes a violent, undesirable effect to block the rewarding effects of alcohol. If the APRN is prescribing disulfiram, the patient should be cautioned to completely avoid not only alcohol consumption but also any substance containing alcohol. These substances include, but are not limited to, prescription medications in oral solution or concentrate, over-the-counter cough and cold preparations in liquid form, various vinegars and sauces, and toiletries such as mouthwash because they too will precipitate nausea, vomiting, and a general undesirable effect. Likewise, naltrexone should be avoided if the patient is coadministered opiate medications because rapid and potentially violent withdrawal symptoms also will occur.

Because of the high incidence of comorbidity between substance abuse and psychiatric illness, caution is advised when the two disorders are treated simultaneously. In the treatment of opiate abuse and dependence with methadone, one must monitor for the risk of serotonin syndrome if the patient is also receiving treatment for depression, anxiety, or psychosis. Additionally, because the agents used to treat opiate addiction also may contribute to dependence, they may be desirable for diversionary purposes. Methadone, buprenorphine, and buprenorphine-naloxone combination all have "street value," and the APRN should counsel the patient about the effect of diversion on their practitioner-patient relationship. Similarly, the consequences of overuse and "loss of prescriptions" should be discussed with the patient before prescribing.

Regarding the medications used to assist with smoking cessation and abstinence, the nicotine replacements, including gum, lozenges, transdermal patch, inhaler, and spray, are contraindicated for use in pregnancy. Bupropion may be a better choice for use in pregnancy because of its Category B rating.

U.S. Food and Drug Administration–Approved Indications and Warnings

The U.S. Food and Drug Administration (FDA)–approved medications for treatment of alcohol, opioid/opiate, and nicotine abuse and dependence are outlined in Tables 7–5, 7–6, and 7–7.

Buprenex, an alternative form of buprenorphine, is not approved for opiate addiction. The Substance Abuse and Mental Health Services Administration recommends using the combination agent buprenorphine-naloxone as the first-line treatment for maintaining abstinence from opiates (Center for Substance Abuse Treatment 2004).

It should also be noted that topiramate (Topamax) may be prescribed off-label by a practitioner for the maintenance of sobriety in alcohol dependence, but the FDA has not yet approved it for the treatment.

In regard to FDA safety alerts, bupropion holds a black box warning for increased risk of suicidality in young adults. Varenicline also has a black box warning for the increased risk of neuropsychiatric events, including depression, psychosis, and suicidal thinking.

Dosing Considerations

Tables 7–5, 7–6, and 7–7 offer in-depth adult dosing information for the medications used to assist patients with maintaining abstinence from alcohol, opioids/opiates, and nicotine. These tables highlight some of the properties of each medication and the recommended dosing schedules. The tables do not provide complete information and are not meant to be a substitute for the package inserts or other drug reference sources used by clinicians. For patient information about these and other drugs, the National Library of Medicine provides MedlinePlus (www.nlm.nih.gov/medlineplus). Whether a medication should be prescribed and in what amount is a matter between individuals and their health care providers. The prescribing information provided here is not a substitute for an APRN's judgment.

Treatment of Special Populations

Pregnant Women

Although all of the agents approved for treatment of substance abuse and dependence are pregnancy Category C (except for bupropion), methadone historically has been used for both detoxification and abstinence maintenance in pregnant women. Bupropion, rated pregnancy Category B, may be the best treatment option to aid women who are pregnant to stop smoking. It also may provide prophylaxis for postpartum depression. Withdrawal from alcohol must be carefully monitored in pregnancy because the potential health risks are grave. Maintaining sobriety is critical, and the nurse and patient should certainly discuss the effect not only on the pregnant woman but also on the unborn child. Fetal alcohol syndrome is a devastating manifestation in children of those women who continue consuming alcohol throughout their pregnancy. For women who continue to abuse other substances, premature delivery, low birth weight of the infant, and neurological deficits and withdrawal in the infant are potential manifestations. When weighing the risks and benefits of treating substance abuse in the pregnant woman, it is imperative to consider the welfare of the fetus and discuss the pros and cons with the woman at the earliest possible time.

Children and Adolescents

Although children and adolescents have been known to experiment with and abuse alcohol, prescription and over-the-counter drugs, and illicit substances, the use of pharmacological agents to treat substance abuse in children and adolescents is not discussed in this chapter. It is a highly specialized area with very unique manifestations. The APRN is advised to seek out references related to the treatment of substance abuse and dependence in children and adolescents.

Older Adults

We often fail to think of the elderly population as potential abusers of substances. Although they may not be found on the street corners purchasing illicit substances, the elderly may be, either knowingly or unwittingly, abusing alcohol and prescription and over-the-counter substances within their own homes. Elderly men are among the largest population of alcohol abusers in the United States. An estimated 11% of hospitalized elderly and 20% of psychiatrically hospitalized elderly patients show symptoms of alcohol dependence. They are also known to have the highest lethality when suicide is attempted (Learn-About-Alcoholism.com 2012). In 2007, the National Institute of Mental Health published the following statistics related to suicide and the elderly:

- People age 65 years or older accounted for 16% of suicides in 2004.
- Non-Hispanic white men age 85 years or older were the most likely to die by suicide, with a rate of 49.8 deaths per 100,000 persons in that age cohort.

In addition, the elderly are vulnerable to substance abuse because of the incidence of polypharmacy. They may not know or understand that a medication was changed or discontinued and inadvertently continue to take the medication. This is especially dangerous if the medication happens to be an opiate or a benzodiazepine because it may lead to withdrawal symptoms, seizures, or possibly death if doses are missed, extra doses are taken, or the drug is discontinued abruptly.

Patients With Comorbid Psychiatric Illness

O'Brien et al. (2004) in the Department of Psychiatry at the University of Pennsylvania School of Medicine suggested that treatment of substance abuse and dependence will lead to improvement in depressive symptoms and improve the care of persons with co-occurring psychiatric illness. The high incidence of comorbidity was discussed earlier in this chapter. Some agents used to treat substance dependence may have an adjunctive effect on mental health symptoms. For instance, buprenorphine has shown effectiveness in treatment-resistant depression and comorbid opiate abuse (Gerra et al. 2006). Medications, such as lamotrigine (Lamictal), used to treat bipolar depression have been helpful in reducing the cravings related to comorbid cocaine abuse (Brown et al. 2006). A myriad of other examples are available, and it behooves the prescribing APRN who works with the patient presenting with comorbid addiction and mental illness to explore the various medication treatment options to maximize the treatment outcomes by using the minimum number of medications.

Summary

I have presented the various pharmacological treatment options available for substance abuse and dependence. In many cases, the patient may have co-occurring psychiatric symptoms, and generally, the substance use disorder should be treated first to establish a baseline of the individual's psychopathology. If this is not possible, or the APRN determines that it is in the patient's best interests to treat the dually occurring disorders simultaneously, pharmacological treatment of depressive and anxiety symptoms during active addiction is relatively safe and may actually reduce cravings and abuse of both drugs and alcohol. Greater caution is advised, however, when treating schizophrenia or bipolar disorder during active addiction because the psychopharmacological medications may have a higher incidence of side effects and drug-drug interactions when coadministered with the medications used in the treatment of substance use disorders.

Clinical Pearls

- Practitioners should entertain the idea that the patient may be self-medicating and explore further.
- APRNs should explore the role and benefit substance abuse serves in their patients' lives.
- Substance abuse and dependence are highly comorbid with psychiatric illness.
- All drugs of abuse target dopamine and the various dopamine pathways.
- The prescriber should discuss the consequences of misuse of prescription medications with the patient before prescribing psychopharmacological therapies.

References

Alcohol Abuse Treatments: Alcohol abuse statistics. 2012. Available at: http://alcoholabusetreatments.com/alcohol-abuse-treatment-guide/alcohol-abuse-statistics. Accessed May 23, 2012.

American Psychiatric Association: Diagnostic and Statistical Manual of Mental Disorders, 4th Edition, Text Revision. Washington, DC, American Psychiatric Association, 2000

Brown ES, Perantie DC, Dhanani N, et al: Lamotrigine for bipolar disorder and comorbid cocaine dependence: a replication and extension study. J Affect Disord 93:219–222, 2006

Center for Substance Abuse Treatment: Clinical Guidelines for the Use of Buprenorphine in the Treatment of Opioid Addiction (DHHS Publ No SMA 04-3939). Rockville, MD, Substance Abuse and Mental Health Services Administration, 2004.

Centers for Disease Control and Prevention (CDC): Vital signs: overdoses of prescription pain relievers—United States, 1999–2008. MMWR Morb Mortal Wkly Rep 60(43):1487–1492, 2011

Coletsos IC, Bursztajn HJ: Self-medication: medicating the doctor, medicating the patient. Psychiatric Times 28(11), November 8, 2011

Comings DE, Gade R, Wu S, et al: Studies of the potential role of the dopamine D1 receptor gene in addictive behaviors. Mol Psychiatry 2:44–56, 1997

Comings DE, Gade-Andavolu R, Gonzalez N, et al: The additive effect of neurotransmitter genes in pathological gambling. Clin Genet 60:107–116, 2001

DrugBank: Disulfiram (DB00822). 2012. Available at: http://www.drugbank.ca/drugs/DB00822. Accessed May 23, 2012.

Duncan DF: Drug abuse as a coping mechanism (letter). Am J Psychiatry 131:724, 1974

Education Specialty Publishing, LLC: Blood alcohol concentration (BAC). 2011. Available at: http://www.intheknowzone.com/substance-abuse-topics/alcohol/bac.html. Accessed January 9, 2013.

Gerra G, Leonardi C, D'Amore A, et al: Buprenorphine treatment outcome in dually diagnosed heroin dependent patients: a retrospective study. Prog Neuropsychopharmacol Biol Psychiatry 30:265–272, 2006

Goodman A: The neurobiological development of addiction: an overview. Psychiatr Times 26(9), August 8, 2009

Kendler KS: A gene for...: the nature of gene action in psychiatric disorders. Am J Psychiatry 162:1243–1252, 2005

Khantzian EJ: The self-medication hypothesis of addictive disorders: focus on heroin and cocaine dependence. Am J Psychiatry 142:1259–1264, 1985

Khantzian EJ, Mack JE, Schatzberg AF: Heroin use as an attempt to cope: clinical observations. Am J Psychiatry 131:160–164, 1974

Köhnke MD, Kolb W, Köhnke AM, et al: DBH*444G/A polymorphism of the dopamine-beta-hydroxylase gene is associated with alcoholism but not with severe alcohol withdrawal symptoms. J Neural Transm 113:869–876, 2006

Kreek MJ, Nielsen DA, Butelman ER, et al: Genetic influences on impulsivity, risk taking, stress responsivity and vulnerability to drug abuse and addiction. Nat Neurosci 8:1450–1457, 2005

Leahy LG: Psycho-social health problems, in Advanced Practice Nursing of Adults in Acute Care. Edited by Foster J, Prevost S. Philadelphia, PA, FA Davis, 2012, pp 127–174

Learn-About-Alcoholism.com: Alcoholism statistics. 2012. Available at: http://www.learn-about-alcoholism.com/alcoholism-statistics.html. Accessed May 23, 2012.

McCance-Katz EF, Sullivan LE, Nallani S: Drug interactions of clinical importance among the opioids, methadone and buprenorphine, and other frequently prescribed medications: a review. Am J Addict 19:4–16, 2010

Mokdad AH, Marks JS, Stroup DF, et al: Actual causes of death in the United States, 2000. JAMA 291:1238–1245, 2004

National Institute of Mental Health: Older adults: depression and suicide facts (NIH Publ No 4593). April 2007. Available at: http://www.nimh.nih.gov/health/publications/older-adults-depression-and-suicide-facts-fact-sheet/index.shtml. Accessed May 23, 2012.

National Institute on Drug Abuse: Drugs, Brains, and Behavior: The Science of Addiction (NIH Publ No 10-5605). April 2007. Available at: http://www.drugabuse.gov/publications/science-addiction. Accessed May 23, 2012.

National Institute on Drug Abuse: DrugFacts: cigarettes and other tobacco products. 2010. Available at: http://www.drugabuse.gov/publications/infofacts/cigarettes-other-tobacco-products. Accessed May 23, 2012.

National Institute on Drug Abuse: Topics in brief: prescription drug abuse. December 2011. Available at: http://www.drugabuse.gov/publications/topics-in-brief/prescription-drug-abuse. Accessed May 23, 2012.

O'Brien CP, Charney DS, Lewis L, et al: Priority actions to improve the care of persons with co-occurring substance abuse and other mental disorders: a call to action. Biol Psychiatry 56:703–713, 2004

Porter SJ, Somogyi AA, White JM: Kinetics and inhibition of the formation of 6β-naltrexol from naltrexone in human liver cytosol. Br J Clin Pharmacol 50:465–471, 2000

Stahl SM: Stahl's Essential Psychopharmacology: Neuroscientific Basis and Practical Applications, 3rd Edition. New York, Cambridge University Press, 2008

Sullivan JT, Sykora K, Schneiderman J, et al: Assessment of alcohol withdrawal: the revised clinical institute withdrawal assessment for alcohol scale (CIWA-Ar). Br J Addiction 84:1353–1357, 1989

Uhl GR, Liu QR, Naiman D: Substance abuse vulnerability loci: converging genome scanning data. Trends Genet 18:420–425, 2002

Vonlaufen A, Wilson JS, Pirola RC, et al: Role of alcohol metabolism in chronic pancreatitis. Alcohol Res Health 30:48–54, 2007

Weinshenker D, Miller NS, Blizinsky K, et al: Mice with chronic norepinephrine deficiency resemble amphetamine-sensitized animals. Proc Natl Acad Sci U S A 99:13873–13877, 2002

8

Sleep-Wake Disorders

Elaine M. Neidert, M.S.N., A.P.R.N., P.M.H.-N.P., B.C.

It appears that every man's insomnia is as different from his
neighbor's as are their daytime hopes and aspirations.

—F. Scott Fitzgerald

Overview of Sleep-Wake Disorders

Sleep disturbances have been identified as a risk factor for the development of
psychiatric disorders, and worse outcomes can be expected among people with
concurrent psychiatric disorders. It is imperative that the psychiatric advanced
practice nurse obtain a thorough history of the patient's sleep habits to determine whether the patient's sleep disturbance is a symptom of a primary psychiatric disorder or a comorbid condition. Rating scales such as the Epworth
Sleepiness Scale (ESS; Johns 1991) and the Pittsburgh Insomnia Rating Scale

215

(PIRS; Moul et al. 2002) are useful tools to guide the clinician's assessment (see Appendix 4, "Psychiatric Rating Scales").

The Sleep in America poll conducted by the National Sleep Foundation (2008) offered astounding results: Americans need restorative sleep! More than half of the approximately 1,500 participants in the study experienced at least one symptom of insomnia; more than one-third woke frequently throughout the night and did not feel refreshed in the morning. One in five of those surveyed reported difficulty falling asleep or waking too early and being unable to fall back to sleep (National Sleep Foundation 2008). The National Institutes of Health estimates that insomnia affects more than 50 million Americans. Almost 3% of Americans take sleep medications in any given year, and of those, about 25% take the medication on a nightly basis for a minimum of 4 months (Duke Medicine News and Communications 2004). Table 8–1 (Nadolski 2005) outlines age-related sleep needs across the life span.

Sleep disorders can be fatal. A 2002 study found that those who slept fewer than 3.5 hours per night had a mortality risk 15% higher than those who slept an average of 7 hours per night ("Sepracor Announces Approvable Action for Estorra [Eszopiclone] for the Treatment of Insomnia and Provides Update on Launch Plans" 2004). Table 8–2 highlights the effects of disrupted sleep, which are often minimized.

Sleep Evaluation

Advanced practice registered nurses, regardless of the practice setting or discipline, are commonly faced with patients who experience difficulty sleeping, but all sleep is not the same. Table 8–3 (Sateia et al. 2000) provides guidelines for evaluating sleep.

The clinical interview is helpful in evaluating for sleep disorders, but laboratory studies such as a complete blood count with differential, comprehensive metabolic profile, thyroid function studies, and Epstein-Barr virus titers also should be completed to rule out any underlying medical disorders. Poor sleep continuity and increased stage 1 and decreased stages 3 and 4 sleep are often shown on polysomnography. This tool is also used to diagnose narcolepsy and sleep-related breathing disorders. An electroencephalogram performed during sleep may reveal variations in muscle tension and increased amounts of alpha and beta activity, which also may disrupt sleep (Stradling et al. 1999).

Table 8–1.   Age-related sleep needs across the life span

Newborns	16–20 hours/day
Toddlers	9–12 hours/day
Adolescents	9–10 hours/day
Adults	7–9 hours/day
Older adults	7–8 hours/day
Short sleepers	4–5 hours/day

Table 8–2.   Effects of disrupted sleep

Insomnia

Loss of work due to absenteeism

Increased health care costs

Increased risk for accidents

Impaired and failed relationships

Impaired cognition and memory

Poor attention and concentration

Irritability

Frustration

Increased medical illnesses

Depression

Anxiety

Other psychiatric illnesses

Stages of Sleep

It is also important to understand the various stages of sleep. Overall, sleep is broken down into two distinct states: rapid eye movement (REM) sleep and non-REM sleep. The entire natural sleep cycle lasts approximately 90 minutes, of which REM sleep constitutes approximately 15–20 minutes per cycle. The non-REM stages of sleep are outlined in Table 8–4.

Table 8–3. Components of a sleep evaluation

Nature of the sleep disturbance

When do you fall asleep and awaken?

Where do you fall asleep?

Quantity of sleep

Quality of sleep

Frequency of insomnia

Rate seriousness of problem on 1–10 scale

Development of the sleep problem

Sleep patterns as a child, adolescent, young adult, before onset of problem

Age at which sleep began to deteriorate

Stressors around time of sleep problems (e.g., birth of child, death of loved one, career change/stress, financial stress)

Traumatic event (e.g., when, where)

Sudden onset vs. gradual onset

Events that have made the sleep problem worse

Events that have improved the problem

Nighttime sleep

Activities before bed (e.g., watching television, reading, exercise, snacking)

Bedtime on weeknights vs. weekends

How long does it take to fall asleep?

Interferences to falling asleep (e.g., noise, light)

What do you do when you cannot sleep?

How many times per night do you wake? Why?

How long does it take to fall back to sleep?

What do you do when you are awake in the middle of the night?

Physical issues (e.g., snoring, urinating, pain)

Morning awakenings

Wake time on weekdays vs. weekends

What wakes you in the morning (e.g., alarm, light, spontaneous, family)?

Rate how easy it is to get out of bed

Rate how rested you feel upon rising

Table 8–3. Components of a sleep evaluation *(continued)*

Daytime functioning

How drowsy are you during the day?

How is your mood (e.g., irritable, anxious, depressed, "moody")?

Any naps? If so,

What time? How long?

Planned vs. spontaneous

Sleep-wake patterns

Trouble falling asleep but have sleep of "normal" quality and duration

Fall asleep early and easily, but do you wake before you would like? Is sleep of "normal" quality and quantity?

Shift work issues

Differences between weeknight and weekend sleep

Recent travel across time zones

Seasonal variation to sleep (e.g., winter vs. summer)

Sleep environment

Type of bed, age of bed, location in room

Noise level, light level, temperature

Sleep-wake schedules of other household members

Who sleeps in the room? In the bed? In the home, and where? Privacy?

Safety/security of home/neighborhood

Sleep patterns of bed partner

What activities are conducted in the bed other than sleep?

How well do you sleep in a hotel or an environment other than your home?

Sleep beliefs

Thoughts about the physical effects of poor sleep

Thoughts about the mental and emotional effects of poor sleep

How worried are you when you are unable to sleep?

What do you think causes your poor sleep?

Source. Adapted from Sateia et al. 2000.

Table 8–4. Stages of healthy non–rapid eye movement (REM) sleep

Stage 1	Drowsiness or light sleep, easily awakened or aroused
Stages 1 and 2	50% of total sleep time
Stage 2	Eye movements stop, brain activity slows
Stage 3	Extremely slow brain waves (delta waves) with some faster waves
Stages 3 and 4	30% of total sleep time
Stage 4	Almost exclusively delta waves, deepest sleep, most restorative

Although moving through the various stages of sleep is essential to one's overall health and well-being, REM sleep is believed to contribute to psychological rest and long-term emotional well-being (National Sleep Foundation 2008). If an individual's sleep quality is compromised, the body will attempt to compensate by moving quickly through non-REM sleep stages 1 and 2, thereby increasing the time spent in stages 3 and 4 as well as REM sleep (Nadolski 2005).

Types of Sleep Disorders

Many factors can influence an individual's sleep patterns, and not all patients meet the criteria for a sleep disorder. The following brief descriptions address the symptoms and criteria for the many sleep disorders that interfere with patients' health, occupations, families, and other relationships. For a list of DSM-IV-TR (American Psychiatric Association 2000) sleep disorders, refer to Table 8–5.

Dyssomnias

Dyssomnias are primary disorders of initiating or maintaining sleep or of excessive sleepiness and are characterized by a disturbance in the amount, quality, or timing of sleep (American Psychiatric Association 2000). Dyssomnias include the following:

Primary insomnia. Patients have difficulty falling asleep or staying asleep for at least 1 month, which causes significant difficulty in the person's life and is not caused by any other medical or psychological problem.

Table 8–5. DSM-IV-TR sleep disorders

Dyssomnias

307.42 Primary insomnia

307.44 Primary hypersomnia

347.00 Narcolepsy

780.57 Breathing-related sleep disorder

327.3x Circadian rhythm sleep disorder

307.47 Dyssomnia not otherwise specified

Parasomnias

307.47 Nightmare disorder

307.46 Sleep terror disorder

307.46 Sleepwalking disorder

307.47 Parasomnia not otherwise specified

Sleep disorders related to another mental disorder

327.02 Insomnia related to another mental disorder

327.15 Hypersomnia related to another mental disorder

Other sleep disorders

327.xx Sleep disorder due to a general medical condition

    Specify type:

    .01 insomnia type

    .14 hypersomnia type

    .44 parasomnia type

    .8 mixed type

Substance-induced sleep disorder

Note. To code, you would use the name of the general medical condition on Axis I along with the type modifier. For example, sleep disorder due to lung carcinoma, insomnia type (327.01).

Source. Adapted from American Psychiatric Association 2000.

Primary hypersomnia.   Patients experience excessive sleepiness for at least a 1-month period, as evidenced by prolonged sleep episodes or daytime sleep episodes that occur almost daily. Hypersomnia causes significant impairment in the person's life and is not caused by any other medical or psychological issue.

Narcolepsy.   Patients have overwhelming attacks of sleepiness ("falling asleep standing up") that occur daily for at least 3 months. The person will have brief, sudden bilateral loss of muscle tone (cataplexy) and/or periods of sleep "hallucinations" or sleep paralysis.

Breathing-related sleep disorder.   Sleep disruption leads to excessive fatigue and insomnia and generally is caused by a sleep-related breathing condition, such as obstructive or central sleep apnea.

Circadian rhythm sleep disorder.   A recurring or persistent pattern of sleep disruption leads to excessive sleepiness or insomnia as a result of a mismatch between the sleep-wake schedule required by a person's environment and his or her circadian sleep-wake pattern (i.e., jet lag, shift work, or having a delayed sleep phase, in which the person goes to sleep late and wakes up late even though he or she may need to be up early).

Dyssomnia not otherwise specified.   The person has excessive sleepiness and fatigue and/or insomnia that do not meet criteria for a specific dyssomnia but are a result of his or her environment (e.g., noise, light), ongoing sleep deprivation, "restless legs syndrome," or periodic limb movements.

Parasomnias

Parasomnias are disorders characterized by abnormal behavioral or physiological events occurring in association with sleep, specific sleep stages, or sleep-wake transitions (American Psychiatric Association 2000). Parasomnias include the following:

Nightmare disorder.   Patients have repeated awakenings during the second half of the sleep period caused by frightening dreams involving threats to security, survival, or self-esteem. The person usually becomes alert and oriented once awake, and the dreams and frequent awakenings cause significant distress and impairment.

Sleep terror disorder. Sleep terror disorder generally is seen more in young children. Recurrent episodes of abrupt awakening from sleep usually occur during the first third of the sleep period and begin with a panicky scream. Patients have intense fear and symptoms of autonomic arousal (e.g., sweating, tachycardia) and are not responsive to efforts of others to comfort them; they have amnesia regarding the event. The events cause significant distress and impairment in areas of daily functioning.

Sleepwalking disorder. Repeated episodes of walking about occur during the first third of the sleep period. The sleepwalking person has a blank face, is relatively unresponsive to others, and wakes only with great difficulty; on awakening, the person has no memory of the episode. Sleepwalking may cause extreme distress and impairment in the person's social, occupational, or other areas of functioning.

Parasomnia not otherwise specified. Abnormal behavioral or physiological events occur during sleep or sleep-wake transitions but do not meet criteria for any of the specific parasomnias (e.g., REM sleep behavior disorder, sleep paralysis).

Sleep Disorder Due to a General Medical Condition

This category includes insomnia, hypersomnia, or a parasomnia that is caused by a medical condition (e.g., insomnia due to lung carcinoma).

Sleep Hygiene

Although I focus in this chapter on the psychopharmacological agents available to treat sleep disorders, pharmacotherapy is by no means the only beneficial intervention. For many who have disturbances of sleep, developing or amending sleep hygiene will markedly improve quality of sleep. Experimenting with relaxation exercises, warm milk, herbal teas, and other sleep hygiene treatments should be attempted prior to prescribing hypnotic medications. Table 8–6 lists healthy sleep habits that will enhance the benefits of psychopharmacotherapy.

Table 8–6. Healthy sleep habits

Sleep homeostatic factors (increased drive for sleep at night)

Avoid napping.

Avoid spending too much waking time in bed.

Exercise regularly, 30–40 minutes per day, at least 3 hours prior to bedtime.

Enjoy a hot bath within 2 hours before bedtime.

Circadian factors (increased regularity of sleep-wake schedule)

Maintain a regular bedtime and wake time 7 days per week (do not deviate more than 1 hour).

Increase your exposure to bright natural light during the day.

Avoid exposure to bright light if you need to get up during the night.

Exercise at a standard time each day.

Medication and drug factors

Avoid the use of tobacco products. If you do smoke, try to avoid smoking after 7:00 P.M.

Avoid caffeinated beverages after 3:00 P.M. Limit beverages and foods containing caffeine.

Restrict or avoid consumption of beverages containing alcohol. Alcohol can fragment the second half of the sleep cycle, disrupting the restorative sleep.

Review prescription and over-the-counter medications as well as supplements with your medical practitioner because many may contribute to sedation or stimulation.

Arousal in the sleep environment

Keep the bedroom dark, quiet, well ventilated, and cool throughout the night.

Develop a bedtime routine.

Try reading prior to "lights out," which may be helpful to induce sleep.

Turn off electronics (computer time, video games, surfing the Internet) within 3 hours of bedtime.

Keep a pad and paper next to your bed to write down thoughts, which may keep you awake.

Avoid eating or drinking heavily for 3 hours before bedtime. A light snack, warm milk, or decaffeinated herbal tea may help to induce sleep.

Table 8–6. Healthy sleep habits *(continued)*

Arousal in the sleep environment *(continued)*

Avoid spicy or acidic foods prior to bedtime if you experience heartburn.

Keep the clock facing away from you and do not attempt to find out the time if you awaken during the night.

Use stress management skills during the day and relaxation techniques at night.

Avoid too many "accoutrements" in the bed (e.g., pets, stuffed animals, pillows).

Use the bedroom for sleep and sexual intercourse *only!* Avoid work and other activities in bed.

Source.   Adapted from Avidan and Zee 2011.

Neurobiology of the Human Sleep Cycle

The human sleep cycle is regulated by serotonin, adenosine, and γ-aminobutyric acid (GABA), whereas the wake cycle is regulated by dopamine, norepinephrine, histamine, acetylcholine, and glutamate. Most of the psychopharmacological agents either antagonize the "wakefulness" neurotransmitters or agonize (stimulate) the "sleepiness" neurotransmitters. A set of neurocircuitry in the hypothalamus basically acts as the "sleep-wake switch," much like an on-off switch. The "wake promotor" or "on" switch and the "sleep promotor" or "off" switch are regulated by the neurotransmitters histamine and GABA. When the switch is on, histamine is released, which increases wakefulness. However, when the switch is off, GABA is released to promote sleep and inhibit wakefulness (Stahl 2008).

Pharmacological Treatment of Insomnia

Herbal Preparations

Herbal dietary supplements have been used since ancient times to treat insomnia, anxiety, and restlessness and are used widely in Europe for this purpose. Multiple combination formulas are commonly available in retail stores, but the two that have been studied and used most frequently are valerian and chamomile. Both work on GABA and have sedative properties in dosages of

600–900 mg. They may be taken as a tea or in capsule form about 1 hour before bedtime. Caution is necessary when combining with other sedative-hypnotics or alcohol and when using chamomile with anticoagulants because it may potentiate their action. Chamomile is well tolerated. Side effects with valerian may include headaches, dizziness, or gastrointestinal upset (Jellin et al. 2009). People with severe allergies to the ragweed family of plants should avoid taking chamomile, and persons with a known diagnosis of schizophrenia or bipolar disorder should avoid taking valerian because some evidence indicates that it may exacerbate their current illness (Kuhn and Winston 2008).

Antihistamines

The antihistamines target histamine type 1 (H_1) receptor antagonists, thereby producing the effect of drowsiness. They are generally very safe and effective and have the advantage of being nonaddicting. In addition, the chief antihistamine used, diphenhydramine (Benadryl), is inexpensive and can be purchased over the counter. Diphenhydramine has a 3- to 12-hour half-life and should be taken 30 minutes before retiring. The usual dose is 25–50 mg, but more can be taken without harmful effects. Side effects include overall drying effect, sedation, and a "foggy feeling," which may last into the next day for some individuals. The prescription antihistamine hydroxyzine (Vistaril) also may be used with the same effects. It also has the advantage of relieving anxiety for individuals whose insomnia may be affected by an anxiety component.

Melatonergic Hypnotics

Melatonin is a naturally occurring hormone produced by the pineal gland, which plays a role in the control of circadian rhythms and sleep. Little is known about its mechanism of action, but it is used to effectively treat insomnia and jet lag. The usual dose is 3–6 mg 30 minutes before bed. It can be bought without a prescription. Side effects include gastrointestinal upset, headache, depression, and "hangover effect." The melatonin receptor agonist ramelteon (Rozerem) is by prescription only and is approved for use in sleep-onset insomnia. It has a half-life of 1–5 hours and is metabolized extensively through the cytochrome P450 (CYP) 3A4, 1A2, and 2C systems. A typical dose is 8 mg at bedtime; however, because it has a highly variable absorption, a substantial dose range may be necessary. It should *not* be administered with or immediately following a high-fat meal because this may delay onset of action or diminish efficacy. Ramelteon may decrease testosterone levels and increase prolactin levels by an unknown mechanism. It should not be used in conjunction with fluvoxamine (Luvox) or in patients with severe liver impairment.

Benzodiazepines

Benzodiazepines are the most commonly prescribed class of medication for insomnia (Table 8–7). They may be extremely helpful for short-term use but are not intended for long-term management of insomnia. Benzodiazepines influence $GABA_A$ receptors to induce relaxation and sleep, but they may cause restlessness and disturbed sleep in some patients. Depending on the half-life of the agent chosen, hangover effect may occur, along with side effects of forgetfulness, depression, ataxia, dizziness, weakness, and rebound insomnia when withdrawn. This class of drug should be used with extreme caution with other central nervous system (CNS) depressants. Potential for addiction and dependence is high; benzodiazepines should not be prescribed to anyone with an addiction history. This type of medication should *not* be stopped abruptly; a gradual taper is necessary to prevent withdrawal and potential seizures. Benzodiazepines should not be used in pregnant or nursing patients and should be used in reduced dosages in the elderly.

Nonbenzodiazepine Hypnotics

Nonbenzodiazepine hypnotics are more commonly prescribed for ongoing management of insomnia when long-term use may be an issue (see Table 8–7). They are safer for long-term use than are benzodiazepines because they do not cause a high degree of tolerance, dependence, or withdrawal. They enhance GABA by acting as modulators at the GABA receptor sites. Nonbenzodiazepine hypnotics should not be used with alcohol or other CNS depressants and should not be taken unless immediately ready for bed because of their rapid action. Their major side effect is "sleep behaviors" such as driving, preparing food, and other complex behaviors in some individuals.

Miscellaneous Agents

The two medications commonly found in this category are trazodone (Desyrel) and doxepin (Silenor), both antidepressants used for their highly sedat-

Table 8–7. Commonly used benzodiazepines and nonbenzodiazepines for sleep

Drug and FDA-approved indication	Dose (mg)	Half-life (hours)	Side effects	Special considerations and cautions
Eszopiclone (Lunesta), sleep onset and sleep maintenance	1–3	6	Unpleasant taste, sedation, dizziness, dose-dependent amnesia, nervousness, dry mouth, headache	Rebound insomnia may occur the first night after stopping; use caution with concurrent use of CYP3A4 inhibitors and inducers; if taking for more than a few weeks, taper to avoid any chance of withdrawal symptoms
Flurazepam (Dalmane), short-term use	15–30	24–150	Because of long half-life, may cause daytime sedation and/or impaired motor and cognitive skills	Effects become cumulative over time
Temazepam (Restoril), short-term use	7.5–30	15–30	Dizziness, sedation, ataxia, weakness, forgetfulness	Slowly absorbed; give 1–2 hours before bedtime, which may improve onset and duration of action
Triazolam (Halcion), short-term use	0.125–0.5	1–3	Anterograde amnesia; same side effects as temazepam; side effects may increase with dose	Do not use if patient is taking potent CYP3A4 inhibitors such as nefazodone; grapefruit juice may increase triazolam levels; for short-term use only (7–10 days)

Table 8–7. Commonly used benzodiazepines and nonbenzodiazepines for sleep (*continued*)

Drug and FDA-approved indication	Dose (mg)	Half-life (hours)	Side effects	Special considerations and cautions
Zaleplon (Sonata), short-term use	5–20	1	Sedation, ataxia, dose-dependent amnesia, hyperexcitability, nervousness	May not be ideal for those who eat just prior to bedtime; cimetidine may increase plasma levels, requiring lower initial dosing (5 mg/day); CYP3A4 inducers such as carbamazepine may reduce the efficacy of zaleplon
Zolpidem (Ambien), short-term use	5–20	1.5–2.5	Sedation, dizziness, ataxia, temporary memory loss (>10 mg)	Designed for short-term use only (<3 weeks); sertraline may increase plasma levels of zolpidem; rifampin may decrease zolpidem levels; may take if waking in middle of night
Zolpidem CR (Ambien CR), continued use	6.25–12.5	2.5–3	Sedation, ataxia, dose-dependent amnesia, hyperexcitability, nervousness	For use in chronic or recurrent insomnia; do not crush, split, or chew controlled-release tablets

Note. CYP=cytochrome P450; FDA=U.S. Food and Drug Administration.

ing side effects. Trazodone has been used off-label for many years for its major side effect of sedation, caused by its H_1 antihistamine and α_1-adrenergic antagonist properties at low doses. It has an 8- to 12-hour half-life and can cause a hangover effect at higher doses. The usual starting dose is 25–50 mg, and the dose should be increased as tolerated to a maximum of 300 mg. Side effects include extreme sedation, nausea, dizziness, dry mouth, and priapism in males. It may interfere with the effects of antihypertensive drugs and increase digoxin or phenytoin levels. It should not be used in the first trimester of pregnancy and should be used with caution in the elderly.

Doxepin has been remarketed at low-dose formulations specifically for insomnia under the name Silenor. Doxepin, also called Sinequan, can be used at slightly higher formulations as well for insomnia (10–50 mg). Doxepin is a tricyclic antidepressant, which is thought to cause drowsiness by its antihistamine effects. Usual dosage of Silenor is 3–6 mg 30 minutes before bedtime. It should not be taken within 3 hours of a meal. Sedation, dizziness, and dry mouth are the most common side effects. It should not be used in the first trimester of pregnancy or in nursing mothers. The suggested dosage in elderly patients is 3 mg/day.

Pharmacological Treatment of Hypersomnia

Psychostimulants

Preparations of methylphenidate (Ritalin, Ritalin-SR, Metadate ER, Methylin ER) and amphetamine (Dexedrine, Adderall) are approved for use in the treatment of excessive sleepiness and narcolepsy. They elevate mood, increase wakefulness, and improve concentration and attention by blocking monoamine reuptake and increasing dopamine release. Various forms and dosages may be necessary according to weight and age of the individual. Side effects may include hyperactivity and jitteriness, elevated blood pressure, anorexia, blurred vision, headache, and insomnia. Weight (especially in the elderly or the young), blood pressure, complete blood count, platelet count, and liver function studies should be monitored periodically. Psychostimulants have a high abuse potential and should not be used in anyone who has an addiction history or severe cardiac issues.

Wakefulness-Promoting Agents

Wakefulness-promoting agents increase wakefulness, improve cognition, and enhance executive functioning by multiple mechanisms, mainly enhancing activity in the hypothalamic wakefulness center. They are approved currently to treat obstructive sleep apnea, shift work sleep disorders, narcolepsy, and other off-label uses such as fatigue in depression and multiple sclerosis.

The two main agents are modafinil (Provigil) and armodafinil (Nuvigil). Both have similar side effects of headache, anxiety, dizziness, and nausea and should be taken once daily in the morning. Most individuals notice an immediate reduction in daytime sleepiness and improved cognitive functioning within 2 hours of the first dose, with continued improvement over several days. Both armodafinil and modafinil may antagonize hormonal contraceptives, are affected by CYP3A4 inhibitors and inducers, and affect other drugs metabolized by CYP1A2 or CYP2B6. They should not be prescribed for patients with severe hypertension or cardiac arrhythmias.

Over-the-Counter Preparations

Many individuals use caffeine or caffeine-based preparations (e.g., energy drinks such as Monster Energy), nicotine, or other substances available without a prescription to help with hypersomnia or related disorders. Caffeine, an adenosine type 2 (A_2) receptor antagonist, increases wakefulness and improves cognition and attention. Caffeine itself has a half-life of 3–7 hours, depending on age, gender, smoking, and other variables. The average cup of coffee contains approximately 125 mg of caffeine. Most individuals consuming daily amounts of more than 300–400 mg experience withdrawal symptoms when they stop using caffeine abruptly. Nicotine has an extremely high risk of addiction as well as multiple risks to physical health. Many individuals with hypersomnia use a combination of these substances to try and obtain more sustained results.

Pharmacological Treatment of Parasomnias

Several medications are currently in use for the treatment of sleep terror disorder, nightmare disorder, and REM sleep behavior disorder, although they are off-label. The antihypertensive drug prazosin (Minipress) has been used successfully for nightmare disorder as well as nightmares associated with post-traumatic stress disorder. Because of its hypotensive effects, individuals should be cautioned to avoid rapid position changes, and their blood pressure should be monitored on a regular basis. It may cause fatigue, headache, cough, and occasional wheezing. It should not be used with trazodone because it may cause priapism in males.

The tricyclic antidepressants imipramine (Tofranil) and clomipramine (Anafranil) have been used for all of the parasomnias described earlier to reduce excessive nightmares, sleep anxiety, and sleepwalking associated with anxiety. Both drugs are extremely sedating and can cause weight gain, sweating, constipation, blurred vision, urinary retention, and cardiac sequelae such as arrhythmias. They should be started only after a baseline electrocardiogram is obtained in patients with a family history of cardiac disease or in those individuals who have prolonged QTc intervals.

The anticonvulsants topiramate (Topamax) and gabapentin (Neurontin) as well as the benzodiazepines clonazepam (Klonopin) and diazepam (Valium) are also used, particularly for sleepwalking and REM sleep behavior disorder. It is unknown why they are effective, but long-term studies have shown that they have been particularly helpful in controlling these behaviors. Clonazepam and diazepam are long-acting benzodiazepines with muscle relaxant properties. They are sedating and have a high potential for dependence, tolerance, and abuse. Other side effects include memory impairment (especially with regular use), ataxia, dizziness, fatigue, and depression. Topiramate may cause kidney stones and should not be used in individuals with renal disease. Both gabapentin and topiramate may cause sedation, dizziness, ataxia, fatigue, and dry mouth.

Summary

Sleep and wakefulness are seen as having not only many interrelated causes but also multiple effects on the body and cognition. The neurobiology is linked to an arousal system and on-off switch in the hypothalamus and the main neurotransmitters histamine, dopamine, norepinephrine, serotonin, and acetylcholine and GABA. When sleep and wake hygiene techniques have been ineffective and the decision is made to prescribe a sleep- or wake-promoting agent, it is important for the advanced practice nurse to initiate the medication at the lowest possible dose and to titrate slowly until relief is obtained. Additionally, given the potential for dependence on many of these agents, caution should be exercised when considering refills on the prescription. The various classes of hypnotics, including benzodiazepines, nonbenzodiazepines, melatonergics, herbals, and miscellaneous drugs used for their sedative properties, were discussed. The use of these substances, their actions, side effects, and use in special populations were covered along with typical dosing for insomnia. The use of stimulants and wakefulness-promoting agents was covered for the treatment of hypersomnia, as well as various common and over-the-counter substances often used for stimulant purposes. The treatments for parasomnias also were outlined.

Clinical Pearls

- Clinicians should always remember to ask patients about caffeine intake if they are complaining of insomnia. Caffeine can be found not only in coffee and tea but also in soft drinks and diet products.
- The clinician should obtain a thorough list of *all* medications and supplements the patient may be taking; many of these medications and supplements or their combination may cause insomnia.
- Sometimes changing sleep hygiene is enough to reestablish normal sleep patterns. The health care provider should determine the patient's sleep hygiene patterns. Does the patient read stimulating material or watch horror movies at bedtime? Does he or she sleep late on weekends or take naps? Is the room too hot or too cold? Are there pets sleeping with the patient?
- For insomnia, sometimes the use of diphenhydramine (Benadryl), 25–50 mg at bedtime, is all that is needed rather than a prescription medication.
- The patient should experiment with alternative treatments such as the use of progressive muscle relaxation, massage, soothing music before bed, or calming herbal teas (e.g., Sleepytime by Celestial Seasonings) before using prescription medications. Often, these are effective if stress is the major factor involved in insomnia.

- The prescriber must remember to use the smallest possible effective dose and to order only a short-term supply with no refill for substances with high addiction potential, such as benzodiazepines and stimulants.

References

American Psychiatric Association: Diagnostic and Statistical Manual of Mental Disorders, 4th Edition, Text Revision. Washington, DC, American Psychiatric Association, 2000

Avidan AY, Zee PC: Handbook of Sleep Medicine, 2nd Edition: Appendix E. Philadelphia, PA, Wolters Kluwer Health, 2011

Duke Medicine News and Communications: New drug proves helpful for treating long-term insomnia. Updated November 3, 2004. Available at: http://www.dukehealth.org/health_library/news/7126. Accessed January 15, 2012.

Jellin JM, Gregory PJ, Batz F, et al: Pharmacist's Letter/Prescriber's Letter Natural Medicines Comprehensive Data Base, 12th Edition. Stockton, CA, Therapeutic Research Faculty, 2009

Johns MW: A new method for measuring daytime sleepiness: the Epworth Sleepiness Scale. Sleep 14:540–545, 1991

Kuhn M, Winston D: Herbal Therapy and Supplements. New York, Lippincott Williams & Wilkins, 2008

Moul DE, Pilkonis PA, Miewald JM, et al: Preliminary study of the test-retest reliability and concurrent validities of the Pittsburgh Insomnia Rating Scale (PIRS). Sleep 25 (Abstract Suppl):A246–A247, 2002

Nadolski N: The quest for a good night's sleep: behavioral change and hypnotics offer effectiveness. Adv Nurse Pract 13(11):20–26, 2005

National Sleep Foundation: Sleep in America Poll summary of findings (press release). March 3, 2008. Available at: http://www.sleepfoundation.org/article/press-release/sleep-america-poll-summary-findings. Accessed November 2012.

Sateia MJ, Doghramji K, Hauri PJ, et al: Evaluation of chronic insomnia: an American Academy of Sleep Medicine review. Sleep 23:243–308, 2000

Sepracor announces approvable action for Estorra (eszopiclone) for the treatment of insomnia and provides update on launch plans. March 1, 2004. Available at: http://www.drugs.com/nda_estorra_040301.html. Accessed November 2012.

Stradling JR, Pitson DJ, Bennett L, et al: Variation in the arousal pattern after obstructive events in obstructive sleep apnea. Am J Respir Crit Care Med 159:130–136, 1999

9

Trauma and Posttraumatic Stress Disorder

Donna Sabella, Ph.D., M.Ed., M.S.N., P.M.H.-C.N.S.

> PTSD is a whole-body tragedy, an integral human event of enormous proportions with massive repercussions.
>
> —Susan Pease Banitt, L.C.S.W., psychotherapist

As a whole, human beings are resilient. For the most part, we are able to deal with a variety of obstacles and unexpected and unsettling aspects of life that confront most, if not all, of us at some point in our lives. Rare is the person who has never faced adversity or experienced some measure of stress. Fortunately, most are able to cope and move on. Yet for a small number, that is not the case, and what they experience posttrauma goes beyond the norm, leading to some serious and life-altering disruptions. I provide an overview of trauma and posttraumatic stress disorder (PTSD), including its history, causes, evidence-based treatments, and suggestions for nurse practitioners working with patients who have PTSD.

Overview of Traumatic Stress Disorders

Background

PTSD was formally acknowledged in 1980 in DSM-III (American Psychiatric Association 1980) in large measure because of the emotional difficulties experienced by many of the veterans returning from the Vietnam War, but the disorder existed well before then and over time has been referred to in various ways. The terms *war syndrome* and *postcombat disorder* were used to refer to unexplained physical and psychological problems soldiers experienced in the line of duty and were associated with various military conflicts. Prior to 1914, some of the terms used to describe various war syndromes were *wind contusion, nostalgia neurasthenia,* and *disordered action of the heart* (Jones 2006). The term used during the American Civil War was *irritable heart.* During World War I, the terms used were *shell shock* and *effort syndrome.* The Second World War also referred to soldiers' combat difficulties as *effort syndrome* or *combat stress reaction* and *battle exhaustion.* Korean War veterans were given the diagnosis *combat exhaustion* or *effort syndrome,* and Vietnam War veterans were labeled as having *combat fatigue, post-Vietnam syndrome,* or *delayed stress response syndrome* (Da Costa 1971; Hyams et al. 1996; Jones 2006).

Although awareness of the disorder in modern times originated because of military activity and conflict, PTSD is not unique to soldiers or to any one population. Basically, PTSD is a debilitating condition that occurs after exposure to a traumatic or terrifying event and that can affect anyone given the right conditions. According to figures from the U.S. Department of Veterans Affairs (2010), approximately 60% of all men and 50% of all women will experience at least one traumatizing event in their lives. Of those experiencing such an event, approximately 8% of the men and 20% of the women will develop PTSD. Other estimates of the incidence of PTSD have ranged from 8%–9% of the population to 9%–15%, but certain populations are believed to be at particular risk (Cukor et al. 2010; Hidalgo and Davidson 2000; Sadock and Sadock 2007; Yule 2001). Many studies indicate that gender influences who will develop PTSD. The findings to date indicate that women are twice as likely to develop PTSD symptoms as men are and that being female increases the risk of developing PTSD (M. B. Stein et al. 2000; Tolin and Foa 2006).

Clinical Characteristics

PTSD is considered an anxiety disorder and part of a spectrum of traumatic stress disorders ranging from acute stress reaction to acute stress disorder (ASD), acute PTSD, and chronic PTSD. Some will experience all parts of the spectrum, whereas others may experience one or two of the disorders (U.S. Department of Veterans Affairs 2004). PTSD symptoms can occur after an individual either directly or indirectly experiences or witnesses a traumatic, life-threatening event that elicits feelings of helplessness, fear, hopelessness, and horror. A traumatic event can include having combat-related experiences, being involved in natural disasters or serious accidents, witnessing terrorist events or acts of violence and abuse, being tortured, being the victim of a violent crime or sexual or physical assault, and witnessing the death of a loved one.

According to DSM–IV-TR (American Psychiatric Association 2000), the following major symptom clusters characterize PTSD: reexperiencing symptoms, avoidance and numbing symptoms, and hyperarousal symptoms. After a traumatic event, it is not unusual for a person to experience a variety of emotions, including fear, sadness, anxiety, guilt, depression, and anger, as well as physical responses such as irritability and increased cardiac and respiratory rates. In trying to cope, individuals often behave in ways that they normally would not, such as sleeping more, drinking more, neglecting their health, or avoiding certain people and places. However, most eventually will be able to make the necessary adjustments and move on with their lives. Some may experience ASD, characterized as occurring within 4 weeks of the event and remitting within 2 days to 4 weeks (American Psychiatric Association 2000). For those whose symptoms do not improve and last more than a month, the possibility of PTSD needs to be considered.

Of note is the plan to change the diagnostic criteria for PTSD in DSM-5 (scheduled for publication in 2013) by separating avoidance symptoms from emotional numbing symptoms (American Psychiatric Association 2012). Current DSM-IV-TR diagnostic criteria for PTSD are shown in Table 9–1 (American Psychiatric Association 2000).

ASD is part of the spectrum of traumatic stress disorders. The current DSM-IV-TR diagnostic criteria for ASD (Table 9–2) are similar to the criteria for PTSD, although the criteria for ASD focus more on dissociative symptoms, and the diagnosis must be given within the first month after a traumatic event.

Table 9–1.   DSM-IV-TR diagnostic criteria for 309.81 posttraumatic stress disorder

A.   The person has been exposed to a traumatic event in which both of the following were present:

(1)   the person experienced, witnessed, or was confronted with an event or events that involved actual or threatened death or serious injury, or a threat to the physical integrity of self or others

(2)   the person's response involved intense fear, helplessness, or horror.   **Note:** In children, this may be expressed instead by disorganized or agitated behavior

B.   The traumatic event is persistently reexperienced in one (or more) of the following ways:

(1)   recurrent and intrusive distressing recollections of the event, including images, thoughts, or perceptions.   **Note:** In young children, repetitive play may occur in which themes or aspects of the trauma are expressed.

(2)   recurrent distressing dreams of the event.   **Note:** In children, there may be frightening dreams without recognizable content.

(3)   acting or feeling as if the traumatic event were recurring (includes a sense of reliving the experience, illusions, hallucinations, and dissociative flashback episodes, including those that occur on awakening or when intoxicated).   **Note:** In young children, trauma-specific reenactment may occur.

(4)   intense psychological distress at exposure to internal or external cues that symbolize or resemble an aspect of the traumatic event

(5)   physiological reactivity on exposure to internal or external cues that symbolize or resemble an aspect of the traumatic event

C.   Persistent avoidance of stimuli associated with the trauma and numbing of general responsiveness (not present before the trauma), as indicated by three (or more) of the following:

(1)   efforts to avoid thoughts, feelings, or conversations associated with the trauma

(2)   efforts to avoid activities, places, or people that arouse recollections of the trauma

(3)   inability to recall an important aspect of the trauma

(4)   markedly diminished interest or participation in significant activities

Table 9–1.   DSM-IV-TR diagnostic criteria for 309.81 posttraumatic stress disorder *(continued)*

(5) feeling of detachment or estrangement from others

(6) restricted range of affect (e.g., unable to have loving feelings)

(7) sense of a foreshortened future (e.g., does not expect to have a career, marriage, children, or a normal life span)

D. Persistent symptoms of increased arousal (not present before the trauma), as indicated by two (or more) of the following:

(1) difficulty falling or staying asleep

(2) irritability or outbursts of anger

(3) difficulty concentrating

(4) hypervigilance

(5) exaggerated startle response

E. Duration of the disturbance (symptoms in criteria B, C, and D) is more than 1 month.

F. The disturbance causes clinically significant distress or impairment in social, occupational, or other important areas of functioning.

Specify if:

Acute: if duration of symptoms is less than 3 months

Chronic: if duration of symptoms is 3 months or more

Specify if:

With Delayed Onset: if onset of symptoms is at least 6 months after the stressor

Risk Factors, Symptom Course, and Comorbidity

As mentioned previously, not everyone who experiences trauma will develop PTSD. The likelihood of developing PTSD depends on several things, including how intense the experience was and its duration, one's level of resilience, how strong one's reaction was, how much help and support was available posttrauma, and the stressor's subjective meaning to the individual (U.S. Department of Veterans Affairs 2010). Known risk factors include being female, having little education, being a minority, having other mental health problems,

Table 9–2. DSM-IV-TR diagnostic criteria for 308.3 acute stress disorder

A. The person has been exposed to a traumatic event in which both of the following were present:

    (1) the person experienced, witnessed, or was confronted with an event or events that involved actual or threatened death or serious injury, or a threat to the physical integrity of self or others

    (2) the person's response involved intense fear, helplessness, or horror

B. Either while experiencing or after experiencing the distressing event, the individual has three (or more) of the following dissociative symptoms:

    (1) a subjective sense of numbing, detachment, or absence of emotional responsiveness

    (2) a reduction in awareness of his or her surroundings (e.g., "being in a daze")

    (3) derealization

    (4) depersonalization

    (5) dissociative amnesia (i.e., inability to recall an important aspect of the trauma)

C. The traumatic event is persistently reexperienced in at least one of the following ways: recurrent images, thoughts, dreams, illusions, flashback episodes, or a sense of reliving the experience; or distress on exposure to reminders of the traumatic event.

D. Marked avoidance of stimuli that arouse recollections of the trauma (e.g., thoughts, feelings, conversations, activities, places, people).

E. Marked symptoms of anxiety or increased arousal (e.g., difficulty sleeping, irritability, poor concentration, hypervigilance, exaggerated startle response, motor restlessness).

F. The disturbance causes clinically significant distress or impairment in social, occupational, or other important areas of functioning or impairs the individual's ability to pursue some necessary task, such as obtaining necessary assistance or mobilizing personal resources by telling family members about the traumatic experience.

G. The disturbance lasts for a minimum of 2 days and a maximum of 4 weeks and occurs within 4 weeks of the traumatic event.

H. The disturbance is not due to the direct physiological effects of a substance (e.g., a drug of abuse, a medication) or a general medical condition, is not better accounted for by brief psychotic disorder, and is not merely an exacerbation of a preexisting Axis I or Axis II disorder.

and having experienced childhood trauma. Other risk factors include genetic vulnerability to mental health disorders; having borderline, paranoid, dependent, or antisocial personality disorder traits; and having had prior or recent stressful or life-threatening experiences (Sadock and Sadock 2007; U.S. Department of Veterans Affairs 2010).

In terms of progression and prognosis, after trauma, symptoms can occur in as quickly as a week or take years to develop. Those whose symptom onset is 6 months posttrauma are said to be experiencing delayed-onset PTSD. In most cases, the disorder appears fairly soon after the individual experiences the trauma and resolves fairly soon as well, often in a matter of months (Shalev 2001). Most who report symptoms at this point recover and go on to do well. However, it is reported that a minority of those experiencing traumatic events will go on to develop PTSD and that some do not do well and may have prolonged symptoms that could last for life; some individuals have had symptoms for as long as 50 years posttrauma (Dubovsky 2011; Shalev 2001). Sadock and Sadock (2007) estimated that 10% of those exposed to trauma who are not treated remain the same or have symptoms that worsen. Of the remaining 90%, 20% are reported to have moderate symptoms, 40% are reported to have mild symptoms, and 30% recover.

Individuals with PTSD often experience other mental health disorders and problems. Comorbid disorders can include depression and depressive disorders, anxiety disorders, substance abuse, psychotic disorders, personality disorders, sleep disorders, and bipolar disorders (Magellan Health Services 2009; Shalev 2001). In fact, those with preexisting disorders are believed to be more susceptible and vulnerable to experiencing PTSD than are those who have no preexisting disorders (Sadock and Sadock 2007). It is important to note that people receiving treatment for PTSD tend to do better and have more successful outcomes when co-occurring disorders are recognized and treated as well (U.S. Department of Veterans Affairs 2010).

Neuroanatomy and Neurochemistry of Fear and Response to Threat

Several psychodynamic and cognitive-behavioral factors may explain the mechanisms of PTSD, but biological components and factors are believed to

242 Manual of Clinical Psychopharmacology for Nurses

play a role in the disorder. According to Van Der Kolk (2006. p. 282), "trauma can be conceptualized as stemming from a failure of the natural physiological activation and hormonal secretions to organize an effective response to threat." It appears that PTSD may in some measure develop in those individuals whose biological response to trauma is atypical, and the atypical biological response causes a maladaptive psychological response in the individual (Shalev 2001). Much of the research on PTSD focuses on how the mind responds to trauma and attempts to understand why some people's minds have difficulty processing feelings and thoughts in a healthy way after exposure to traumatic events. Brain regions that create intense emotions are believed to be activated when people recall past traumatic events, while the activity of brain structures that inhibit emotions is decreased. The end result is that some people react to trauma with subcortically initiated responses that are harmful (Van Der Kolk 2006).

Because of modern advances in technology, more is becoming known about the mind, its structure, and neurochemicals in regard to PTSD. Research has implicated and proposed many possible causes of PTSD, although results across studies often have been inconsistent or contradictory (Etkin and Wager 2007; Ravindran and Stein 2009). No one factor therefore can be thought of as being responsible for the development of the disorder. However, several brain structures are believed to be involved in the neurocircuitry of PTSD. Among them are the hippocampus, amygdala, thalamus, hypothalamus, posterior cingulate, parietal and motor cortex, and medial prefrontal cortex (Nemeroff et al. 2009; Shin et al. 2006; U.S. Department of Veterans Affairs 2009).

The amygdala, part of the limbic system, plays an important role in processing our emotions. The amygdala is one of the structures responsible for determining the emotional significance of incoming stimuli (Van Der Kolk 2006). Of special significance to PTSD is how the amygdala processes the emotion of fear because the structure may become overactive and create excessive fear in those with PTSD, although some neuroimaging studies have found this not to be the case (Shin et al. 2006). The amygdala also connects the experienced traumatizing event from the past with a nontraumatizing event in the present. In doing so, the individual then is triggered or primed to feel fear from a situation or an event that before the pairing had been a safe and nonthreatening experience, thus losing the ability to distinguish what is safe from what is unsafe (Lanius 2007). Connected to the amygdala is the medial prefrontal cortex, which plays an important role in the process of extinction of fear conditioning. Those experiencing PTSD show constant and disproportionate fear responses, leading some to believe that abnormalities in the medial prefrontal cortex may exist, including decreased activation, although research findings have not been consistent (Shin et al. 2006). The hippocampus, also a part of the limbic system, plays an important role in emotional response, forming and consolidating memories, and connecting emotions to various sensory input (Shin et al. 2006). The hippocampus is believed to decrease in mass and volume in those with PTSD, which may explain the memory loss often associated with the disorder (Pitman 2001; Shin et al. 2006; Yehuda 2001).

PTSD also is associated with changes in levels of stress hormones and various neurotransmitters. Cortisol, known as the stress hormone, is released as a response to stress that one experiences. One would expect those with PTSD to have higher levels of cortisol because of the stress they are experiencing, but the opposite has been found in some instances. Results are not consistent across studies, but some patients with PTSD have been found to have lower levels of cortisol compared with those who do not have PTSD (Ravindran and Stein 2009). Conversely, some evidence shows that those with PTSD have higher levels of epinephrine and norepinephrine, the hormones associated with stress and fight or flight (Ravindran and Stein 2009).

Another area of exploration centers on the hypothalamic-pituitary-adrenal (HPA) axis, which is believed to malfunction in those with PTSD, leading to a disruption of the system, which results in a "false alarm" when the individual is hyperaroused unnecessarily. The HPA axis plays a role in managing stress. Responding to a stressor, the hypothalamus releases certain stress hormones, which then cause the pituitary gland to release several things, including corticotropin (Yehuda 2001). That stimulates the adrenal glands, which release cortisol and epinephrine, the hormones responsible for the fight-or-flight reaction mentioned previously. Although research findings are inconsistent, the HPA axis is believed to be hyperregulated in those with PTSD, and alterations and abnormalities in HPA axis function are thought to be associated with the disorder (Kanter et al. 2001; Ravindran and Stein 2009; Yehuda 2001).

Even though more is known about the disorder than in earlier times, more research needs to be done. At present, studies often yield inconsistent or opposing results, and whether the abnormalities identified thus far are preexisting or are a result of the disorder is often unclear (Shin et al. 2006).

Biological Underpinnings of Trauma- and Stressor-Related Disorders

PTSD is a complex disorder and, like other emotional disorders, can be viewed as consisting of biological, psychological, and social components. In prescribing medications, it is useful to have an understanding of the biological underpinnings to better appreciate how the medications act on the neurotransmitters and fear and anxiety circuitry of the brain (Jeffereys 2009). Biological dysregulation among opioid, glutamatergic, γ-aminobutyric acid (GABA)ergic, serotonergic, noradrenergic, adrenergic, and neuroendocrine pathways has been and continues to be associated with and implicated in PTSD (Hageman et al. 2001; Ravindran and Stein 2009; U.S. Department of Veterans Affairs 2009).

The opioid system is believed to be connected with the avoidance and hyperarousal symptoms of PTSD. When exposed to stress, the individual may experience an endogenous opioid release, which then manifests itself as withdrawal symptoms such as sleep disturbances, irritability, and instances of aggressive behavior (Hageman et al. 2001). A possible hyperregulation of the opioid system in some individuals may be responsible for their developing PTSD (Sadock and Sadock 2007).

The glutamatergic and GABA pathways play a role in encoding emotional and fear memory. Investigators believe that possible increased activation of the glutamate system allows for the creation of memory traces of the event. Ideally, medications given as close to the event as possible have a better chance of preventing the formation of the memory traces (Hageman et al. 2001). Glutamate also has been implicated in causing hippocampal damage. The use of N-methyl-D-aspartate receptor antagonists, one of the two types of glutamate receptors, could play a role in inhibiting traumatic memories and fear conditioning (Ravindran and Stein 2009; Vaiva et al. 2004).

The concept of *kindling* also has been suggested as a possible factor in PTSD. Kindling was first developed to explain how subthreshold electrical stimulation could and in fact did lead to full-blown seizures. Repeated traumatization to an individual might kindle or spark limbic nuclei to cause some of the behavior changes associated with PTSD (Hageman et al. 2001).

Serotonin has not been studied extensively in relation to PTSD but is believed to have a possible indirect effect on PTSD and to be related to central nervous system functions such as irritability, mood and anxiety symptoms, suicidality, and impulsivity, all common symptoms in PTSD (Ravindran and Stein 2009). The serotonin system is known to interact with the adrenergic, HPA, glutamate, GABA, and dopamine systems (U.S. Department of Veterans Affairs 2009).

Observations of individuals showing signs of hypervigilance, palpitations, sweating, increased blood pressure, exaggerated startle reflexes, and trouble sleeping indicate that noradrenergic function in PTSD is hyperactive (Ravindran and Stein 2009; Sadock and Sadock 2007). Adrenergic mechanisms also play a role in PTSD-related symptomatology. By working through the adrenergic system to inhibit excessive α_1- and β-adrenergic receptor activation, the expectation is that a decrease in amygdala activation would result, an important outcome because disinhibition of the amygdala is associated with recurrent fear conditioning, whereby the individual loses the ability to distinguish between harmless and harmful stimuli, judging all to be threatening (U.S. Department of Veterans Affairs 2009).

Treatment Approach to Traumatic Stress Disorders

As is the case with other psychiatric disorders, pharmacotherapy plays a role in treating PTSD. However, the role of psychotropics in PTSD has been questioned and even debated at times. Pharmacotherapy is viewed as helping to address some of the neurochemical imbalances associated with the disorder, but medications are not yet able to fix the underlying problems responsible for the disorder (Van Der Kolk 2006). Furthermore, although it is recognized that a wide variety of psychotropic medications are used to treat various aspects of PTSD symptomatology, systematic research on many of them is lacking (Hageman et al. 2001).

As recently as 2008, the Institute of Medicine's report on the efficacy of both psychotherapy and pharmacotherapy in treating PTSD stated that evidence was insufficient to support the efficacy of pharmacological treatment in those with PTSD (Institute of Medicine 2008). However, several studies suggest that cognitive-behavioral therapy (CBT) provides greater relief from PTSD symptoms than do medications (Jefferys 2009; Norrholm and Jovanovic 2010). To date, numerous studies indicate the efficacy of various psychotherapies either alone or in conjunction with medications, particularly the SSRIs (Benedek et al. 2009; Kozaric-Kovacic 2008; Norrholm and Jovanovic 2010) In fact, CBT and exposure therapy both have been reported to be effective in treating PTSD (Cukor et al. 2010).

However, we do know that in many cases medication helps, and guidelines for the psychopharmacological management of PTSD are available (Institute of Medicine 2008). In addition to the secondary symptoms of PTSD, which include poor coping skills, impaired functioning, and psychiatric morbidity, treatment is directed at the three core symptom clusters of PTSD: reexperiencing, avoidance, and hyperarousal (Jeffereys 2009).

Psychopharmacological Treatment of PTSD

Antidepressants

Selective serotonin reuptake inhibitors.　Although medications used in treating various aspects of PTSD symptomatology include almost every group of psychotropic agents, the selective serotonin reuptake inhibitors (SSRIs) are the first choice of treatment for PTSD. All of the SSRIs have been and continue to be used, but sertraline (Zoloft) and paroxetine (Paxil) are the only two with U.S. Food and Drug Administration (FDA) approval for treating PTSD. Fluoxetine (Prozac), fluvoxamine (Luvox), citalopram (Celexa), and escitalopram (Lexapro), although not FDA approved, have shown some promise in treating PTSD (Benedek et al. 2009; Kozaric-Kovacic 2008; Magellan Health Services 2009). Table 9–3 lists the pharmacological properties of the SSRIs (Fuller and Sajatovic 2009; Keltner and Folks 2005; Stahl 2009).

On the whole, the SSRIs are the most researched and the most frequently prescribed class of medications for treating PTSD (Hageman et al. 2001; Jeffereys 2009; Ravindran and Stein 2009). They are considered efficacious, safe, and tolerable, with few side effects (Sadock and Sadock 2007). They are thought to target broad-spectrum symptoms across the three clusters mentioned earlier (Hageman et al. 2001; Norrholm and Jovanovic 2010). However, recent research suggests that combat-related PTSD and non-combat-related PTSD differ and that SSRIs may not be as effective among the former group as was originally thought (Benedek et al. 2009). Thus, it is not possible to recommend SSRIs for individuals with combat-related PTSD with the same level of confidence as was done previously (Hageman et al. 2001).

Other antidepressants.   Other antidepressants used in treating PTSD include the serotonin-norepinephrine reuptake inhibitors (SNRIs), tricyclic antidepressants (TCAs), and monoamine oxidase inhibitors (MAOIs) (Hageman et al. 2001; Jeffereys 2009; Kozaric-Kovacic 2008; Ravindran and Stein 2009). Among the SNRIs, venlafaxine (Effexor, Effexor XR) was found to be effective in treating symptoms. Among the TCAs, nortriptyline (Pamelor), amitriptyline (Elavil), and imipramine (Tofranil) have shown some promise (Magellan Health Services 2009). Among the MAOIs, two that were studied—moclobemide (Manerix; a reversible inhibitor of monoamine oxidase A) and brofaromine (Consonar)—are not available on the U.S. market (Hageman et al. 2001). The latter also showed no difference in symptom reduction when compared with placebo (Kozaric-Kovacic 2008). However, phenelzine (Nardil) was found to be effective in some cases but not others (Kozaric-Kovacic 2008); thus, both its efficacy and its safety are in question given the risk of hypertensive crisis if foods high in tyramine are consumed while taking an MAOI. The TCAs and MAOIs are thought to be less effective in targeting various symptoms in the three clusters than are the SSRIs (Sadock and Sadock 2007). However, several studies found that TCAs helped to alleviate symptoms of intrusion and hyperarousal (Davidson et al. 2009; Hageman et al. 2001; Kozaric-Kovacic 2008). Table 9–4 describes the pharmacological properties of various non-SSRI antidepressants used in treating PTSD (Fuller and Sajatovic 2009; Keltner and Folks 2005; Stahl 2009).

Antidepressant efficacy in PTSD.   Overall, current thinking is that the SSRIs are best in treating core PTSD symptoms. They have efficacy for all three symptom clusters and work better than other drugs on the avoidance and numbing that accompany the disorder (Hageman et al. 2001). In addition, they are effective in treating depression and panic disorder, which often accompany PTSD. They are relatively safe and have fewer side effects than older psychopharmacological agents. Second-line medications include the TCAs because they are believed to play a role in alleviating intrusive symptoms and anxiety and depressive symptoms (Hageman et al. 2001; Kozaric-Kovacic 2008; Magellan Health Services 2009; Ravindran and Stein 2009).

Table 9–5 provides an overview of the antidepressant medications commonly used in treating PTSD (Davidson et al. 2009; Fuller and Sajatovic 2009; Isaacs 2005; Keltner and Folks 2005; Schatzberg et al. 2010; Stahl 2009).

Table 9–3.   Pharmacological characteristics of selective serotonin reuptake inhibitors (SSRIs)

SSRI	Pharmacodynamics	Pharmacokinetics
Sertraline (Zoloft): FDA approved for PTSD	Inhibits CNS neuronal uptake of serotonin (+++) Boosts neurotransmitter serotonin Inhibits dopamine reuptake (+) Blocks acetylcholine (+) and α_1-adrenergic (+) receptors	Parent drug half-life: 22–36 hours Peak plasma level: 6–8 hours Protein binding: 99% Excreted in urine Inhibits CYP2D6 and CYP3A4
Paroxetine (Paxil): FDA approved for PTSD	Inhibits CNS neuronal uptake of serotonin (+++) and norepinephrine (+) Antagonizes acetylcholine (+) and histamine (+) receptors Mild anticholinergic actions	Parent drug half-life: 21 hours Peak plasma level: 2–8 hours Protein binding: 95% Renal (64%) and hepatic (36%) elimination Inhibits CYP2D6
Citalopram (Celexa)	Inhibits neuronal reuptake of serotonin Minimal effects on norepinephrine and dopamine reuptake inhibitors Mild antagonist actions at histamine type 1 receptors	Parent drug half-life: 23–45 hours Peak plasma level: 3–4 hours Protein binding: 80% Metabolized by liver; excreted in urine Inhibits CYP2D6
Escitalopram (Lexapro)	Blocks serotonin reuptake inhibitors on the presynaptic neuron Desensitizes serotonin receptors, especially type 1A receptors	Parent drug half-life: 30 hours Peak plasma level: 3–4 hours Protein binding: 54% No significant action on CYP enzymes

Table 9–3.   Pharmacological characteristics of selective serotonin reuptake inhibitors (SSRIs) *(continued)*

SSRI	Pharmacodynamics	Pharmacokinetics
Fluoxetine (Prozac)	Inhibits CNS neuronal uptake of serotonin Desensitizes serotonin receptors, especially type 1A receptors Antagonizes acetylcholine (+), histamine (+), and α_1-adrenergic (+) receptors Antagonist properties on serotonin type 2C receptors, which may increase norepinephrine and dopamine neurotransmission	Parent drug half-life: 48–72 hours Peak plasma level: 6–8 hours Protein binding: 95% Metabolized by liver; excreted in urine Inhibits CYP2D6 and CYP3A4
Fluvoxamine (Luvox)	Inhibits CNS neuronal uptake of serotonin Desensitizes serotonin receptors, especially type 1A receptors	Parent drug half-life: 9–28 hours Peak plasma level: 2–8 hours Protein binding: 80%

Note.   CNS=central nervous system; CYP=cytochrome P450; FDA=U.S. Food and Drug Administration; PTSD=posttraumatic stress disorder. +=mild affinity; ++=moderate affinity; +++=high affinity.

Source.   Fuller and Sajatovic 2009; Keltner and Folks 2005; Stahl 2009.

Table 9–4. Pharmacological characteristics of non-selective serotonin reuptake inhibitor antidepressants

Category	Drug	Pharmacodynamics	Pharmacokinetics
SNRI	Venlafaxine (Effexor, Effexor XR)	Inhibition of serotonin (++) and norepinephrine (+) uptake Increases levels of serotonin, norepinephrine, and dopamine Weak inhibitor of dopamine reuptake at higher doses	Half-life: 3–7 hours Peak plasma levels: 1–2 hours Protein binding: 27% Excreted in urine
TCA	Amitriptyline (Elavil)	Blocks reuptake of norepinephrine (+) and serotonin (++) into presynaptic neurons Antagonist for acetylcholine (++), histamine (+++), and α_1-adrenergic (++) receptors Can increase dopamine neurotransmission in frontal cortex	Half-life: 10–28 hours Peak plasma levels: 2–12 hours Protein binding: >95% Metabolized by liver; excreted in urine and feces
TCA	Imipramine (Tofranil)	Blocks reuptake of norepinephrine (+) and serotonin (++) into presynaptic neurons Antagonist for acetylcholine (++), histamine (++), and α_1-adrenergic (++) receptors Can increase dopamine neurotransmission in frontal cortex	Half-life: 8–16 hours Peak plasma levels: 2–5 hours Protein binding: 89%–95% Excreted in urine and feces

Table 9–4. Pharmacological characteristics of non–selective serotonin reuptake inhibitor antidepressants *(continued)*

Category	Drug	Pharmacodynamics	Pharmacokinetics
TCA	Nortriptyline (Pamelor)	Blocks reuptake of norepinephrine (–+) and serotonin (+) into presynaptic neurons Antagonist for acetylcholine (+), histamine (+), and α_1-adrenergic (++) receptors Can increase dopamine neurotransmission in frontal cortex	Half-life: 18–28 hours Peak plasma levels: 7–8.5 hours Protein binding: >90% Metabolized by liver; excreted in urine and feces
MAOI	Phenelzine (Nardil)	Inhibits MAO by binding to MAO-A and MAO-B, thereby blocking it from breaking down norepinephrine, serotonin, and dopamine Increases endogenous epinephrine, norepinephrine, serotonin, and dopamine in CNS storage sites	Half-life: 11 hours Metabolized by liver; excreted in urine

Note. CNS=central nervous system; MAOI=monoamine oxidase inhibitor; PTSD=posttraumatic stress disorder; SNRI=serotonin-norepinephrine reuptake inhibitor; TCA=tricyclic antidepressant. +=mild affinity; ++=moderate affinity; +++=high affinity.
Source. Fuller and Sajatovic 2009; Keltner and Folks 2005; Stahl 2009.

Table 9–5. Overview of antidepressants used to treat posttraumatic stress disorder (PTSD)

	SSRIs	TCAs	MAOIs
General	• First-line treatment for PTSD • FDA approved: sertraline and paroxetine • Full benefits in 4–8 weeks • Considered a safe category of medications with limited risk of serious drug interactions	• Considered second-line agents for PTSD • Therapeutic effectiveness in about 2–4 weeks	• Considered second- or third-line agents in treating PTSD • Therapeutic effectiveness in 2–4 weeks
Pharmacokinetics	• Serum half-life: 20–168 hours • Can be given once daily • Tolerance does not develop • Low potential for overdose	• Serum half-life: 20–126 hours • Can be taken once daily	• Unknown serum half-life
Contraindications	• Seizures • Hepatic or renal disease • Pregnancy or breast-feeding	• Cardiovascular disease • Glaucoma • Benign prostatic hyperplasia • Liver or renal disease • Pregnancy or breast-feeding	• Cardiovascular disease • History of stroke • Hyperthyroidism • Pheochromocytoma • Pregnancy or breast-feeding

Table 9–5.   Overview of antidepressants used to treat posttraumatic stress disorder (PTSD) *(continued)*

	SSRIs	TCAs	MAOIs
Drug-drug interactions	• Additive serotonergic effects may occur when combined with other antidepressants such as TCAs and MAOIs • Need a 5-week washout period when switching to an MAOI • Can increase levels of haloperidol and clozapine (fluvoxamine), TCA levels (paroxetine and fluoxetine), and carbamazepine and phenobarbital	• Possible fatal interactions when used with MAOIs, SSRIs, and antiarrhythmics • Additive hypotensive effects when combined with drugs that lower blood pressure • Additive anticholinergic effects when taken with antihistamines, antipsychotics, and antiparkinsonian drugs	• Foods containing high levels of tyramine • Hypertensive crisis possible with bupropion, carbamazepine, and mirtazapine • Increased serotonergic effects when taken with other antidepressants • Additive anticholinergic effects when taken with medications also having anticholinergic effects
Common side effects	• Gastrointestinal such as nausea, diarrhea, and heartburn • Headache • Insomnia • Weight loss • Sexual dysfunction • Agitation • Tremors	• Anticholinergic effects such as dry mouth, constipation, urinary retention, and blurred vision • Weight gain • CNS effects of sedation and fatigue • Cardiovascular effects including cardiac conduction abnormalities, tachycardia, heart failure, prolonged QRS complex, and hypotension or hypertension	• Anticholinergic side effects • Weight gain • Orthostatic hypotension • Headache • Agitation • Sexual dysfunction • Dietary restriction • Restlessness and insomnia/somnolence • Need to watch diet and cold remedies such as decongestants and antihistamines

Table 9–5. Overview of antidepressants used to treat posttraumatic stress disorder (PTSD) *(continued)*

	SSRIs	TCAs	MAOIs
Serious concerns/ side effects	• Serotonin syndrome • Discontinuation syndrome	• Narrow safety margins • Lethal in overdose • Serotonin syndrome • Agranulocytosis • Seizures	• Can be lethal in overdose or life-threatening drug-drug interactions • Should be discontinued several weeks prior to surgery to avoid decline in blood pressure related to anesthesia • Hypertensive crisis • Stroke • Myocardial infarction • Agranulocytosis • Hepatic toxicity

Note. CNS=central nervous system; FDA=U.S. Food and Drug Administration; MAOIs=monoamine oxidase inhibitors; SSRIs=selective serotonin reuptake inhibitors; TCAs=tricyclic antidepressants.

Source. Davidson et al. 2009; Fuller and Sajatovic 2009; Isaacs 2005; Keltner and Folks 2005; Schatzberg et al. 2010; Stahl 2009.

Other Agents

Mood stabilizers and anticonvulsants. Several other drugs have been used to help alleviate and minimize symptoms, although their use is somewhat questionable at this point, and more research needs to be done. Open and randomized controlled trials (RCTs) have shown questionable, conflicting, or varying levels of efficacy in some cases for the medications mentioned here, including mood stabilizers and anticonvulsants (Davidson et al. 2009; Jeffereys 2009; Kozaric-Kovacic 2008; Ravindran and Stein 2009). The *American Psychiatric Association Guideline Watch* noted limited efficacy of mood stabilizers and anticonvulsants in the treatment of PTSD, although several studies did report some effectiveness (Benedek et al. 2009; Hageman et al. 2001). Among those researched were valproate (Depakote), carbamazepine (Tegretol), and lamotrigine (Lamictal) (Benedek et al. 2009; Magellan Health Services 2009).

Atypical antipsychotics. Atypical antipsychotics are used when psychosis accompanies PTSD but are not typically and routinely recommended for use as monotherapy for PTSD, although some reports indicated that they reduced intrusive symptoms such as flashbacks in several trials (Hageman et al. 2001; Jeffereys 2009; Norrholm and Jovanovic 2010; Ravindran and Stein 2009). Risperidone (Risperdal), a second-generation atypical antipsychotic medication, has shown some effectiveness in several studies, as has olanzapine (Zyprexa), but typically in limited contexts. These antipsychotics are thought to be useful in treating PTSD in patients with aggressive, overwhelming, and self-destructive behaviors and are viewed as adjunctive forms of medication (Benedek et al. 2009; Hageman et al. 2001; Magellan Health Services 2009; Norrholm and Jovanovic 2010; Ravindran and Stein 2009). However, some argue that current evidence is insufficient to recommend any atypical antipsychotic as an adjunctive agent for treating PTSD, including risperidone (Jeffereys 2009).

Benzodiazepines. Benzodiazepines are addictive, and studies have shown that they are unable to target core PTSD symptoms, but they are used to treat acute anxiety posttrauma (Davidson et al. 2009; Hageman et al. 2001; Jeffereys 2009; Ravindran and Stein 2009). However, they are not intended to be used long term in the treatment of the disorder.

Alpha- and beta-blockers.   Of note in more recent findings are the drugs prazosin (Minipress) and propranolol (Inderal) (Davidson et al. 2009; Norrholm and Jovanovic 2010; Ravindran and Stein 2009). Prazosin, an α_1-adrenergic receptor blocker medication, is commonly used to treat hypertension and benign prostatic hyperplasia. However, it is showing effectiveness and is a reliable adjunct in helping to decrease PTSD trauma nightmares (Cukor et al. 2010; Jeffereys 2009; Norrholm and Jovanovic 2010; Ravindran and Stein 2009). Propranolol is also being explored as a possible treatment to alleviate some of the symptoms of PTSD. This beta-blocker may reduce the consolidation or interrupt the reconsolidation of traumatic memories through protein synthesis inhibition. Several studies have shown that a single dose of the drug helps to block the ability to recall and retrieve traumatic memories but not neutral memories; thus, propranolol is a promising treatment option for the adverse memories associated with PTSD (Ravindran and Stein 2009).

Some reviews of clinical studies designed to test the effectiveness of various pharmacological agents in the treatment of PTSD noted that the studies had limitations because of their small sample size, a lack of blinding and randomization, and small effect size (Benedek et al. 2009; Institute of Medicine 2008; Kozaric-Kovacic 2008; Norrholm and Jovanovic 2010; Ravindran and Stein 2009). Future research needs to be more rigorously designed, with more comparative studies to determine the efficacy, tolerability, and usefulness of medications.

Pharmacotherapy for Acute Stress Disorder

Little is known about the pharmacotherapy for ASD. The widely held belief is that if one intervenes quickly enough posttrauma to treat ASD, then perhaps PTSD could be prevented altogether or at least have reduced symptoms. Several studies have been done with various medications, but as with PTSD studies, the results vary, and further studies are needed (Davidson et al. 2009). As reported in the *Guideline Watch,* while intervention studies have been in progress since 2004, no major research on ASD has been published (Benedek et al. 2009).

Medication Safety and Efficacy

All medications have potential side effects. Most of the drugs in the arsenal to treat PTSD have been in existence long enough that we are well informed of their risks and benefits and their safety and efficacy in treating PTSD. Although the TCAs and MAOIs were among the first to be studied in controlled trials of PTSD treatment, the SSRIs have come to be viewed as the most effective and safest pharmacological agents for PTSD, making them the accepted first-line treatment (Davidson et al. 2009).

The SSRIs have been extensively studied in the treatment of PTSD, more so than any other class of medications (Hageman et al. 2001). In fact, the SSRIs are the most extensively studied and have the largest body of pharmacological PTSD treatment literature of all other drugs used to treat the disorder (Ravindran and Stein 2009). Findings from various studies indicate that they are better than placebo in helping to diminish symptoms (Benedek et al. 2009; Hageman et al. 2001; Jeffereys 2009). They are believed to be helpful in treating core symptoms, to have efficacy for all three symptom clusters of the disorder, and to be more effective than other drugs in alleviating the avoidance and numbing cluster symptoms (Hageman et al. 2001). Also, evidence from several studies indicated that the extended use of SSRIs beyond the initial acute phase can continue to ameliorate symptoms and prevent relapse (Davidson et al. 2009; Ravindran and Stein 2009). SSRIs have fewer and less problematic side effects than do other antidepressants and, on the whole, are well tolerated (Hageman et al. 2001). A welcome feature of these medications is that they have a low fatality rate related to overdose. Of the more than 55,000 overdoses in the United States in 2003, 106 fatalities were reported (Davidson et al. 2009). Furthermore, the risk of serious drug interactions with the SSRIs is limited (Davidson et al. 2009).

The SNRI venlafaxine, which has shown some efficacy in treating PTSD in a few studies, has similar uses, characteristics, and side effects to the SSRIs (Benedek et al. 2009; Davidson et al. 2009; Ravindran and Stein 2009). It is also considered a first-line treatment for PTSD on the basis of findings from large multisite RCTs (Jeffereys 2009). This drug has been noted to alleviate symptoms that have not responded to an SSRI (Schatzberg et al. 2010). The most notable side effects, which tend to occur immediately but then eventually subside, include headache, nervousness, nausea, diarrhea and decreased appetite, hyponatremia, and sedation. Serious side effects such as seizures are rare (Stahl 2009). Contraindications include the use of MAOIs, and caution should be taken in patients with cardiovascular disease, hypertension, a history of seizure, and renal or hepatic impairment. This drug is not as safe with regard to overdose as the SSRIs because overdose can be lethal (Stahl 2009).

In summary, findings from studies done to date indicate that both the SSRIs and the SNRIs improve symptoms and result in sustained improvement over time, even preventing remission in some cases (Benedek et al. 2009; Davidson et al. 2009).

The TCAs, considered a second-line treatment, are believed to be effective on the whole in alleviating intrusive, anxious, and depressive symptoms (Hageman et al. 2001). Numerous studies point to modest efficacy rates related to intrusion and hyperarousal symptoms and general PTSD symptoms (Davidson et al. 2009; Hageman et al. 2001; Kozaric-Kovacic 2008). However, the TCAs can be lethal in overdose. They also can have an antiarrhythmic effect and other contraindications.

Studies of the MAOIs have shown some positive effects on PTSD-related symptoms. However, they, like the TCAs, are not the first line of treatment. The MAOIs are generally avoided because of their safety and side-effect profiles, particularly regarding the need to limit tyramine-rich foods such as aged wines and beers, aged cheeses, cured meats, soy sauce, and similar products because of the life-threatening risk of hypertensive crisis if one does not (Hall-Flavin 2010).

U.S. Food and Drug Administration–Approved Indications and Warnings

As previously stated, the only medications specifically approved for the treatment of PTSD by the FDA are the SSRIs sertraline, which was approved in December 1999, and paroxetine, approved in December 2001. Although other SSRIs and other medications are commonly used in treatment of PTSD as well, they are done so off-label. However, being approved does not mean that no risk is involved. In 2005, the FDA adopted a black box warning label on all antidepressants related to the possible increased risk of suicidal ideation and attempts in children and adolescents taking these medications. In May 2007, the FDA requested that drug companies extend their warnings to include young adults ages 18–24 years prescribed these medications for initial treatment, usually for the first month or two they are taking the medication. The intent of the warning is to stress the need to monitor those taking these medications, particularly during the beginning of treatment, and to assess for any increased risk of suicidal thoughts or behaviors (U.S. Food and Drug Administration 2007).

Dosing for Titration, Augmentation, and Discontinuation

Table 9–6 offers guidelines on how to dose and augment some medications used in treating PTSD. This table also offers other considerations to act as guidelines when prescribing for the symptoms of PTSD.

Treatment Issues in Specific Populations

One of the complexities of treating PTSD is that it is heterogeneous in its presentation and its outcome. What might be the case for combat-related PTSD does not necessarily apply to non-combat-related PTSD. Noted differences in PTSD risk factors and outcomes are related to variables such as age, gender, race, educational level, abnormal personality traits, and past traumatic experience (Hidalgo and Davidson 2000).

Women's reactions to various traumas can be and often are different from men's reactions to similar traumas. PTSD is more common in women than in men, even when excluding sexual trauma (M.B. Stein et al. 2000; Tolin and Foa 2006). Also, exposure to certain types of trauma such as rape or combat is associated with an increased risk of developing PTSD (M.B. Stein et al. 2000). For example, a study of women involved in prostitution in nine countries found a PTSD prevalence rate among them of 68% because many of the women had been raped and brutalized while on the job (Farley et al. 2003). Even when exposed to similar traumas, women still are more likely to develop PTSD and experience symptoms longer than are men (Tolin and Foa 2006).

It is now acknowledged that children also experience PTSD, although this is a relatively new observation. In the past, it was believed that children

Table 9–6. Dosing of medications commonly used in the treatment of posttraumatic stress disorder (PTSD)

Drug	Dosing range	Dosing strategies	Considerations
Selective serotonin reuptake inhibitors			
Sertraline (Zoloft): FDA approved	25–200 mg once daily	Increase dose by 25 mg weekly based on effect and tolerance	Augment with bupropion
Paroxetine (Paxil): FDA approved	10–40 mg once daily	Increase dose by 5–10 mg weekly; discontinue *very* slowly	Augment with bupropion, mirtazapine, or trazodone
Citalopram (Celexa): off-label	10–40 mg once daily	Increase dose by 5–10 mg weekly	Augment with bupropion, mirtazapine, or trazodone
Escitalopram (Lexapro): off-label	5–20 mg once daily	Increase dose by 5 mg weekly; maximum dose=20 mg/day	Augment with bupropion, mirtazapine, or trazodone
Fluoxetine (Prozac): off-label	10–80 mg once daily	Increase dose by 5–10 mg weekly; tapering for discontinuation is generally not required because of long half-life	Augment with bupropion, mirtazapine, or trazodone

Table 9–6. Dosing of medications commonly used in the treatment of posttraumatic stress disorder (PTSD) *(continued)*

Drug	Dosing range	Dosing strategies	Considerations
Serotonin-norepinephrine reuptake inhibitors			
Venlafaxine XR (Effexor XR): off-label	75–375 mg once daily	Increase by 37.5 mg (XR) weekly; taper slowly	Augment with bupropion, nortriptyline, or desipramine (with caution because of potential for cardiac arrhythmias)
Tricyclic antidepressants			
Amitriptyline (Elavil): off-label	25–300 mg/day; dose may be divided	Increase dose by 25 mg every 3–7 days as tolerated	
Imipramine (Tofranil): off-label	25–300 mg/day; dose may be divided	Increase dose by 25 mg every 3–7 days as tolerated	
Nortriptyline (Pamelor): off-label	10–300 mg/day; dose may be divided	Increase dose by 10–25 mg every 3–7 days as tolerated	
Monoamine oxidase inhibitors			
Phenelzine (Nardil): off-label	15 mg twice to three times daily; target 60–90 mg/day	Increase dose by 15 mg weekly	Tyramine-free diet required

Table 9–6. Dosing of medications commonly used in the treatment of posttraumatic stress disorder (PTSD) (*continued*)

Drug	Dosing range	Dosing strategies	Considerations
Other medications			
Propranolol (Inderal)	10–240 mg/day divided into 2 doses	Increase dose by 10–20 mg weekly as tolerated	May reduce PTSD-related flashbacks; monitor for hypotension
Prazosin (Minipress)	2–10 mg at bedtime	Increase dose by 2 mg weekly as tolerated	May reduce PTSD-related nightmares; monitor for hypotension

Note.　FDA=U.S. Food and Drug Administration.
Source.　Adapted from Scharzberg et al. 2010; Stahl 2009.

bounced back from having a transient reaction to a single adverse event (Yule 2001). Today it is recognized that children and teenagers can and do develop PTSD, although their reactions may be different from those of adults and may include behaviors that can be characterized as being aggressive, impulsive, disruptive, disrespectful, and destructive (National Institute of Mental Health 2008; Norrholm and Jovanovic 2010; U.S. Department of Veterans Affairs 2007). However, as is the case with many adults, for many children symptoms resolve on their own within several months (National Institute of Mental Health 2008). Studies also indicate that certain populations are at great risk for being exposed to traumatic events and PTSD, such as African American people living in urban environments with low income (Norrholm and Jovanovic 2010).

Regardless of what population category the patient may fit into, prescribers need to be mindful of the potential problems, contraindications, and concerns associated with any of the medications prescribed. With all patients, the clinician must be aware of past experiences with any of the medications, possible allergies, what other medications are being taken, current health status and medical conditions, and contraindications. If a woman is pregnant or breastfeeding, the prescriber must weigh the risks and benefits of these medications because these medications are either risk Category C or risk Category D. With the elderly, the advice is to "start low and go slow." For young children, medication may not be indicated, and CBT may be considered, although medications may be indicated with adolescents and teenagers (Yule 2001). For all patients taking antidepressants, one needs to remember that despite the relative safety and popularity of the antidepressants, especially the SSRIs, they are accompanied by black box warnings (National Institute of Mental Health 2008). Because some PTSD patients may be very sensitive to somatic reactions, it is advised to start low and go slow with all patients to improve patient adherence by minimizing side effects (Jeffereys 2009). Also, it is important to assess for substance abuse in prescribing various medications (Jeffereys 2009). Table 9–5 includes concerns for the SSRIs, TCAs, and MAOIs.

Pretreatment Assessment and Treatment Monitoring

Prior to treating PTSD, clinicians must ensure that it is not another disorder that is related to anxiety and hyperarousal, such as panic disorder and generalized anxiety disorder. One needs to have been exposed to a dangerous or frightening event either directly or indirectly. Although it is normal to feel stressed and upset afterward, symptoms that remit after a few weeks are indicative of ASD. Symptoms that last for more than a month may indicate PTSD. The individual may experience hyperarousal symptoms such as being easily startled, being tense, and having trouble sleeping. Avoidance symptoms can include having trouble remembering the event, feeling emotionally numb, avoiding places that are reminders of the experience, and feeling guilt and depression. Reexperiencing symptoms include having bad dreams, frightening thoughts, and flashbacks in which the trauma is relived, accompanied by physical symptoms. Several screening tools can be used by clinicians in helping to properly diagnose symptoms when they suspect PTSD (Deployment Health Clinical Center 2011; U.S. Department of Veterans Affairs 2011). These screening tools also may be helpful in assessing a patient's progress with treatment. Once treatment has begun, patients should be monitored for any potential side effects related to their medication as well as how their symptoms are responding. All medications that are not proving efficacious need to be discontinued by the prescriber (Jeffereys 2009). To avoid the potential for withdrawal symptoms, it is suggested that the dose be reduced by 50% every 3–7 days until the drug is discontinued. Because comorbidity is frequently an issue among those with PTSD, patients also should be monitored for comorbid conditions.

Summary

I have provided an overview of the causes of PTSD and its psychopharmacological treatment. No hard and fast guidelines exist for treating PTSD pharmacologically. The need for ongoing research is recognized by all. Several medications have been studied, but limitations related to randomization, study size, replicability, and generalizability have been cited (Benedek et al.

2009; Kozaric-Kovacic 2008; Norrholm and Jovanic 2010). Many consider the data not very convincing and believe that much more needs to be done before clinicians can formulate solid and evidence-based therapeutic recommendations (Vasile and Vasiliu 2010). In fact, some question the value of pharmacotherapy in treating PTSD altogether and cite sources that indicate that treatment guidelines recommend psychotherapy as the most effective treatment for PTSD (Cukor et al. 2010; Jeffereys 2009; Institute of Medicine 2008; D.J. Stein et al. 2009). Various modalities of psychotherapy have long been considered a valuable tool in the treatment arsenal for PTSD, for both children and adults—specifically, CBT, prolonged exposure therapy, and cognitive processing therapy (Benedek et al. 2009; Cukor et al. 2010; Davidson et al. 2009; Jeffereys 2009; Nemeroff et al. 2009; National Institute of Mental Health 2008; Norrholm and Jovanovic 2010; Yule 2001). Clinicians should provide their patients with information about cognitive-behavioral approaches to the treatment of PTSD along with psychopharmacological approaches. Ideally, the clinician and patient will work together to decide on a plan of action regarding pharmacological, psychotherapeutic, or combined treatment depending on the patient's symptoms, co-occurring disorders, and preferences.

Clinical Pearls

- Not everyone exposed to trauma will develop PTSD.

- Most children and adults recover on their own.

- Symptoms do not always appear soon after the event and can take months or even longer to manifest.

- The medications do not cure the disorder. In fact, in some patients medications do not work at all.

- Some studies suggest that behavioral therapies have greater effects on improving symptoms than do medications alone.

- Response to treatment differs, depending on various personal factors and characteristics.

- More research on both biological and psychological approaches is needed and is under way.

References

American Psychiatric Association: Diagnostic and Statistical Manual of Mental Disorders, 3rd Edition. Washington, DC, American Psychiatric Association, 1980

American Psychiatric Association: Diagnostic and Statistical Manual of Mental Disorders, 4th Edition, Text Revision. Washington, DC, American Psychiatric Association, 2000

American Psychiatric Association: DSM-5 Development: G 03 posttraumatic stress disorder. May 11, 2012. Available at: http://www.dsm5.org/ProposedRevision/Pages/proposedrevision.aspx?rid=165. Accessed November 2, 2011.

Benedek DM, Friedman MJ, Zatzick D, et al: American Psychiatric Association Guideline Watch: Practice Guideline for the Treatment of Patients With Acute Stress Disorder and Posttraumatic Stress Disorder. Washington, DC, American Psychiatric Association, March 2009

Cukor J, Olden M, Lee F, et al: Evidence-based treatments for PTSD, new directions, and special challenges. Ann NY Acad Sci 1208:82–89, 2010

Da Costa JM: On irritable heart: a clinical study of a form of functional cardiac disorder and its consequences. Am J Med Sci 61:17–52, 1971

Davidson JRT, Connor KM, Zhang W: Treatment of anxiety disorders, in The American Psychiatric Publishing Textbook of Psychopharmacology, 4th Edition. Edited by Schatzberg AF, Nemeroff CB. Washington, DC, American Psychiatric Publishing, 2009, pp 1171–1200

Deployment Health Clinical Center: Clinicians: Standard Health Assessment Tools. Bethesda, MD, U.S. Department of Defense, 2011. Available at: http://www.pdhealth.mil/clinicians/assessment_tools.asp. Accessed November 18, 2011.

Dubovsky S: Why don't all traumatized people develop PTSD? Journal Watch Psychiatry October 3, 2011. Available at: http://psychiatry.jwatch.org/cgi/content/full/2011/1003/1?eaf. Accessed October 11, 2011.

Etkin A, Wager TD: Functional neuroimaging of anxiety: a meta-analysis of emotional processing in PTSD, social anxiety disorder, and specific phobia. Am J Psychiatry 164:1476–1488, 2007

Farley M, Cotton A, Lynnes J, et al: Prostitution and trafficking in nine countries: an update on violence and posttraumatic stress disorder. Journal of Trauma Practice 2(3/4):33–74, 2003

Fuller MA, Sajatovic M: Drug Information Handbook for Psychiatry, 7th Edition. Hudson, OH, Lexi-Comp, 2009

Hageman I, Andersen HS, Jorgensen MB: Post-traumatic stress disorder: a review of psychobiology and pharmacotherapy. Acta Psychiatr Scand 104:411–422, 2001

Hall-Flavin DK: MAOIs and diet: is it necessary to restrict tyramine? 2010. Available at: http://www.mayoclinic.com/health/maois/HQ01575. Accessed January 8, 2013.

Hidalgo RB, Davidson JR: Posttraumatic stress disorder: epidemiology and health-related considerations. J Clin Psychiatry 61 (suppl 7):5–13, 2000

Hyams K, Wignall S, Roswell R: War syndromes and their evaluation: from the U.S. Civil War to the Persian Gulf War. Ann Intern Med 125:398–405, 1996

Institute of Medicine: Treatment of Posttraumatic Stress Disorder: An Assessment of the Evidence. Washington, DC, National Academy of Science, 2008

Isaacs A: Mental Health and Psychiatric Nursing, 4th Edition. New York, Lippincott Williams & Wilkins, 2005

Jeffereys M: Clinician's Guide to Medications for PTSD. Washington, DC, U.S. Department of Veterans Affairs, 2009

Jones E: Historical approaches to post-combat disorders. Philos Trans R Soc Lond B Biol Sci 361:533–542, 2006

Kanter ED, Wilkinson CW, Radant AD, et al: Glucocorticoid feedback sensitivity and adrenocortical responsiveness in posttraumatic stress disorder. Biol Psychiatry 50:238–245, 2001

Keltner NL, Folks DG: Psychotropic Drugs, 4th Edition. St. Louis, MO, Elsevier Mosby, 2005

Kozaric-Kovacic D: Psychopharmacotherapy of posttraumatic stress disorder. Croat Med J 49:459–475, 2008

Lanius R: Complex adaptations to traumatic stress: from neurobiological to social and cultural aspects. Am J Psychiatry 164:1628–1630, 2007

Magellan Health Services: Magellan Clinical Practice Guideline for the Assessment and Treatment of Patients With Posttraumatic Stress Disorder and Acute Stress Disorder. Columbia, MD, Magellan Health Services, 2009. Available at: https://www.magellanprovider.com/MHS/MGL/providing_care/clinical_guidelines/clin_prac_guidelines/ptsd_asd.pdf. Accessed October 15, 2011.

National Institute of Mental Health: Post-Traumatic Stress Disorder (PTSD) (NIH Publ No 08 6388). Bethesda, MD, U.S. Department of Health and Human Services, National Institutes of Health, 2008. Available at: http://nimh.nih.gov/health/publications/post-traumatic-stress-disorder-ptsd/nimh_ptsd_booklet.pdf. Accessed November 6, 2011.

Nemeroff C, Bremner JD, Foa E, et al: Posttraumatic stress disorder: a state-of-the-science review. Focus: The Journal of Lifelong Learning in Psychiatry 7(2):254–273, Spring 2009

Norrholm SD, Jovanovic T: Tailoring therapeutic strategies for treating posttraumatic stress disorder symptom clusters. Neuropsychiatr Dis Treat 6:517–532, 2010

Pitman RK: Investigating the pathogenesis of posttraumatic stress disorder with neuroimaging. J Clin Psychiatry 62:47–54, 2001

Ravindran LN, Stein MB: Pharmacotherapy of PTSD: premises, principles, and priorities. Brain Res 1293:24–39, 2009

Sadock BJ, Sadock VA (eds): Posttraumatic stress disorder and acute stress disorder, in Kaplan and Sadock's Synopsis of Psychiatry: Behavioral Sciences/Clinical Psychiatry, 10th Edition. Philadelphia, PA, Lippincott Williams & Wilkins, 2007, pp 612–621

Schatzberg AF, Cole JO, DeBattista C: Manual of Clinical Psychopharmacology, 7th Edition. Washington, DC, American Psychiatric Publishing, 2010

Shalev AY: What is posttraumatic stress disorder? J Clin Psychiatry 62 (suppl 17):4–10, 2001

Shin LM, Rauch SL, Pitman RK: Amygdala, medial prefrontal cortex, and hippocampal function in PTSD. Ann NY Acad Sci 1071:67–79, 2006

Stahl SM: The Prescriber's Guide: Stahl's Essential Psychopharmacology, 3rd Edition. New York, Cambridge University Press, 2009

Stein DJ, Ipser J, McAnda N: Pharmacotherapy of posttraumatic stress disorder: a review of meta-analyses and treatment guidelines. CNS Spectr 14 (1 suppl 1):25–31, 2009

Stein MB, Walker JR, Forde DR: Gender differences in susceptibility to posttraumatic stress disorder. Behav Res Ther 38:619–628, 2000

Tolin DF, Foa EB: Sex differences in trauma and posttraumatic stress disorder: a quantitative review of 25 years of research. Psychol Bull 132:959–992, 2006

U.S. Department of Veterans Affairs: VA/DoD Clinical Practice Guideline for the Management of Post-Traumatic Stress. Version 1.0. January 2004. Available at: http://www.healthquality.va.gov/ptsd/ptsd_full.pdf. Accessed October 24, 2011.

U.S. Department of Veterans Affairs: National Center for PTSD: PTSD in children and teens. January 1, 2007. Available at: http://www.ptsd.va.gov/public/pages/ptsd-children-adolescents.asp. Accessed November 14, 2011.

U.S. Department of Veterans Affairs: National Center for PTSD: Pharmacological treatment of acute stress reactions: a neurobiological systems approach. June 29, 2009. Available at: http://www.ptsd.va.gov/professional/pages/pharmacological-treatment-acute-stress.asp. Accessed October 28, 2011.

U.S. Department of Veterans Affairs: National Center for PTSD: Understanding PTSD. October 6, 2010. Available at: http://www.ptsd.va.gov/public/pages/understanding_PTSD.asp. Accessed November 2, 2011.

U.S. Department of Veterans Affairs: National Center for PTSD: List of all measures. December 20, 2011. Available at: http://www.ptsd.va.gov/professional/pages/assessments/all_measures.asp. Accessed November 17, 2011.

U.S. Food and Drug Administration: Antidepressant use in children, adolescents, and adults. May 2, 2007. Available at: http://www.fda.gov/Drugs/DrugSafety/InformationbyDrugClass/UCM096273. Accessed October 30, 2011.

Vaiva G, Thomas P, Ducrocq F, et al: Low posttrauma GABA plasma levels as a predictive factor in the development of acute posttraumatic stress disorder. Biol Psychiatry 55:250–254, 2004

Van Der Kolk BA: Clinical implications of neuroscience research in PTSD. Ann NY Acad Sci 1071:277–293, 2006

Vasile D, Vasiliu O: Matching psychotropics to neurobiological mechanisms in the aftermath of a traumatic event: a literature review, in Proceedings of the World Medical Conference, Malta, September 15–17, 2010, pp 287–293. Available at: http://www.wseas.us/e-library/conferences/2010/Malta/MEDICAL/MEDICAL-39.pdf. Accessed October 31, 2011.

Yehuda R: Biology of posttraumatic stress disorder. J Clin Psychiatry 62 (suppl 17):41–46, 2001

Yule W: Posttraumatic stress disorder in the general population and in children. J Clin Psychiatry 62 (suppl 17):23–28, 2001

10

Delirium and Dementia

Richard Pessagno, D.N.P., A.P.R.N.,
P.M.H.-C.N.S./N.P., B.C.

One person caring about another represents life's greatest value.

—Jim Rohn, motivational speaker

The field of neuropsychiatry is complex. This area of specialty works at connecting the relation between human behavior and brain functioning. The main tenets within this area of practice are to articulate concise assessment, formulate an accurate diagnosis, and identify evidence-based treatment plans for patients with a wide array of physical, cognitive, behavioral, and emotional symptoms. The aims of advanced practice psychiatric nursing addressing neuropsychiatric dysfunction are to develop a solid clinical understanding of the underpinnings of the symptoms to formulate a thoughtful clinical conceptualization based on psychosocial and neurobiological factors (Sachdev 2005). Neuropsychiatric disorders are complex and often underdiagnosed, but they are treatable, and symptom abatement is achievable.

Overview of Neurocognitive Disorders

Delirium

Delirium is a severe and sudden brain dysfunction in the setting of medical illness that can cause an individual to present with an often underrecognized constellation of symptoms. This constellation of symptoms can be subtle or fluctuate over time, creating a clinical presentation that may lead practitioners to attribute a patient's behavioral and cognitive changes to a variety of other etiologies such as dementia, anxiety, depression, and hypomania. Although delirium is most often associated with older adults, it can occur in patients at any age (Burns et al. 2010). The importance of remaining cognizant that delirium can occur at any period within the life span will enhance the practitioner's ability to successfully identify and rapidly treat delirium and its symptoms.

The neuroanatomy of the occurrence of delirium involves the cortical and the subcortical structures and pathways within the brain, yet the exact mechanism and neuropathophysiology have not been established and are not clearly understood. Alagiakrishnan and Blanchette (2011) noted various abnormalities among multiple neurotransmitters, as well as the occurrence of cerebral oxidative metabolism. Various neurotransmitters that mediate or are associated with the onset of delirium have been identified. Those most frequently noted include dopamine, serotonin (5-HT), acetylcholine, histamine, and cortisol.

Delirium is considered a medical emergency and is often associated with high morbidity and mortality rates. The rapid onset of delirium over hours to days is typically hallmarked by the individual's confusion and alterations in attention (Alagiakrishnan and Blanchette 2011). DSM-IV-TR (American Psychiatric Association 2000) outlines a spectrum of symptoms associated with the disorder, which include disorientation, confusion, changes in consciousness, and difficulty with recall. Also common are changes in speech and the onset of psychosis.

Three clinical subtypes of delirium have been identified, each associated with the onset of different symptomatology:

1. *Hyperactive* delirium is most illustrative of patients who are highly confused, agitated, hyperaroused, and at times hallucinating. Hyperactive delirium is most commonly identified because the clinical presentation often warrants immediate intervention.
2. *Hypoactive* delirium is the most commonly missed diagnosis. These patients are often quiet, at times docile, and even lethargic, presenting with symptoms of changes in cognition and level of consciousness that frequently go unnoticed and undetected.
3. Patients with *mixed states* of delirium present with a combination and fluctuation of symptoms that denote a lability of symptoms and are often more easily identified in the hyperactive states of delirium, prompting health care providers to intervene.

Approximately 30% of all patients admitted for inpatient medical treatment have comorbid delirium (Boustani and Buttar 2007). It should be remembered that postoperative delirium is very common, especially among the older adult population. Multiple risk factors are associated with the predisposition of patients to delirium. Common risk factors are listed in Table 10–1 and include advanced age, physical illness, electrolyte changes, and immobility. Various medications also have been linked to the onset of delirium, including opiates, anxiolytics, antidepressants, and steroids (Alexander 2009).

The rate of occurrence and morbidity of delirium have been closely associated with a variety of issues but are most often related to an increased length of stay within the acute care setting and an increase in the need for long-term care placement among older adults. Long-lasting cognitive and physical effects of delirium have been noted up to 6 months after discharge from acute care settings, with about 18% of patients still experiencing sequelae of delirium symptoms.

Cognitive dysfunction in some form is another sequela of delirium, especially when symptoms were unidentified or treatment was delayed. Persistent delirium is associated with increased long-term morbidity and mortality (Cole et al. 2009), which underscores the need for early detection and intervention.

Table 10–1.   Risk factors for delirium

Older age

Male sex

Sensory impairment

Cognitive impairment

Dehydration

Substance abuse

Immobility

Depression

Urinary tract infection

Physical restraints

Metabolic imbalance

Various medication use

The health care costs associated with delirium could be reduced by millions of dollars annually if hospital stays could be reduced by just 1 day. This could be accomplished by more rapid identification of delirium and more timely implementation of treatment.

Dementia

Dementia is a neurocognitive disorder that affects individuals in many ways. Individuals diagnosed with dementia will have a noted decline in reasoning capabilities, memory functioning, cognitive skills, and language (Hale and Frank 2011). Dementia is not a normal part of aging, but the occurrence of the disorder is common in older adults, affecting nearly 50% of those older than 85 and about 13% of those older than 65 (Alzheimer's Association 2012). The progressive and chronic nature of the illness eventually causes individuals to become completely dependent on others for care.

In the United States, an estimated 5 million persons have some form of dementia (Alzheimer's Association 2012). The number of patients with dementia is expected to increase as the number of older adults in the population increases. Today, dementia is one of the main factors leading to the institutionalization of older adults in assisted living and long-term-care facilities (Hale and Frank 2011). Dementia may result from many factors. These causative factors are linked to either damage to or alteration in the functioning of the brain (Hale and Frank 2011). Common causes of dementia within the United States and Europe include neurodegenerative disorders, vascular dementia, chronic drug use, infections, hydrocephalus, depression, and hormonal and vitamin deficiencies. Many causes of dementia have no cure, but the progression of the symptoms often associated with the condition can be slowed. With early identification and early intervention, abatement and amelioration of symptoms are possible, often allowing individuals to maintain independent functioning for longer periods in the earlier stages of the disease (Brodaty 2008).

Dementia has a variety of subtypes (Table 10–2). Alzheimer's dementia, which is the most common type of dementia, has been linked to nearly half of all cases of the illness. The etiology of this type of dementia is linked to protein deposits that occur within the brain, causing a decline in memory and other cerebral functions. Vascular dementia is another subtype of dementia, which has been linked to plaque buildup within the vascular system; this interrupts blood flow to the brain and its structures, causing cognitive changes. Lewy body dementia also has been linked to protein deposits within the brain that can lead to a host of physical and neurophysiological changes, including tremors, muscle weakness, and changes in attention and focus. Parkinsonism is a neurological disorder that, during the later stages, also has been connected to the onset of dementia, affecting a variety of cognitive and cerebral functions.

The symptoms of dementia vary depending on the type of dementia and the progression of the illness. In the early stages of dementia, individuals may have difficulty identifying words in conversation. Another common symptom is forgetfulness, which might be noticed in simple tasks such as forgetting names or appointments or misplacing objects. Often, individuals with dementia may find themselves becoming lost in familiar places or forgetting how to complete simple tasks such as turning on home appliances. Symptoms associated with later progression of the disease can present as personality changes, mood swings, behavioral changes, confusion, and exercising poor judgment. Hallucinations, disorientation, and aggressive behavior may indicate the intermediate stage of the disease. Toward the end of the disease, language skills are often lost, and individuals lose the ability to care for themselves.

Diagnosis of dementia can be complex because the symptoms of the illness may mimic a variety of other disorders. Practitioners should complete a

Table 10–2. Common types of dementia

Type of dementia	Usual onset age	Risk factors	Symptoms	Treatment
Alzheimer's disease	65 years and older	Age; family history	Memory impairment; poor judgment; mood changes; repetitive questions	Acetylcholinesterase inhibitors; symptom management; behavioral management
Vascular dementia	65 years and older	Hypertension; diabetes; history of myocardial infarction or cerebrovascular accident; high cholesterol	Memory changes; cognitive changes; aphasia; apraxia; agnosia; executive function changes	Acetylcholinesterase inhibitors; cardiovascular management; behavioral management
Lewy body dementia	50–80 years	Age	Memory loss; confusion; changes in judgment; apathy; depression; delusions	No FDA-approved treatments; acetylcholinesterase inhibitors; antipsychotics typically not used; behavioral management
Frontotemporal dementia	40–65 years	Presence of motor-neural disease (e.g., amyotrophic lateral sclerosis)	Flat affect; loss of empathy; impaired judgment; loss of insight; compulsive behavior	Serotonergic medications can be helpful to manage affective symptoms

Table 10–2.   Common types of dementia *(continued)*

Type of dementia	Usual onset age	Risk factors	Symptoms	Treatment
HIV dementia	Varies	HIV infection	Memory changes; apathy; social withdrawal; decreased concentration	Symptom management with antidepressants and antipsychotics
Huntington's dementia	30–40 years	Huntington's disease	Cognitive changes; mood changes; behavioral changes	Symptom management to improve function, including antidepressants

Note.   FDA=U.S. Food and Drug Administration.

comprehensive medical and psychiatric examination, including a full mental health examination; laboratory tests, such as comprehensive metabolic panel, thyroid function tests, vitamin B_{12} levels, sedimentation rate, and screens for syphilis, HIV, and autoimmune disorders; and, possibly, brain imaging with computed tomography or magnetic resonance imaging scanning to rule out potentially reversible medical conditions before a diagnosis of dementia is made. Neuropsychological testing also may be indicated, depending on clinical presentation and symptom presentation.

Dementia is a difficult diagnosis for patients and their families to face. The longer-term effect on patients and their caregivers creates a very challenging terrain for families to navigate. The loss of memory, intellectual functioning, and capacity to function independently can be horrific. Early detection and intervention, as well as amelioration of symptoms during the course of the illness, can make the progressive deterioration of the disease easier on patients and their families.

Biological Underpinnings of Neurocognitive Disorders

Delirium

Today, much of the research associated with delirium focuses on an investigation of the numerous factors that contribute to disease development. Although no distinct or single cause has been associated with the onset of delirium, undergoing surgery, medications, infection, metabolic changes, and various conditions associated with augmentation of stress play a significant role in the onset of delirium. Fricchione et al. (2008) articulated seven potentially life-threatening presentations of delirium that require immediate intervention: 1) hypoglycemia, 2) hypoxia, 3) poisoning, 4) Wernicke's encephalopathy, 5) intracerebral hemorrhage, 6) hypertensive encephalopathy, and 7) meningitis.

Physical stress conditions such as stroke, pain, and infection can increase the production of glucocorticoids. The abnormal shutoff of the hypothalamic-pituitary-adrenal axis causes an inadequate suppression, thereby increasing levels of cortisol, which disturbs an individual's declarative memory and attention; this triggers hypercortisolism, which can lead to delirium.

According to Fricchione et al. (2008), the influences of anesthesia on vasodilation postsurgery lead to the onset of delirium in many postsurgical patients and in more than 80% of postsurgical older adults. Delirium resulting from infection is associated with a high production of cytokines, which contributes to an increase in the permeability of the blood-brain barrier, which then alters neurotransmission. This increase in blood-brain barrier permeability is often associated with the cognitive impairment that has been linked to the onset of delirium (Fricchione et al. 2008). The main neurochemical correlate associated with the onset of delirium is a decrease in cholinergic activity. A significant portion of delirium research has focused attention on the muscarinic-cholinergic system, in which the neurotransmitter acetylcholine is the key arouser of the cortical levels that affect various functions, including attention, memory, learning, the rapid eye movement associated with induction of sleep, mood, thought, perception, and orientation. As the processes begin to alter, the subtle changes of delirium begin.

Significant dysfunction within the brain stem, amygdala, hippocampus, thalamus, and prefrontal cortex occurs during the onset of delirium (Fricchione et al. 2008). The purpose of rapid identification, diagnosis, and treatment is protection of the brain from long-standing insult and reduction of symptoms to regain regulation of neuronal and brain functioning.

Dementia

Neuroanatomically, a brain with Alzheimer's dementia is characterized by the variance noted in the cerebral cortex, which is primarily associated with atrophic processes. Atrophy within a brain affected by dementia will be noted in areas of the frontal and temporal lobes, but only minimal atrophy occurs within the centrum semiovale. The ventricles are also typically enlarged.

One brain alteration that occurs as a result of Alzheimer's dementia is neuritic plaque formation. Others include selective neuron loss and shrinkage, loss of synapses, and the alteration of neuritic processes. A positive relation has been shown among the level of dementia severity, the occurrence of senile plaque density, and the decline of cholinergic markers. Most patients with dementia have abundant plaque accumulation and a decrease of cholinergic markers such as somatostatin. A distinct microscopic feature of Alzheimer's dementia is the selective nature of neuron loss or decline. This loss has been shown to be greatest in the neocortex pyramidal neurons of both the temporal and the frontal lobes of the brain.

The most consistent neurotransmitter alteration found in the Alzheimer's dementia brain is the loss of cholinergic markers. Biopsy of the brain in the earlier stages of Alzheimer's dementia shows that choline acetyltransferase is lower than normal. A high-affinity uptake of chlorine is seen, whereas acetylcholine synthesis is reduced in the Alzheimer's dementia disease process.

Postmortem examination shows presynaptic noradrenergic deficits in the neocortex of patients with Alzheimer's dementia. Apart from these deficits, Alzheimer's dementia disease progression depletes neurotransmitters such as serotonin, somatostatin, corticotropin-releasing factor, and glutamate. Evidence obtained from animals with dementia-like states showed lesions of the cholinergic tracks, which caused severe deficits in cognition. This combination of evidence has prompted investigators to develop means to intervene in the damage and losses caused by acetylcholinesterase inhibitors. Other research has suggested that the loss of other neurotransmitters may limit the potential benefits of the cholinergic symptomatic approach.

Clinical Assessment of Delirium and Dementia

Effective treatment of neurocognitive disorders is dependent on accurate assessment, and a complete history and examination are paramount for correct diagnosis. The use of various screening tools can provide additional clinical information in the identification of the disorder.

The Mini Mental State Examination (Folstein et al. 1985), the Confusion Rating Scale (Williams 1991), the Delirium Symptom Interview (Albert et al. 1992), the Delirium Rating Scale (Trzepacz et al. 1988), and the Confusion Assessment Method (Inouye et al. 1990) all have been shown to be effective instruments for identifying and diagnosing delirium (Fricchione et al. 2008).

Screening tools available for standardized assessment of cognitive dysfunction in dementia include the Mini Mental State Examination, the Abbreviated Mental Test (Hodkinson 1972), the Montreal Cognitive Assessment (Nasreddine et al. 2005), and the clinical and neuropsychological batteries developed by the Consortium to Establish a Registry for Alzheimer's Disease (CERAD; Fillenbaum et al. 2008).

Medications Used to Treat Psychiatric Symptoms in Delirium and Dementia

Delirium

The treatment of delirium involves two main strategies. First, the underlying causes that are affecting the brain should be treated, and then the brain must be optimized for proper functioning. The pharmacological management of delirium includes administration of first- and second-generation antipsychotics. For long-standing delirium, antidepressants and mood stabilizers may be indicated. These medications have different functions and are used for different purposes. The side effects of these various medications are listed in Table 10–3.

Antipsychotics tend to be lipophilic in nature and are well absorbed within the body. Antipsychotics are high plasma-binding protein agents that are typically widely distributed and then metabolized by the liver. Antipsychotics as a class, including both first- and second-generation antipsychotics, are known for blocking dopamine D_1-like receptors (which stimulate adenylate cyclase) and dopamine D_2-like receptors (which inhibit adenylate cyclase) at the cortical synapses and the basal ganglia (Keck and McElroy 2002).

The U.S. Food and Drug Administration (FDA) has not yet approved any drug for the treatment of delirium. The American Psychiatric Association (1999) and the Society of Critical Care Medicine (Jacobi et al. 2002) have recommended the use of haloperidol for the treatment of delirium because the potential benefits of the medication outweigh the potential risks associated with this use. Other medications, including anxiolytic and mood-stabilizing agents, also have been used in the treatment of delirium. These medications are prescribed according to the signs and symptoms of the clinical presentation. It should be noted again that all antipsychotics have a black box warning regarding their use in patients with dementia because of the increased incidence of and risk for myocardial infarction and stroke. If antipsychotics are used in this patient population, patients and families should be made aware of the risks associated with the specific agent, and the patient should be closely monitored, including glucose monitoring. The risk-benefit ratio should be carefully evaluated, and thorough psychoeducation should be provided.

Haloperidol (Haldol), often considered the gold standard in the treatment of delirium, has been shown to be highly effective in treating the symptoms of both active and mixed states of delirium. Administration of haloperidol can be

Table 10–3. Side effects of medications commonly used in the treatment of delirium

Drug group	Generic (trade name)	Side effects
First-generation antipsychotics (first-line medication)	Haloperidol (Haldol)	QT interval prolongation, cardiac arrhythmia, sedation, neuroleptic malignant syndrome, extrapyramidal symptoms
Second-generation antipsychotics (second-line medication)	Olanzapine (Zyprexa); Risperidone (Risperdal); Quetiapine (Seroquel)	QT interval prolongation, cardiac arrhythmia, drowsiness/sedation, lower risk of neuroleptic malignant syndrome and extrapyramidal symptoms
Benzodiazepines (used in some circumstances for alcohol and benzodiazepine withdrawal)	Lorazepam (Ativan); Clonazepam (Klonopin); Chlordiazepoxide (Librium); Oxazepam (Serax)	Drowsiness, dizziness, hypotension, blurring of vision
Mood stabilizers (rarely used)	Lithium (Lithobid); Valproic acid (Depakote)	Cardiac arrhythmia, increased urination and thirst, hypothyroidism

oral, intravenous, or intramuscular. Intravenous haloperidol has been shown to cause fewer extrapyramidal side effects (EPS; noted as muscle movements such as akathisia or akinesia, which occur as a result of taking antipsychotic medications) and may be more advantageous to patients in an intensive care unit or critical care step-down unit, where intravenous medication can be closely observed (Menza et al. 1987).

Also used in the treatment of delirium are risperidone (Risperdal), olanzapine (Zyprexa), and quetiapine (Seroquel). Risperidone binds at the D_2 receptor and at several 5-HT receptor sites. Risperidone has been shown to be effective in the treatment of delirium and has a linear pharmacokinetic effect, with the patient reaching the stable state of the drug within 24 hours with both oral and intramuscular administration. Risperidone is rapidly absorbed in the body when administered orally. On reaching the liver, one-third of the medication is metabolized prior to arriving in the systemic circulation. Like haloperidol, risperidone can be very effective for treating hyperactive and mixed states of delirium. In addition, risperidone can contribute to improving both cognition and behavior in delirious patients. Incidents of drowsiness, oversedation, hypotension, and tachycardia, as well as EPS, also have been linked to risperidone (Keck and McElroy 2002).

Olanzapine is a thienobenzodiazepine that has a very similar structure to clozapine (Clozaril), another antipsychotic. Olanzapine has an affinity for $5-HT_2$ and, to a lesser extent, D_2 receptors. Histamine H_1 and α_1-adrenergic receptors are also shown to have an affinity to olanzapine (Keck and McElroy 2002). The drug has a bioavailability as high as 80%. Because it affects the α_1-adrenergic receptors, olanzapine brings about the effect of sedation, which can be highly desirable in cases of active or mixed states of delirium. Because of the effects associated with its procholinergic properties, olanzapine has been shown to be useful in improving cognitive functioning in patients as well. Olanzapine is readily available in tablets, intramuscular formulations, and disintegrating tablets. The drug is well absorbed and reaches peak plasma concentrations within 6 hours (Keck and McElroy 2002). Elimination is rapid, and the drug achieves first-pass metabolism with about 40% having been metabolized before arriving in systemic circulation. Because the drug has linear kinetics, the half-life elimination is about 30 hours, and a stable condition is attained in about 5–7 days.

Quetiapine is a derivative of dibenzothiazepine that also has shown efficacy in the management of psychosis. Quetiapine has a weak affinity for D_1, muscarinic M_1, and $5-HT_{1A}$ receptors and a moderate affinity for H_1, $5-HT_{2A/2C}$, and α_1- and α_2-adrenergic receptors. This medication shows antagonism to the D_2 receptor. After oral administration of quetiapine, rapid absorption occurs, and peak concentrations in the plasma are reached within 1–1.5 hours. Administration of quetiapine with food reduces the bioavailability, which should be taken into account for those patients who do not have adequate oral intake (Keck and McElroy 2002). Quetiapine is noted to be highly plasma protein bound. Metabolism of quetiapine occurs in the liver, and the mean half-life is 2–3 hours. Those patients with renal impairment experience reduced elimination by about 25% without any significant change in clinical plasma concentration.

Dementia

Individuals with dementia have a variety of symptoms that require careful assessment. Because the clinical presentation of dementia varies, clinicians can best assess symptoms by categorizing them into cognitive dysfunction, mood disorders, and behavioral disruption related to aggression, psychosis, anxiety, depression, and sleep changes.

In regard to cognitive decline in dementia, no specific medications are available to stop brain-cell loss; however, medications are available that aim to slow the progression of brain-cell loss. The FDA has approved two types of drugs for the treatment of the cognitive symptoms of dementia: acetylcholinesterase inhibitors and N-methyl-D-aspartate (NMDA) antagonists. The side effects of these cognition-enhancing agents are listed in Table 10–4. These agents are described later in this chapter (see "Dementia" section under "Dosing Guidelines").

Pharmacological treatment of the behavioral and mood symptoms associated with dementia involves psychotropic medications commonly used to treat other psychiatric disorders, including antidepressants, mood stabilizers, and antipsychotics (detailed information on the use and monitoring of these agents can be found in Chapter 3, "Depressive Disorders," Chapter 4, "Bipolar Disorders," and Chapter 5, "Psychotic Disorders," respectively). Treatment efficacy is maximized by correctly identifying and addressing the underlying causes of the patient's symptoms (Caselli and Windle 2011).

Underlying mood disorders are often found in patients with dementia, and these require the use of antidepressants (Caselli and Windle 2011). Stahl (2011) noted that depression can occur before the onset of dementia. The management of depression and dementia that also may coexist with delirium can be difficult among the older adult population. For patients with dementia, there may be improved efficacy with serotonin-norepinephrine reuptake inhibitors (SNRIs) targeting the symptoms of both depressed mood and cognitive decline (Stahl 2011). Medications such as duloxetine (Cymbalta) have shown some positive efficacy in such cases. SNRI antidepressants in these cases will block proteins within the presynaptic neurons that function as the reuptake mechanism. The function augments the concentration of both neurotransmitters at the synaptic cleft.

Table 10–4.   Side effects of medications commonly used in the
treatment of dementia

Drug group	Generic (trade name)	Side effects
Acetylcholinesterase inhibitors	Donepezil (Aricept); Galantamine (Razadyne); Rivastigmine (Exelon)	Anorexia, nausea, vomiting, diarrhea, abdominal pain
N-methyl-D-aspartate antagonists	Memantine (Namenda)	Constipation, fatigue, drowsiness

Anticonvulsants have some use in the treatment of mood stabilization in patients with dementia, specifically among those patients with behavior problems, such as are seen in aggression or disinhibition. Common anticonvulsants used in these cases include divalproex sodium (Depakene, Depakote), carbamazepine (Tegretol), and gabapentin (Neurontin). These medications have shown positive effects in the management of mood related to agitation and some aggressive behaviors. Although anticonvulsants are well tolerated, clinicians should monitor for skin changes associated with rash, sedation, gait alterations, weight gain, and thrombocytopenia.

The treatment of behavioral symptoms of aggression or psychosis in dementia patients is an important concern because behavioral disruptions can decrease the quality of life for patients, families, and caregivers. Nonpharmacological interventions should be the first line of approach because of the various complications that often occur when pharmacological interventions are introduced to patients with dementia. Nonpharmacological interventions such as behavioral management, environmental changes, sensory changes relative to sound and light, and social interaction can all play a role in the shifting of stimulation for the individual with dementia (Aupperle 2006).

First- and second-generation antipsychotics have been shown to be effective when used for aggression and psychosis, yet both categories of medications have potentially negative effects on patients. Aupperle (2006) reported that first-generation antipsychotics may reduce symptoms associated with aggressive behavior in patients but have little effect on agitation. In addition, the incidence of EPS is high in older adults, so caution and monitoring are necessary when first-generation antipsychotics are used. Second-generation antipsychotics cause fewer EPS when used in patients with psychotic spectrum symptoms, but caution is needed because of black box warnings for patients with dementia resulting from increased death rates among patients with dementia taking second-generation antipsychotics. Careful and detailed documentation is required when prescribing second-generation antipsychotics to patients with dementia to ensure a clear justification for the use; to articulate relative dosing and how monitoring will be conducted; and to record the patient's and/or family members' agreement with the explanation, justification, and dosing of the medication, including their understanding of the black box warning.

Dosing Guidelines

Delirium

First-Generation Antipsychotics

According to the American Psychiatric Association (1999) guidelines, haloperidol is the drug of choice for delirium in most patients because it has fewer anticholinergic side effects and EPS compared with other antipsychotics and has shown to be highly effective. The dose of haloperidol should be started at 1–2 mg every 2–4 hours and should be titrated to a higher dose if the patient remains agitated after a few hours. Patients who require multiple doses of haloperidol should be closely monitored for side effects. Generally, 2–20 mg/day is required for haloperidol to bind to 60% of the D_2 receptors, which is necessary to achieve the antipsychotic effect, but high doses of haloperidol may be excessive in treatment of delirium and produce side effects.

Generally, symptoms of delirium can persist from 1 week to 2 months. In most cases, however, patients recover within 10–12 days. Haloperidol should be continued during that period to avoid further complications.

Second-Generation Antipsychotics

The starting dosage of olanzapine should be 2.5–5 mg at bedtime. The dosage can be increased to 20 mg/day if symptoms persist. The ideal starting dosage of risperidone is 0.25–0.5 mg twice daily for symptomatic relief, which can be increased to 4 mg/day if the symptoms fail to clear. In clinical medicine, 0.25–0.5 mg of risperidone every 4 hours is used for patients with agitation and increased delirium. For quetiapine, 25–50 mg twice daily is considered the ideal starting dosage; this can be increased to 100 mg twice daily based on the condition of the patient. Usually, these drugs are continued for 7–10 days, even after the patient returns to baseline (Schwartz and Masand 2002).

Benzodiazepines

Benzodiazepines are not recommended in the treatment of delirium, unless the delirium is related to alcohol or benzodiazepine withdrawal. A long-acting benzodiazepine dose can be given initially and then tapered. Clinicians should remember that alcohol withdrawal typically peaks at 1–3 days, and withdrawal can last 5–7 days. Benzodiazepine withdrawal varies. Short-acting benzodiazepine peak withdrawal is between 2 and 4 days, and longer-acting benzodiazepine peak withdrawal lasts 4–7 days. The duration of benzodiazepine withdrawal for long-acting sedatives is between 7 and 14 days, with short-acting sedatives lasting 4–7 days. Predictive factors that can indicate the possible onset of delirium related to alcohol and benzodiazepine withdrawal include a history of delirium tremens or withdrawal seizures.

Dementia

The treatment protocol for dementia consists of mainly symptomatic treatment. Patients with dementia can present with memory impairment and other cognitive dysfunction, mood changes such as depression and anxiety, behavioral symptoms such as aggression and agitation, and sometimes hallucinations, paranoia, and delusions.

Two classes of drugs are approved for the treatment of cognitive symptoms in dementia: acetylcholinesterase inhibitors and *N*-methyl-D-aspartate (NMDA) antagonists.

Caprylidene, a medical food, has show efficacy in the stabilization of memory and cognitive function associated with mild to moderate Alzheimer's disease. It does not, however, reverse the degenerative process or reverse the cognitive decline existing prior to beginning this therapy.

The first- and second-generation antipsychotic medications (e.g., haloperidol, risperidone, quetiapine) have been used to treat agitation and aggressive behaviors associated with dementia. Additionally, the antidepressants (e.g., escitalopram, citalopram) have been used to relieve the associated symptoms of depression and anxiety that may occur comorbidly with dementia.

Acetylcholinesterase Inhibitors

Symptoms related to the dementia disease process, such as decline in memory, impaired awareness, and altered cognitive functioning, are often best treated by medications from the class of drugs known as acetylcholinesterase inhibitors. Commonly prescribed acetylcholinesterase inhibitors include donepezil (Aricept), rivastigmine (Exelon), and galantamine (Reminyl, Razadyne). The function of this class of drugs is to augment the neurotransmitter acetylcholine within the brain itself. Increased levels of acetylcholine have been linked to improved cognitive functioning (Caselli and Windle 2011). Acetylcholinesterase inhibitors are absorbed within the gastrointestinal tract, with varying concentration peaks cited, depending on the specific medication (Jann et al. 2002).

Tacrine (Cognex), the first-ever drug in this group, was approved by the FDA in 1993, but it is not used currently because it has been linked to significant liver damage. Donepezil, rivastigmine, and galantamine received FDA approval in 1996, 2000, and 2001, respectively. These agents, which tend to be well tolerated with few side effects, are widely utilized in Alzheimer's-type dementia (Table 10–5).

Donepezil is initiated at 5 mg/day for 30 days before increasing to 10 mg/day. For patients with moderate to severe Alzheimer's disease, the dosage can be increased to 23 mg/day after 3 months.

Rivastigmine is started at 1.5 mg twice a day, which can be increased in increments of 3 mg/day every 2 weeks to a maximum dosage of 12 mg/day. Rivastigmine is also available in transdermal administration of a 4.6 mg/24 hour patch, which can be increased after 30 days to the larger patch of 9.5 mg/24 hours.

Galantamine is available in an immediate-release formulation (which requires twice-a-day dosing) and a daily extended-release formulation. Dosage is started at a total of 8 mg/day, which can be increased every 30 days to a maximum dosage of 24 mg/day.

NMDA Antagonists

In 2003, the FDA approved memantine (Namenda), an NMDA antagonist that modifies the functioning of NMDA brain receptors, for use in the treatment of Alzheimer's disease. The starting dose for memantine is 5 mg once daily. The dosage can be increased to 10 mg/day after 1 week.

Table 10–5. Acetylcholinesterase inhibitors

Drug	Starting dosage	Titration	Recommended target dosage	Minimum therapeutic dosage	Formulations
Donepezil (Aricept)	5 mg/day	Every 4 weeks	10 mg/day	5 mg/day	5- and 10-mg tablets
Galantamine IR (Razadyne IR)	4 mg twice daily	Every 4 weeks	12 mg twice daily	8 mg twice daily	4-, 8-, and 12-mg tablets
Galantamine ER (Razadyne ER)	8 mg/day	Every 4 weeks	24 mg/day	16 mg/day	8-, 12-, and 24-mg tablets
Rivastigmine (Exelon)	1.5 mg twice daily	Every 4 weeks	6 mg twice daily	3 mg twice daily	1.5-, 3-, 4.5-, and 6-mg tablets

Note.   ER=extended release; IR=immediate release.

Medical Foods

In 2009, the FDA approved caprylidene (Axona) for the clinical dietary management of the metabolic processes associated with mild to moderate Alzheimer's disease. Caprylidene is a medical food that increases the concentration of ketone bodies in the blood and brain and is hypothesized to help counter the effects of impaired cortical glucose metabolism in Alzheimer's disease. The drug is formulated as a powder (supplied in 40-g packets) to be dissolved in water. The recommended dosage is one packet taken once per day, as tolerated, with monitoring of intestinal side effects. Laboratory tests such as blood urea nitrogen (BUN), creatinine, uric acid, and triglycerides may also be used in monitoring.

First- and Second-Generation Antipsychotics

Haloperidol, a first-generation antipsychotic, can be dosed at less than 1.5 mg/day, showing a variable effect in lower doses. Monitoring for EPS, anticholinergic effects, oversedation, tardive dyskinesia, neuroleptic malignant syndrome, changes in blood pressure, and prolonged QT time is required. Second-generation antipsychotics, which have a black box warning, must be used with caution. Prescribers must provide a detailed explanation of the increased mortality risk to patients and families and ensure clear documentation of all explanations, dosing, and the patients' acknowledged understanding of risk, dosing, and monitoring.

Dosing for risperidone is between 0.5 and 1 mg typically at bedtime to improve both agitation and psychosis. Its hypnotic effects are an added benefit, which may aid in sleep. Quetiapine can be started as low as 12.5 mg twice daily for reduction in psychosis and agitation. Hypnotic effects and reduction in some anxiety symptoms also have been noted when dosed at bedtime. Olanzapine dosing starts at 2.5–10 mg to improve aggressive symptoms and psychosis; typically, the dose is given at bedtime because of its hypnotic effects, which may improve sleep. Although the incidence of EPS is decreased with second-generation antipsychotics, monitoring for EPS, QT prolongation, sedation, blood pressure changes, tardive dyskinesia, and neuroleptic malignant syndrome should be ongoing among older adults receiving this class of medication.

Antidepressants

Serotonin specific antidepressants are well tolerated and commonly prescribed for patients with dementia. The selective serotonin reuptake inhibitor

(SSRI) citalopram is widely used in this population because of its high tolerability and efficacy and limited medication interactions. The starting dosage of citalopram (Celexa) is 10–20 mg/day, with titration up to 40 mg/day. Citalopram has shown efficacy for depression symptoms and some reduction in agitation among patients with dementia. Side effects typically are gastrointestinal, such as nausea and constipation, with dry mouth, headache, and fatigue also noted.

Duloxetine, an SNRI, has been shown to be effective in the treatment of depression among dementia patients (Stahl 2011). Dosing for duloxetine typically begins at 30 mg/day, with augmentation after 7 days based on tolerance. The recommended target dosage is 60 mg/day. Common side effects include nausea, dry mouth, constipation, fatigue, and headache. Duloxetine also has been effective for pain associated with diabetic peripheral neuropathy and fibromyalgia.

The serotonin antagonist and reuptake inhibitor trazodone (Desyrel) has antidepressant effects, yet the sedation often associated with administration promotes its use for hypnotic effects. Trazodone also shows some benefit in reducing verbal aggression. Dosing starts at 25 mg/day, typically taken at bedtime, with augmentation up to 300 mg/day based on tolerance and reduction of symptoms.

Anticonvulsant Mood Stabilizers

Off-label use of anticonvulsants for mood-stabilizing effect should be explained to patients and families and should be well documented. Divalproex can be dosed off-label for mood management to reduce agitation in dementia patients over time. Typically, the dosage starts at 5–12.5 mg/kg/day and may be slowly increased based on tolerance, side effects, and reduction in symptoms. Clinicians must remember to start low and go slow in the older population. Monitoring blood levels for toxicity and for elevation in liver enzymes is necessary.

Dosing for carbamazepine also varies depending on the patient's height, weight, medical stabilization, and level of aggression. Typically, the starting dosage is 100 mg/day in chewable form or 200 mg/day in tablet form, with augmentation based on symptom control, tolerance, and side-effect profile. Monitoring blood levels for toxicity is key. Laboratory values for liver dysfunction, decreases in sodium levels, and decreases in white blood cell count must be monitored.

Anxiolytics

Buspirone (BuSpar) has been shown to reduce anxiety symptoms among patients with dementia. Dosing starts at 5 mg two to three times per day, with augmentation based on tolerance and reduction of symptoms. Side effects associated with buspirone include drowsiness, nausea, constipation, headache, and dry mouth. Patients can experience gait changes, so monitoring of ambulation should be considered. Caution should be used when prescribing buspirone for patients with hepatic or kidney disease.

Benzodiazepines can be considered in the management of anxiety symptoms in dementia, yet great caution must be observed when prescribing this class of medications. Because of greater sensitivity to benzodiazepines among older adults, the potential for increased confusion, increased agitation, gait and balance problems, cognitive changes, and slowed motor functioning may outweigh any potential benefit to be gained in prescribing this class of medication to patients with dementia with an anxiety presentation. If benzodiazepines are prescribed, the lowest dose should be considered after a careful evaluation is made.

Treatment of Special Populations

Delirium

Even though delirium is thought to predominantly affect elderly populations, it can also occur in children and adolescents. The main causes are infections, neoplasms, and drug-mediated delirium. The main symptoms in pediatrics include impaired attention, poor concentration, confusion, and impaired responsiveness. Children and adolescents are given haloperidol, with a dosage range of 0.25–1 mg/day, by oral or intravenous route. Low-potency antipsychotic agents (chlorpromazine) are used in a few cases (Turkel and Tavaré 2003).

Critically ill or medically compromised patients may experience hallucinations and delusions and may become agitated. Some analgesics (e.g., meperidine [Demerol]) have strong anticholinergic properties and must be replaced with drugs without anticholinergic effects to prevent central nervous system excitation and other symptoms of delirium. Then medications such as typical antipsychotics (e.g., haloperidol) and atypical antipsychotics should be started (American Psychiatric Association 1999). In terminal delirium, the patient is actively dying as a result of other comorbid factors and may experience delirium during that period. To lessen the distress of the patient, sedative drugs such as benzodiazepines are used. Common preparations are lorazepam (Ativan) 1–2 mg predissolved in 3–4 mL of water and then placed along the buccal mucosa.

Dementia

Dementia usually occurs in elderly patients, but certain medical conditions— such as infection, poisoning, Niemann-Pick disease, Batten disease, and Lafora disease—can lead to dementia in children. Symptoms of childhood dementia include confusion, speech and language problems, difficulty performing simple tasks, and changes in mood and behavior. Childhood dementia usually requires psychotherapy instead of pharmacological intervention. Following proper guidelines can alleviate symptoms in most patients (Mace and Peter 2006).

Medically compromised patients with dementia may have anxiety, depression, and paranoia. In addition to routine psychotherapy and pharmacological intervention, electroconvulsive therapy can be used to treat depression in the setting of dementia (Oudman 2012). Lewy body dementia can be ameliorated with acetylcholinesterase medications, as they have a favorable side-effect profile and may also benefit delusions, hallucinations, and apathy (Overshott et al. 2004).

Nonpharmacological Treatment

Several factors other than the usual medications play a vital role in treating symptoms of delirium and dementia. Behavioral adaptations are of great importance in treating delirium and dementia. Given the strain of delirium and dementia on family members and caregivers, education and counseling should be offered as ancillary treatments as well.

Environmental and psychological factors can affect the outcome of a patient with delirium or dementia. Actions that can assist in the patient's recovery are as follows:

- Clearly communicate with the patient.
- Remind the patient about date and time.

- Help the patient to identify individuals.
- Minimize number of staff working with the patient.
- Help the patient in regaining orientation.
- Encourage family members to bring objects from home that are familiar to the patient.
- Move delirious patients to a private room with minimal noise and proper lighting.
- Avoid understimulation.
- Adjust lighting to daytime-nighttime patterns.
- Provide a sitter if the patient is agitated to help the patient calm down (Emanuel et al. 2005).

Summary

Delirium and dementia are often considered diseases of old age and hospitalized patients, but the onset of both conditions can strike individuals at various times across the life span. Effective psychopharmacological management can help a patient reestablish his or her normal life more rapidly, thus effectively increasing quality of life and potentially reducing health care costs. Medications have been developed to treat the symptoms of these disorders, and these medications have become a vital part of the treatment plan.

Clinical Pearls

- Delirium is common among critically ill patients.
- Delirium is associated with increased rates of morbidity and mortality.
- Delirium can be managed with coadministration of antipsychotics and anxiolytics; however, benzodiazepines given as monotherapy tend to contribute to increased agitation.
- Caregivers should be alert to harbingers (e.g., sudden neurological decline and day-night reversal).
- Dementia impairs previously acquired neurological functions.
- Dementia cannot be cured.

- Disease progression in dementia of the Alzheimer's type can be slowed with acetylcholinesterase inhibitors.
- Comorbid symptoms of anxiety and depression can be treated with antidepressants.
- Family members should be counseled that behavior associated with delirium is not related to the patient's personality.
- The patient and his or her family members should be offered counseling. In particular, family members should be advised that behavior associated with delirium is not related to the patient's personality.
- Dementia should be identified as early as possible to mitigate morbidity and mortality.

References

Alagiakrishnan K, Blanchette P: Delirium treatment and management. 2011. Available at: http://emedicine.medscape.com/article/288890-treatment. Accessed December 10, 2011.

Albert MS, Levkoff SE, Reilly C, et al: The delirium symptom interview: an interview for the detection of delirium symptoms in hospitalized patients. J Geriatr Psychiatry Neurol 5:14–21, 1992

Alexander E: Delirium in the intensive care unit: medications as risk factors. Crit Care Nurs 29:85–87, 2009

Alzheimer's Association: 2012 Alzheimer's disease facts and figures. Alzheimers Dement 8:131–168, 2012

American Psychiatric Association: Practice guideline for the treatment of patients with delirium. Am J Psychiatry 156:1–20, 1999

American Psychiatric Association: Diagnostic and Statistical Manual of Mental Disorders, 4th Edition, Text Revision. Washington, DC, American Psychiatric Association, 2000

Aupperle P: Management of aggression, agitation, and psychosis in dementia: focus on atypical antipsychotics. Am J Alzheimers Dis Other Demen 21:101–108, 2006

Boustani M, Buttar A: Delirium, in Primary Care Geriatrics, A Case-Based Approach, 5th Edition. Edited by Ham R, Sloane P, Warshaw G, et al. St. Louis, MO, Mosby, 2007, pp 210–218

Brodaty H: Overview of dementia. 2008. Available at: http://www.cmglinks.com/cmg/lectures_dementia/part1/001.htm. Accessed December 10, 2011.

Burns A, Gallagley A, Byrne J: Delirium. J Neurol Neurosurg Psychiatry 75:362–367, 2004

Caselli RJ, Windle ML: Dementia medication overview. 2011. Available at: http://www.emedicinehealth.com/dementia_medication_overview/page2_em.htm. Accessed December 10, 2011.

Cole MG, Ciampi A, Belzile E, et al: Persistent delirium in older hospital patients: a systematic review of frequency and prognosis. Age Ageing 38:19–26, 2009

Emanuel L, Ferris D, Gunten V, et al: Education in Palliative and End of Life Care. Chicago, IL, Thompson Press, 2005

Fillenbaum GG, van Belle G, Morris JC, et al: Consortium to Establish a Registry for Alzheimer's Disease (CERAD): the first twenty years. Alzheimers Dement 4:96–109, 2008

Folstein M, Anthony JC, Parhad I, et al: The meaning of cognitive impairment in the elderly. J Am Geriatr Soc 33:228–235, 1985

Fricchione G, Nejad S, Esses J, et al: Postoperative delirium. Am J Psychiatry 167:803–812, 2008

Hale KL, Frank J: Dementia overview. 2011. Available at: http://www.emedicine-health.com/dementia_overview/page3_em.htm. Accessed December 11, 2011.

Hodkinson HM: Evaluation of a mental test score for assessment of mental impairment in the elderly. Age Ageing 1(4):233-238, 1972

Inouye SK, van Dyck CH, Alessi CA, et al: Clarifying confusion: the confusion assessment method. A new method for detection of delirium. Ann Intern Med 113:941–948, 1990

Jann M, Shirley K, Small G: Clinical pharmacokinetics and pharmacodynamics of cholinesterase inhibitors. Clin Pharmacokinet 41:719–739, 2002

Jacobi J, Fraser GL, Coursin DB, et al: Clinical practice guidelines for the sustained use of sedatives and analgesics in the critically ill adult. Task Force of the American College of Critical Care Medicine (ACCM) of the Society of Critical Care Medicine (SCCM), American Society of Health-System Pharmacists (ASHP), American College of Chest Physicians. Crit Care Med 30:119–141, 2002; erratum in: Crit Care Med 30:726, 2002

Keck PE Jr, McElroy SL: Clinical pharmacodynamics and pharmacokinetics of antimanic and mood-stabilizing medications. J Clin Psychiatry 63 (suppl 4):3–11, 2002

Mace L, Peter R: The 36-Hour Day: A Family Guide to Caring for Persons With Alzheimer Disease, Related Dementing Illness, and Memory Loss in Later Life. Baltimore, MD, Johns Hopkins Press, 2006

Menza MA, Murray GB, Holmes VF, et al: Decreased extrapyramidal symptoms with intravenous haloperidol. J Clin Psychiatry 48:278–280, 1987

Nasreddine ZS, Phillips NA, Bédirian V, et al: The Montreal Cognitive Assessment, MoCA: a brief screening tool for mild cognitive impairment. J Am Geriatr Soc 53:695–699, 2005

Oudman E: Is electroconvulsive therapy (ECT) effective and safe for treatment of depression in dementia? A short review. J ECT 28:34–38, 2012

Overshott R, Byrne J, Burns A: Nonpharmacological and pharmacological interventions for symptoms in Alzheimer's disease. Expert Rev Neurother 4:809–821, 2004

Sachdev PS: Whither neuropsychiatry? (editorial). J Neuropsychiatry Clin Neurosci 17:140–141, 2005.

Schwartz T, Masand P: The role of atypical antipsychotics in the treatment of delirium. Psychosomatics 43:171–174, 2002

Stahl SM: The Prescriber's Guide: Stahl's Essential Psychopharmacology, 4th Edition. New York, Cambridge University Press, 2011

Trzepacz PT, Baker RW, Greenhouse J: A symptom rating scale for delirium. Psychiatry Res 23:89–97, 1988

Turkel SB, Tavaré CJ: Delirium in children and adolescents. J Neuropsychiatry Clin Neurosci 15:431–435, 2003

Williams MA: Delirium/acute confusional states: evaluation devices in nursing. Int Psychogeriatr 3:301–308, 1991

PART II

Special Issues in Clinical Psychopharmacology

Psychopharmacology in Psychiatric Emergencies

Mary Kay Dollard, M.S.N., A.P.R.N., P.M.H.-N.P., B.C.

> Days spent idle in an emergency room represent wasted opportunities to prevent suicide, assault, and suffering. Someone in the midst of a psychiatric crisis needs to be surrounded by safety, not chaos.
>
> —Dr. Jeffrey Fetter, President,
> New Hampshire Psychiatric Society

Patients in psychiatric *crisis* (a term used interchangeably with *emergency*) present to medical emergency departments, dedicated psychiatric emergency departments, crisis centers, and jails. They may be alone or escorted by family, caregivers, community-based crisis intervention teams, ambulance, or police officers. The accepting sites can serve as holding facilities until an agitated patient calms down, detoxification centers until an inebriated person sobers up, or psychiatric hospital gateways for a person needing longer-term mental health care. The models of response in these settings are variable, and new ones are constantly being studied and implemented. The details of each are beyond the scope of this chapter, but common to all is the necessity of rapid evaluation and management. This can best be done by developing a therapeutic alliance with the patient and accompanying personnel, containment of danger, diligent triage, ruling out of medical etiology, and providing supportive measures and treatment in the least restrictive manner (Di Fiorino et al. 2005; Lee et al. 2003; Ramadan 2007; Sadock and Sadock 2007; Zeller 2010). Some models go on to use strategies of aftercare, such as referral to appropriate community services, in hopes of minimizing or mitigating future crises. In these, arguably more thorough, models, behavioral control at presentation is made within the context of the greater disorder, and pharmacological interventions are usually chosen with discharge in mind.

Although the settings to which patients in psychiatric crisis present are varied, and the models of care and protocols for response many, the incidence of mental health emergencies is unquestionably on the rise (Jayaram and Triplett 2008; Lee et al. 2003; Sadock and Sadock 2007; Selverston 2004; Zeller 2010). In the United States, psychiatric emergency services continue to evolve, driven by "treatment advances, fiscal constraints, and changes in mental health paradigms" (Lee et al. 2003, p. 1590). The number of documented psychiatric emergency episodes has more than doubled since 1970, according to Di Fiorino et al. (2005). Zeller (2010) reported that 53 million mental health–related emergency department contacts were made in the United States annually between 1992 and 2001, which represents an increase from 4.9% to 6.3% of all emergency department visits during that period.

Some argue that this rise can be attributed to deinstitutionalization, inadequate community resources (Di Fiorino et al. 2005; Zeller 2010), and privatization of mental health care (Lester 2009). Others attribute the increase to the accessibility and convenience of emergency departments as health care costs rise and fewer are adequately insured to maintain regular psychiatric care (Lester 2009; Zeller 2010). Whatever the reason, the results are clear, and our proper understanding of what constitutes these crises, as well as appropriate treatment of them, is most important.

Approach to Psychiatric Crisis Intervention

According to Selverston (2004, p. 507), a *crisis* is "the painful, frightening human experience that occurs when [a person] is faced with an overwhelming threat to (his or her) equilibrium or familiar state of being." A psychiatric emergency, specifically, can be defined as "any disturbance in thoughts, feelings, or actions for which immediate therapeutic intervention is necessary" (Sadock and Sadock 2007, p. 907). The most common presentations of these emergencies are exacerbations of mood, psychotic, or substance abuse disorders. Sadock and Sadock (2007) contended that 20% of these patients present as suicidal and 10% as violent.

The standard evaluation of a psychiatric emergency includes history gathering, physical evaluation, and a mental status examination. However, the volatile nature of these cases often necessitates situational modifications in both procedure and ethics. The rules of thorough evaluation and strict confidentiality that apply to most outpatient procedures often need to be put aside for the quickest and least harmful intervention. Moreover, consent for treatment can be difficult to obtain because the patient may lack insight into his or her condition or show impaired reality testing or diminished capacity to make sound decisions for himself or herself. In these instances, measures are taken that can be seen as limiting the patient's freedom, but Sadock and Sadock (2007) stated that the emergency clinician must be pragmatic and use every available mode of therapeutic intervention to resolve a crisis, with "less concern than usual about diluting a therapeutic relationship" (p. 911).

In these situations, collateral history attained from accompanying parties can be of paramount importance in determining the ultimate plan of care. These individuals may have a unique perspective on precipitating events, which can be as helpful as laboratory tests in surmising etiology. Known medical history, a recent assault to the patient's person or psyche, illicit or prescribed substance intake, expressed suicidal or homicidal ideation, and threats of harm to self or others are vital components of a thorough history. Because the patient may be reluctant (or unable) to report this information at the time of crisis, the clinician is wise to use this resource.

Also noteworthy is the state of these accompanying parties because they are likely to have been traumatized to an extent before arriving to you as well. The roles of caregivers and security personnel are associated with extraordinary stressors, and a crisis is sure to have exacerbated the situation. In these situations, collateral emotions can run high. Providing a calm, safe, controlled environment for all parties can be a necessary first step in ensuring safety, as well as in attaining historical information. The clinician must seek assistance when necessary but maintain vigilance regarding the manner in which that assistance is given to minimize the volatility of the situation. Although the patient may require immediate treatment, the other parties also may need care, and the clinician must take this into careful account.

To best understand the patient's presentation and perception, an empathetic approach can be a nurse practitioner's most valuable clinical resource. Selverston (2004) argued that the common nursing goal "to understand the person as a whole by assessing both internal and external factors" is particularly important in crisis intervention. Nurse practitioners are expected to delve as deeply into the biological as the psychological and social aspects of each presenting problem. The patient in psychiatric distress is fragile and may lack insight into his or her condition. Perhaps because of impairment or previously negative experiences in such settings, some patients will be untrusting and wary of the psychiatric services they are receiving (Sadock and Sadock 2007). Here, empathy and a nonthreatening, collaborative approach can go a long way. The clinician must be clear in communication and have the patient's best interest in mind at all times.

Differential Diagnosis in Psychiatric Emergency Assessment

When approaching treatment, the emergency clinician must prioritize symptomatic treatment according to codified psychiatric diagnoses because even reimbursement is in direct proportion to the patient's dangerousness at presentation rather than severity of mental illness (Di Fiorino et al. 2005). Mechanisms that lead to agitation also may predispose to impulsivity, aggression, and psychosis. These symptoms are not limited to any specific psychiatric disorders. Thus, differential diagnosis of nonpsychiatric causes for new onset of these behaviors is important. Organic etiology must be ruled out before starting psychopharmacological treatment because one-third of medical conditions present with psychiatric manifestations (Sadock and Sadock 2007).

Some common nonpsychiatric causes for these crises include medication side effects, head trauma, delirium, diabetes mellitus, organ failure, neurological and endocrine or metabolic disturbances, infection, intoxication, and withdrawal (Preston and Johnson 2012; Ramadan 2007; Sadock and Sadock 2007; Schatzberg et al. 2010). Many of these conditions can be life-threatening if missed.

The delineation of causality necessitates diligent observation, proper history taking, and a sound knowledge of this cluster of syndromes. The observant clinician is wise to note if the presentation has had an acute onset, if this is the patient's first similar episode, if recent trauma has occurred (especially to the head), or if known medical comorbidity or substance abuse exists. Additionally, clues such as older age, nonauditory perceptual disturbances, signs of intoxication or withdrawal, pupillary size, and measurement of vital signs should not be missed, because they are keys to etiology and treatment. Important results can come from urine drug screens; complete blood counts; electrolytes; glucose levels; and liver, renal, and thyroid function tests (Fischbach 2004; Ramadan 2007). The clinician also should consider testing for syphilis, HIV, and hepatitis. Pregnancy testing also should be done as appropriate. Electrocardiogram, chest X ray, and computed tomography (CT) scans, or preferably magnetic resonance imaging (MRI) scans, are also helpful tools in the process (American Psychiatric Association 2004).

History and laboratory testing are critical in these emergencies. Likewise, symptom management must be prioritized when psychiatric comorbidity exists. For example, a patient with schizophrenia may present with akathisia, an unfortunate side effect of antipsychotic treatment, which can cause extreme discomfort and restlessness. Although the patient has mental illness, the presenting problem is the motor restlessness and likely agitation from his or her medication. Failure to gather the proper history here could result in a dangerous cascade of events because the clinician could administer more of the precipitating factor to calm the restlessness. Likewise, delirium, which is frequently accompanied by psychomotor disturbances and impulsivity (Piechniczek-Buczek 2010), can present in a known substance user. It also can be the result of an infection or head trauma, however, and lifesaving interventions could be neglected if the onset was not discovered, if proper laboratory testing was not done, or if the presentation was assumed to be part of the

Table 11–1. Medical conditions that may present as psychiatric emergencies

Autoimmune	Metabolic
Lupus	Anoxia/hypoxia
AIDS	Electrolyte disturbances
Endocrine	**Neurological**
Hyper- and hypoglycemia	Tumor
Hyper- and hypothyroidism	Huntington's disease
Hyper- and hypoparathyroidism	Multiple sclerosis
Hyper- and hypopituitarism	Epilepsy
Hypoadrenocorticism	Migraine
Cushing's disease	Central nervous system infection
Pheochromocytoma	Neurosyphilis
Cardiopulmonary	**Others**
Angina	Organ failure
Pulmonary embolus	Trauma
Arrhythmias	Infections
Chronic obstructive pulmonary disease	Toxins
	Vitamin deficiency
	Medications
	Intoxication
	Withdrawal

Source. Adapted from Ramadan 2007; Sadock and Sadock 2007; Townsend 2005.

larger psychiatric diagnosis. Careful observation, history taking, and physical testing are crucial elements of the differential diagnosis in each of these cases.

The reader is referred to the standard reference sources for full diagnostic criteria for the various disorders that include psychosis as an associated or defining feature. Some of the most common medical conditions that may present as psychiatric emergencies are listed in Table 11–1. Conditions to be considered in the differential diagnosis of delirium are shown in Table 11–2.

Table 11–2. Differential diagnosis of delirium

	Delirium	Dementia	Depression	Psychotic illness
Onset	Acute	Gradual	Variable	Variable
Course	Fluctuating	Progressive	Recurrent	Chronic
Consciousness	Altered	Normal	Normal	Normal
Attention	Impaired	Normal (until late)	May be impaired	May be impaired
Orientation	Fluctuating	Impaired	Normal	Normal
Hallucinations	Common	Rare (until late)	Rare	Common

Source. Adapted from Piechniczek-Buczek 2010.

Psychiatric Conditions Requiring Emergency Intervention

Agitation, a common symptom in persons presenting for emergency assessment, may be a manifestation of a patient's underlying depression, anxiety, psychosis, or withdrawal. (The neurobiological underpinnings of depression, anxiety, psychosis, and addiction have been covered in earlier chapters within the text, and the reader is referred to those chapters for discussion of these concepts.) In this section I discuss extreme disturbances of thoughts, mood, and behaviors, particularly as exhibited by restlessness, aggression, or expressed suicidal or homicidal ideation with plan. Table 11–3 lists psychiatric disorders with acute manifestations.

Psychosis

Stahl (2008, p. 1) wrote that "there is perhaps no area of psychiatry where misconceptions are greater than in that of psychotic illness." He contended that psychosis is a term that is misused as often by mental health professionals as by the lay public. Best understood as a syndrome, psychosis is "a mixture of symptoms that can be associated with many different psychiatric conditions, and not a specific disorder in itself. Instead, it is determined by the psychotic patient's mental capacity, affective responses, capacity to recognize reality, communicate, and relate to others" (Stahl 2008, p. 2). Ultimately, the "degree of withdrawal from objective reality" constitutes psychosis (Sadock and Sadock 2007, p. 910). Presenting symptoms include disorganized speech or behavior and distorted reality testing. Aggression is also usually a factor (Stahl 2008).

A history is imperative when determining etiology, especially because acute onset can be life-threatening and necessitates immediate medical intervention. Symptom presentation, including aggression, can require seclusion, restraint, or other rudimentary security measures. Psychopharmacological intervention is called for when medical etiologies have been safely ruled out and calming, assurance, and empathetic listening are initiated. The medications used in these instances include oral and intramuscular formulations of first-generation antipsychotics (FGAs) or second-generation antipsychotics (SGAs), and suppository formulations of the FGA chlorpromazine (Thorazine) are also available. Oral and intramuscular formulations of anticholinergic and antihistaminic medications also can be initiated as a precaution against side effects. Adjunctive

Table 11–3. Psychiatric disorders that may have acute manifestations

Adjustment disorders

Anxiety disorders

Attention-deficit and disruptive behavior disorders

Bereavement

Bipolar disorders

Conversion disorder

Depressive disorders

Impulse-control disorders

Malingering

Personality disorders

Pervasive developmental disorders

Schizophrenia and other psychotic disorders

Sleep disorders

Substance-related disorders

---

oral or intramuscular benzodiazepine treatment also may be initiated. These choices are discussed later in this chapter.

Anxiety

Disorders involving anxiety are among the most common mental disturbances presenting for emergency management. For our purposes, anxiety is specified by the symptoms that predominate. Restlessness and aggression can be manifestations of the aforementioned medical etiologies (Schatzberg et al. 2010) or the exacerbations of psychiatric conditions, including mood disorders, schizophrenia, or substance use (Schatzberg et al. 2010). As with other presentations, ruling out medical causes and applying therapeutic interventions are the clinician's first line of treatment. If the patient is in such distress that he or she becomes combative or otherwise dangerous, however, pharmacological intervention may be initiated. Oral lorazepam (Ativan; 1–3 mg) can be used for less severe presentations of anxiety and repeated hourly until symptoms are improved. This can be increased as needed with a maximum daily dose of 10 mg. In more extreme cases, intramuscular injection is indicated. Commonly, lorazepam 1–3 mg in repeated hourly doses is effective (Schatzberg et al. 2010).

Substance Intoxication and Withdrawal

Substance dependence can be described as both behavioral and physical, the latter including tolerance and withdrawal. The "reversible, nondependent experience" (Sadock and Sadock 2007) of intoxication produces impairment that frequently requires emergent psychiatric intervention. In 2004, an estimated 22.5 million persons older than 12 (10% of the total U.S. population) had a substance-related disorder; 15 million of this group were said to abuse or be dependent on alcohol. Data from this study indicated that heroin dependence or abuse affected 0.3 million in this group, marijuana dependence or abuse affected 4.5 million, cocaine dependence or abuse affected 1.6 million, and prescription drug dependence or abuse affected 1.4 million (Sadock and Sadock 2007).

The DSM-IV-TR (American Psychiatric Association 2000) criteria for substance intoxication and withdrawal include the development of reversible, substance-specific syndromes resulting from recent exposure to or cessation of said substance, respectively. The resulting behaviors can cause clinically significant distress or impairment and are not due to a general medical condition or concomitant psychiatric disorder.

Alcohol

Approximately 1.2 million hospital admissions occur each year for problems related to alcohol abuse, and nearly 5% of these patients go on to develop delirium tremens (McKeown 2010). Although alcohol depresses the central nervous system, like other depressants, it can cause agitation and aggressiveness in some intoxicated people. These symptoms can prompt psychiatric referrals, but subsequent treatment is mostly medical.

As previously suppressed excitatory neurotransmission is unmasked, acute intoxication is overshadowed only by withdrawal after heavy use (McKeown 2010). This can cause minor withdrawal syndromes such as headache, nausea, and dizziness. More troubling and potentially fatal is the severe withdrawal syndrome of delirium tremens, which is a neurological disturbance that can present as psychosis and, if untreated, may be lethal. The person may sweat and tremble uncontrollably and have high blood pressure and temperature. In addition, severe anxiety, insomnia, feelings of terror, and hallucinations (usually nonauditory) may precede grand mal seizures. It is important to treat these symptoms with benzodiazepines to prevent seizures. The benzodiazepines are tapered once withdrawal symptoms are controlled. Dosages are frequently much higher than what is commonly used for treatment of anxiety. Longer-acting formulations like chlordiazepoxide (Librium) are generally thought to provide a smoother, safer withdrawal than other benzodiazepines (Miller and Gold 1998). It is also helpful to initiate supportive measures, including hydration, vitamin B_1 replacement, and pain-relieving medications when not contraindicated.

Benzodiazepines

Benzodiazepine intoxication requires no specific pharmacological intervention (Giannini 2000). Flumazenil (Romazicon), a benzodiazepine antagonist, can be used in critical situations, but caution is necessary because of the potential for sedation and seizures associated with its use. However, withdrawal symptoms are similar in manifestation to those of alcohol. Blood pressure, heart rate, and body temperature should be monitored and other supportive measures initiated. In addition, a precautionary benzodiazepine supplementation and taper should be administered to prevent withdrawal seizures. Long-acting formulations are preferred in these cases as well (Miller and Gold 1998).

Opiates

Heroin intoxication generally produces pleasure, drowsiness, and slowed breathing. The last effect is responsible for most deaths by overdose, and perhaps the only reason for emergency presentation in heroin intoxication. First responders are often equipped with naloxone hydrochloride (Narcan), a pure opioid antagonist, to counter the severe respiratory, sedative, or hypotensive effects caused by opioid overdose (Narcan 2006).

As with other injectable substances, injection heroin users additionally face the risk of numerous blood-borne pathogens from the use of shared and dirty needles. Endocarditis, hepatitis C, HIV, tetanus, and botulism are among the risks. This information should be taken into clinical account for screening and treatment of these patients.

Heroin withdrawal can look like a bad case of influenza, and although it is not fatal in itself, patients report horrific psychic and physical distress. Calming and supportive measures and clonidine (Catapres) can be used in cases of autonomic instability to attenuate withdrawal symptoms of heroin (Stahl 2009).

Stimulants

Intoxication with stimulants like cocaine increases dopamine levels and can cause psychosis. Short-term effects of this drug can include pleasure and alertness at best and paranoia and other forms of psychosis at worst. Cocaine constricts the blood vessels, which can lead to heart damage, stroke, and death. Intoxication with cocaine can cause elevated heart rate and blood pressure, pupillary dilation, chills, muscle cramps, stomach cramps, anorexia, psychomotor agitation or retardation, confusion, seizures, dyskinesias, dystonia, or coma (American Psychiatric Association 2000). When a person experiences cocaine withdrawal, they are said to "crash," which can be accompanied by extreme disturbances in mood. Patients can become severely depressed, complain of extreme fatigue, become irritable, and have outbursts of anger. Physically, the withdrawing patient may have watery eyes, a runny nose, sweating, and vomiting.

Phencyclidine

Phencyclidine (PCP), a dopamine, serotonin, and norepinephrine reuptake inhibitor (Mycek et al. 2000), is a powerful drug that was first used as an anesthetic in veterinary medicine. Very unique, it shares properties with hallucinogens, stimulants, and depressants. The anesthetic properties often lead to extraordinary physical damage to the patient because he or she can feel no pain. Intoxicated patients often have a staggered gait, slurred speech, vertical nystagmus, and muscle rigidity. PCP intoxication can impair memory and attention and cause depression, dissociative amnesia, paranoia, hallucinations, and difficulty breathing. PCP intoxication can also mimic schizophrenia and manifest as symptoms of psychosis, flat affect, agitation, and withdrawal. Hostile and aggressive behavior can occur, but fairly rapid cycling of behavior is also common. Intoxication causes hypersalivation as well as anticholinergic properties (Mycek et al. 2000). Management of this intoxication is mostly limited to seclusion, hydration, and watchful waiting. However, this potentially extreme psychiatric presentation may require psychopharmacological intervention with antipsychotics if aggressive behaviors are not responsive to supportive measures.

Withdrawal from PCP is not in itself fatal, but supportive measures must be taken to control associated impulsivity. The patient may experience anxiety, insomnia, paranoia, panic, irritability, and nausea. Anecdotally, when PCP intoxication has run its course, the patient often returns to a baseline level of functioning without much psychiatric intervention. If he or she is a chronic user, however, the baseline already may be altered and the executive functioning in the prefrontal cortex of the brain compromised.

Societal Perspectives on Substance Use

Acute substance intoxication can require emergent psychiatric interventions. However, the broad implications for drug misuse in itself are grave. Users are predisposed to countless negative dynamics in a society that criminalizes the disease of addiction to substances that mimic many of those we legally prescribe. This reality introduces a unique component to the presentation of many psychiatric emergencies and the treatment that must be offered.

Aggression and Violent Behavior

Aggression can be associated with countless conditions, including disturbances associated with neurological problems, substance intoxication, personality disorders, or suicidal ideation. Clinicians must delineate risk of harm, calm and reassure, and sometimes proceed to pharmacological intervention more rapidly than in other cases. These patients may need to be secluded or restrained, and intramuscular formulations of medication are usually preferred because of their rapidity of onset. The use of both antipsychotic medication and benzodiazepines given at regular intervals to treat target symptoms is common (Ramadan 2007; Schatzberg et al. 2010). Table 11–4 offers an overview of the risk factors for violence against self or others in psychiatric emergencies.

Suicidal Ideation, Threats, and Attempts

Suicidal patients are among the most common presenting to the emergency psychiatric clinician. The patient who verbalizes suicidal ideation remains a potential threat to him- or herself. The acuity of this crisis presentation is

Table 11–4. Factors predictive of suicidal or violent behavior

Extreme calm after attempt

Recent acts of violence

Lethality of threats

Possession of means (e.g., weapons)

Substance intoxication

Psychomotor agitation

Psychosis: poor reality testing, paranoia, presence of command-type auditory hallucinations

Affective instability: lability (tearfulness, lack of verbal restraint)

Impulsivity

Hopelessness

Fearfulness

Guilt

Source. Adapted from American Psychiatric Association 2003; Sadock and Sadock 2007.

overshadowed only by the individual who states a clear plan or one who has made a real attempt on his or her life. In these cases, the clinician must consider all of the likely contributing influences. These can include biological, psychiatric, social, spiritual, and existential factors.

Approximately 30,000 suicides occur each year in the United States (Schatzberg et al. 2010), making it the ninth leading cause of death in this country. Suicide ranks as the third leading cause of death in the 15- to 25-year-old age group. The risk of completed suicide increases with aging of the population, with elderly men being at the highest risk (Ramadan 2007). Rates range from 27.5% in those with previous suicide attempts, to 14.6%–15.5% in the presence of mood disorders, to 6% in people with schizophrenia (American Psychiatric Association 2003).

Other risk factors for suicide include prior attempt(s), depressed mood, hopelessness, psychosis, recent trauma, and substance abuse (see American Foundation for Suicide Prevention Web site at www.afsp.org). The reader is referred to Table 11–5 for an inventory of suicide risk factors.

Table 11–5. Risk factors for suicide

Stated suicidal ideation, threat, intent, or plan

Stated hopelessness or helplessness

Recent threat to self-esteem (real or symbolic)

History of psychiatric illness and/or violence

History of trauma or abuse

History of poor impulse control or poor coping (self-mutilation, recent attempt)

Demographic factors (related to gender, age group, race)

Family history of suicide

Source. Adapted from American Psychiatric Association 2003; Sadock and Sadock 2007.

Few of the medications indicated for the treatment of depression or other mood disorders work quickly enough to be used in the emergency setting; therefore, the emphasis must be on providing a safe environment until behavioral improvement occurs. Longer-term treatment of the underlying disorder is recommended, but in emergency intervention for the acutely suicidal patient, benzodiazepines are most often used (Schatzberg et al. 2010).

Psychotropic Medications Used in Emergency Settings

The pharmacodynamics and pharmacokinetics of the various psychotropic medications—antipsychotics, benzodiazepines, and anticholinergics—used in psychiatric emergencies are addressed in the chapters associated with those specific agents. Please refer to Chapter 2, "Anxiety Disorders," and Chapter 5, "Psychotic Disorders," for additional information on these processes.

Clinical efficacy is directly related to the ability to calm the symptoms that bring the patient into the emergency setting. Medication choices in these situations are limited by factors such as availability and expense, rapidity of intended action, and the patient's history and preference if known. FGAs such as chlorpromazine and haloperidol (Haldol) and SGAs such as risperidone (Risperdal) and olanzapine (Zyprexa) are often used alone or in combination with an antihistaminic or anticholinergic medication for side-effect prophylaxis. Additionally, benzodiazepines such as lorazepam and chlordiazepoxide are used in emergency settings when sedation and seizure prevention are indicated. Benzodiazepines are said to have a wide margin of safety and are extensively used in the treatment of psychiatric emergency.

Both the risks and the benefits of FGA use in the emergency setting should be clear. The choice of SGAs is valuable because of the more favorable side-effect profile and the procognitive therapeutic effects. However, little evidence indicates that SGAs are actually more effective (Schatzberg et al. 2010; Swartz et al. 2007). Moreover, the issues of availability and cost are often of practical significance, and SGAs are often prohibitively expensive. In fact, prescribing practices with these medications have been shown to be directly correlated with marketing and less with clinical outcomes or U.S. Food and Drug Administration (FDA) approvals (Sernyak and Rosenheck 2007).

A limited number of medications are approved for use in psychiatric emergencies, and treatment is generally based on the patient's presenting symptoms. Over the past few decades, clinicians have prescribed haloperidol for psychosis and agitation, lorazepam for anxiety, and benztropine (Cogentin) to ward off potential extrapyramidal symptoms. This combination is better known as "the cocktail," and, for the most part, it is effective in decreasing agitation and aggression. The newer SGAs are just beginning to be used in psychiatric emergencies; however, because of the excessive cost of these drugs, "the cocktail" is often the first-line treatment. Please refer to Table 11–6 for the most commonly prescribed medications in psychiatric emergencies. More detailed information on these and other psychotropic medications is available in the other chapters in this manual.

Treatment of Special Populations

Incarcerated Persons

Presenting to jail may be as likely as to an emergency department when aggressive or psychotic behaviors predominate, especially when a perceived danger to others exists. Often referred to as the criminalization of the mentally ill, the increased number of people with mental illness entering the criminal justice system is astounding (Scott 2010). In 2006, the Human Rights Watch found that 1.25 million American inmates had mental health problems, and most estimates of the total inmate prison/jail population requiring mental health care are around 20% (Fellner 2006). The number of jail and prison beds has increased proportionally to the decrease in state inpatient psychiatric hospital beds since 1955 (Scott 2010). These numbers are attributed to deinstitutionalization, rigid criteria for civil commitment, inadequate community resources, and societal attitudes toward this population (Lamb and Weinberger 1998).

A significant number of psychiatric emergencies also arise within prisons and jails. The unique environment of a correctional facility predisposes to exacerbations of preexisting mental illness, as well as the first psychotic break for some. In others, mood or psychotic disorders can develop, and behavior problems are common. The latter may be an act of last resort to communicate or achieve a sense of control, otherwise limited in such a restrictive environment.

Although the research on this subject is limited (Scott 2010), substance abuse rates in prison are thought to mirror those of greater society; however, obtaining intoxicants is somewhat unique. Inmates trade prescription drugs and ferment foods to make alcohol, and third parties smuggle and mule illicit substances. The psychiatric clinician is wise to take this reality into account when faced with an abrupt mental status change in this population.

Suicide is the third leading cause of death in this environment. The risk of suicide in county jails is said to be four times greater than in the general population and highest during the first 24–48 hours of being detained (Scott 2010). A thorough suicide risk assessment and prevention policy is vitally important in correctional facilities. To treat this patient population properly, familiarity with the unique environmental factors facing them is necessary, along with a solid base of psychiatric knowledge.

Patients With Personality Disorders

DSM-IV-TR defines a personality disorder as an "enduring pattern of inner experience and behavior that deviates markedly from the expectations of the individual's culture [and] is pervasive and inflexible" (American Psychiatric Association 2000, p. 685). Patients with these disorders are said to manifest dysfunction in areas related to cognition, affectivity, interpersonal relationships, and impulse control (American Psychiatric Association 2000). In acute phases, patients may present with brief psychotic episodes or combative, sus-

Table 11–6.   Medications commonly used in psychiatric emergencies

Drug	Target symptoms	Dosing	Potential acute adverse events
Chlorpromazine (Thorazine)	Agitation, aggressive behaviors, psychosis	Severe: 50–75 mg im every 4 hours prn Moderate: 50–100 mg po every 4 hours prn	Sedation, hypotension, orthostasis, ataxia, dystonia, EPS, NMS (rare), black box warning for risk of death when used in elderly with dementia-related psychosis
Haloperidol (Haldol)	Psychosis, agitation, aggressive behaviors, acute delirium	Severe: 2–5 mg im every 4 hours prn Moderate: 1–5 mg po every 4 hours prn Acute delirium: 0.25–2 mg iv every 4 hours until clear (typically administered with lorazepam and benztropine or diphenhydramine)	Sedation, dystonia, EPS, NMS (rare), black box warning for elderly
Olanzapine (Zyprexa)	Psychosis, agitation, aggression	Severe: 20 mg im (≤3 injections in 24 hours) Moderate: 5–10 mg po every 6 hours prn (orally disintegrating tablet)	Sedation, glucose intolerance, EPS (rare), NMS (rare), ataxia, hypotension, black box warning in elderly

Table 11–6.   Medications commonly used in psychiatric emergencies *(continued)*

Drug	Target symptoms	Dosing	Potential acute adverse events
Risperidone (Risperdal)	Agitation, aggression, psychosis, irritability in children	Moderate: 0.5–2 mg po every 6 hours prn (children and adolescents may require lower dose given more frequently)	Sedation, fatigue, EPS, dystonia, lactation, NMS (rare), black box warning in elderly
Lorazepam (Ativan)	Anxiety, panic, agitation, withdrawal from alcohol or benzodiazepines	Moderate: 0.5–1 mg po every 4–6 hours prn Severe: 1–2 mg po or im every 4 hours prn Withdrawal: 1–2 mg iv every 2–4 hours prn (breakthrough symptoms)	Sedation, ataxia, paradoxical agitation (especially in elderly), dizziness, confusion, slurred speech, poor reflex timing

Note.   EPS=extrapyramidal side effects; im=intramuscularly; iv=intravenously; NMS=neuroleptic malignant syndrome; po=orally; prn=as needed.

picious behaviors. People with borderline and antisocial personality disorders often present as emergencies because of repeated attempts at or threats of suicide. Pascual et al. (2007) found that a diagnosis of borderline personality disorder accounted for 9% of psychiatric emergency service visits.

The 2001 American Psychiatric Association *Practice Guideline for the Treatment of Patients With Borderline Personality Disorder* emphasizes hospitalization when the patient has made a serious suicide attempt, is an imminent danger to others, or has had a transient psychotic episode that severely limited his or her functioning. No medications are currently approved by the FDA for the treatment of personality disorders themselves, but pharmacotherapy is increasingly emphasized in the treatment of the component dimensions of the disorders with "demonstrable neurobiological correlates" (Triebwasser and Siever 2007). Pharmacology should be symptom specific in emergency treatment, and SGAs seem most effective because of their mood-stabilizing and anti-impulsivity properties.

Patients with borderline personality disorder are sometimes difficult to accurately assess and treat because of their impulsivity and demanding, manipulative behaviors. It is very important for the clinician to remain aware of the high risk of countertransference with these patients, symptomatically treat, and provide the same care as to any other patient group.

Elderly Patients

Mental illnesses can present differently in the elderly than in younger patients because of different psychosocial stressors, comorbidities, and increased likelihood of side effects from medications (Piechniczek-Buczek 2010). Ramadan (2007) argued that depression, substance abuse, and agitation are common in the elderly and are the products of the interaction of neurobiological, cognitive, and environmental factors. Suicide rates are highest in this age group (Cotter and Strumpf 2002), and withdrawal from substances can be more complicated (Piechniczek-Buczek 2010).

Aggression precipitates many psychiatric emergencies in the elderly, and care needs to be taken to rule out the nonpsychiatric precipitants. The irreversible condition of dementia is sometimes confused with delirium in this population. The crucial differences are rapidity of onset, constancy of symptoms, and degree to which memory is impaired. The DSM-IV-TR diagnostic criteria for delirium include a disturbance of consciousness and a change in cognition that develops over a short period and fluctuates during the course of the day (American Psychiatric Association 2000). If the underlying cause of delirium is properly identified and treated, recovery is more likely to be complete and rapid. This likelihood is compounded if premorbid cognitive and physical functioning were high.

Environmental interventions can be as important as pharmacological interventions with the elderly population. However, after the underlying cause has been diagnosed and treated, supportive measures initiated, and attempts at orientation made, small doses of high-potency FGAs (such as haloperidol) or of benzodiazepines (such as lorazepam) can be used (Schatzberg et al. 2010). Of note, elderly patients with dementia-related psychosis are at increased risk for cardiovascular disease and death while taking antipsychotic medications, according to the black box warning (Stahl 2008).

Children and Adolescents

Although I focus mainly on the psychiatric emergencies in adults, children also can present for emergency care. Suicidal behaviors, abuse, and aggressive or homicidal behaviors can present in children, especially in the context of attention-deficit/hyperactivity disorder, conduct disorder, or any of the pervasive developmental disorders (Ramadan 2007). Less commonly, emergencies are exacerbations of serious psychiatric disorders (Sadock and Sadock 2007). In many of these cases, chronic problem care is initiated in the emergency setting.

With this population, the escorting adult may perceive the child's behavior as a greater emergency than does the clinician. In these cases, when no diagnostically emergent situation is obvious, the clinician's skill at eliciting collateral information via assessment of the family or system involved with the child is imperative (Sadock and Sadock 2007). History can shed light on the child's presentation. In many cases, an underlying family or situational stressor can be teased out of the interview and serve as a platform for future care. However, caution needs to be exercised because it is not always the "parent's fault" or a "problem at home" that is the culprit. Without proper empathy and problem-solving skills, clinicians may be too quick to make a judgment call in these cases, leading to faulty information, improper treatment choices, or alienation of the very person who brought the child to the clinician's attention.

Likewise, care should be taken in medication choices for children. If antipsychotic medication is indicated, SGAs are recommended because of their more favorable side-effect profile and efficacy in treatment of aggression (Bailey 2003). Risperidone is the most commonly used medication in this group and is approved for use as early as age 5 years. Oral forms of olanzapine are not officially recommended in patients younger than 18 years, although clinical data show that olanzapine is probably safe. Intramuscular formulations are not recommended (Stahl 2008). If only an FGA is available, chlorpromazine is safest and can be used cautiously (Stahl 2008).

Substance Users

Because many psychiatric emergencies involve substance intoxication or withdrawal, this population requires special attention in our clinical lexicon. The horrors of substance dependence and the lifestyles that plague addicted individuals are beyond the scope of this chapter. Long-term treatment is not possible in emergency settings, but empathy and overall facilitation of a positive experience during this time are critical. How interventions are enacted can have a significant effect on the patient's decision to continue care.

Medically Compromised Individuals

Anxiety, depression, delirium, and suicidal ideation are the most common psychiatric presentations in end-of-life care as well as in patients with terminal illness and chronic pain (Foti 2003). This can be related to the stress of the illness itself or of its treatment. A chronic disorder also can be exacerbated, particularly in the context of poor pain management, because treatment compliance can be compromised when intense feelings impair the individual's functioning. Proper pain management often can alleviate these symptoms, and psychopharmacological intervention may not be indicated.

Pregnant or Breast-Feeding Women

As with all psychiatric emergencies, the goal is always to treat the presenting symptomatology and weigh the risk of harm against potential benefits of medication use. It is widely agreed that psychiatric symptoms can worsen during pregnancy. A pregnant woman who is experiencing serious psychiatric symptoms requires psychopharmacological treatment; failure to provide such intervention can have long-standing repercussions for both the woman and her unborn child, such as preterm delivery, low birth weight, and/or postpartum depression or psychosis.

In pregnancy, the fewer potential side effects associated with SGAs appear significant if antipsychotic treatment is warranted. Early studies of infants exposed to olanzapine or risperidone in utero showed no adverse events, whereas both chlorpromazine and haloperidol have been associated with negative effects. Most antipsychotic medications are in risk Category C (Stahl 2008).

There is direct evidence of risk to the fetus when the mother takes benzodiazepines during pregnancy, especially during the first trimester. Both chlordiazepoxide and lorazepam are in pregnancy risk Category D (Stahl 2008). If the mother is already taking one of these agents, it should be gradually tapered, not abruptly discontinued, because this can cause seizures that may result in significant harm to the fetus (Stahl 2008).

It is widely accepted that all psychotropic medication is excreted in breast milk. FGAs have been observed to cause dystonia, tardive dyskinesia, and sedation in nursing infants, and benzodiazepines have been reported to cause sedation, feeding difficulties, and weight loss (Stahl 2008).

Treatment Monitoring

Treatment in emergency situations requires close monitoring. This begins with thorough assessment of baseline signs, symptoms, and laboratory values. When seclusion or physical restraint must be used, the patient must be attended to by trained personnel, have his or her vital signs regularly monitored, and be reassured. The same is true when the patient is given psychotropic medications.

Patients administered antipsychotic medication may develop motor symptoms requiring the addition of a benzodiazepine or an anticholinergic agent to their regimen. If a patient is inadvertently given a life-threatening overdose of benzodiazepine, flumazenil can be administered. In patients requiring chlordiazepoxide injection, respiratory functioning must be monitored for up to 3 hours.

Summary

A crisis may best be understood as an internal state that may happen to both healthy and unhealthy individuals, in normal or abnormal circumstances, that is acutely painful, frightening, and often demoralizing (Selverston 2004). In psychiatric crisis, patients present with psychosis, anxiety, substance intoxication or withdrawal, and suicidal or homicidal behaviors (Ramadan 2007). Alone or in combination, these conditions can predispose the patient to emotional disturbances such as fear, anxiety, irritability, and euphoria (American Psychiatric Association 2000) and result in hostility, aggression, combativeness, or impulsivity (Ramadan 2007). Because various causes can trigger these events, which may present in the same way, Ramadan (2007) argued that the emergency clinician assumes the concurrent roles of diplomat, detective, and anthropologist. Being familiar with the situational stressors and medical factors involved in the presentations is as important as being familiar with psychiatric diagnoses.

Nurse practitioners are uniquely suited to provide this care. Nurses are taught to deal with the whole person—the precursors of and precipitants to their presenting problem. Nurses are charged with the de-escalation of the crisis at hand, and a holistic approach is most useful in these settings that are usually chaotic and that do not afford patients the traditional therapeutic relationships they can find in other psychiatric environments (Olsen et al. 2008).

The diagnosis and management of every psychiatric emergency are unique. For example, a well-known 30-year-old schizophrenic patient who has not been taking her medication, but historically responds well to Haldol therapy, should be handled differently from an elderly man who is presenting for the first time, severely depressed, suicidal, and nonviolent. Likewise, an acutely alcohol-intoxicated teenager with no known psychiatric history who has just been arrested for assaulting his mother needs different treatment from a patient in a PCP-induced anesthetized rage who just jumped out of a window in front of his children. The homeless, heroin-addicted person who has been sitting in a police precinct for days undergoing detoxification without sleep, adequate food, or medication requires a different approach from the patient with personality disorders and malingering. The security measures, escorting personnel, and treatment choices in each of these cases speak to the necessity for diligent observation, proper history, and a sound knowledge of this cluster of syndromes.

In these situations, clinicians first must ensure the safety of all involved. This may require seclusion of the patient or even physical restraints when other interventions are not sufficient to prevent harm. Rapid assessment and triage of psychosocial, medical, and basic human necessities are imperative before pharmacological intervention is warranted. When medication is needed, an understanding of fast-acting, appropriate pharmacology is crucial. The clinician's empathetic approach to the situation, development of rapport, timeliness of intervention, and addressing of the basic needs of both the patient and the accompanying parties can have significant effect on ultimate clinical outcomes. Establishment of the patient's general trust in "the system" can facilitate learning from the event and active willingness to continue care. Attempts to minimize the risk of relapse are met by ensuring that the patient is connected with proper community resources. Finally, anticipatory teaching is important because psychiatric symptoms can reemerge after the crisis is over.

Although the focus in psychiatric emergencies is on brief intervention and stabilization (Lee et al. 2003), psychopharmacology in itself is not curative. The truest measure of crisis treatment is long-term effectiveness, which can be measured by the patient's experience during the arguably most difficult time in his or her life. This is of paramount importance to overall mental health care in the practice of emergency psychiatry.

The reader is referred to Table 11–7 for general guidelines for approaching psychiatric emergencies.

Table 11–7. General approach to psychiatric emergency intervention

Gather information

Learn as much historical information as possible before seeing the patient.
If available, medical records and collateral information can facilitate treatment decisions.

Ensure security

Agitated patients and escorts can pose a threat to themselves and others.
If physical restraints are needed, identify trained personnel to implement (monitor closely).
Seclusion may be necessary to reduce stimuli.

Observe clues

General appearance, hygiene, motor activity, pupillary size, nystagmus, age, and evidence of trauma.

Monitor yourself

The clinician's approach to the patient in psychiatric crisis can alter the entire experience.
Apprehension, anger, and defensiveness can set off a cascade of additional clinical problems, but establishment of rapport, trust, and a therapeutic alliance can make the crisis easier for all involved.
Avoid behaviors that can induce shame, guilt, or intimidation.
Do not confront or threaten.

Do not forget basic human needs

Food, hydration, and comfort can facilitate a more positive experience for all involved.
Accompanying parties also may need a degree of care.

Rule out medical etiology

Many medical conditions can present as psychiatric emergencies and can be life-threatening.

Plan for aftercare

Anticipatory teaching, facilitation of a positive experience for the patient, medication choices, and referral to proper community resources can facilitate continuation of the stability achieved.

Clinical Pearls

- Many medical conditions may present with significant psychiatric symptoms. It is important to rule out underlying medical etiology prior to initiating psychiatric treatment.

- One of the most important tasks in psychiatric emergency situations is to assess the patient's level of danger toward self and/or others.

- The first-generation antipsychotic medications continue to be used to decrease aggression, agitation, and psychosis in people presenting to emergency departments and psychiatric crisis centers.

- Maintaining a calm, nonthreatening posture is critical when evaluating a patient in psychiatric crisis. Maintaining the safety of patient, staff, and oneself is imperative throughout a psychiatric emergency.

- A more positive experience can be facilitated by remembering to address the patient's basic human needs for comfort, safety, nutrition, and hydration.

References

American Psychiatric Association: Diagnostic and Statistical Manual of Mental Disorders, 4th Edition, Text Revision. Washington, DC, American Psychiatric Association, 2000

American Psychiatric Association: Practice Guideline for the Treatment of Patients With Borderline Personality Disorder. October 2001. Available at: http://psychiatryonline.org/content.aspx?bookid=28&sectionid=1672600#55256. Accessed October 4, 2011.

American Psychiatric Association: Practice Guideline for the Assessment and Treatment of Patients With Suicidal Behaviors. November 2003. Available at: http://psychiatryonline.org/content.aspx?bookid=28&sectionid=1673332#56021. Accessed October 4, 2011.

American Psychiatric Association: Practice Guideline for the Treatment of Patients With Schizophrenia, 2nd Edition. Arlington, VA, American Psychiatric Association, 2004

Bailey S: Young offenders and mental health. Curr Opin Psychiatry 16:581–591, 2003

Cotter VT, Strumpf NE: Advanced Practice Nursing With Older Adults: Clinical Guidelines. New York, McGraw-Hill, 2002

Di Fiorino M, Danielyan A, Gemignani A: Guidelines for behavioral emergencies. Psychiatr Serv 56:1159–1160, 2005

Fellner J: U.S.: number of mentally ill in prisons quadrupled: prisons ill equipped to cope. September 6, 2006. Available at: http://www.hrw.org/news/2006/09/05/us-number-mentally-ill-prisons-quadrupled. Accessed May 20, 2011.

Fischbach F: A Manual of Laboratory and Diagnostic Tests, 7th Edition. Philadelphia, PA, Lippincott Williams & Wilkins, 2004

Foti ME: Managing psychiatric emergencies in the terminally ill. August 11, 2003. Available at: www.promotingexcellence.org/downloads/.../Psychiatric_Emergencies.ppt. Accessed August 8, 2011.

Giannini AJ: An approach to drug abuse, intoxication and withdrawal. Am Fam Physician 61:2763–2774, 2000

Jayaram G, Triplett P: Quality improvement of psychiatric care: challenges of emergency psychiatry. Am J Psychiatry 165:1256–1260, 2008

Lamb HR, Weinberger LE: Persons with severe mental illness in jails and prisons: a review. Psychiatr Serv 49:483–492, 1998

Lee TS, Renaud EF, Hills OF: An emergency treatment hub-and-spoke model for psychiatric emergency services. Psychiatr Serv 54:1590–1594, 2003

Lester D: Preventing Suicide. New York, Nova Science Publishers, 2009

McKeown N: Withdrawal syndromes. November 16, 2010. Available at: www.emedicine.medscape.com/article/819502-overview#a0104. Accessed September 4, 2011.

Miller NS, Gold MS: Management of withdrawal syndromes and relapse prevention in drug and alcohol dependence [published erratum appears in Am Fam Physician 58:866, 1998]. Am Fam Physician 58:139–146, 1998

Mycek MJ, Harvey RA, Champe PC: Pharmacology, 2nd Edition. Philadelphia, PA, Lippincott Williams & Wilkins, 2000

Narcan. June 2006. Available at: www.drugs.com/pro/narcan.html. Accessed April 17, 2012.

Olsen JC, Cutcliffe B, O'Brien BC: Emergency department design and patient perceptions of privacy and confidentiality. J Emerg Med 35:317–320, 2008

Pascual JC, Córcoles D, Castaño J, et al: Hospitalization and pharmacotherapy for borderline personality disorder in a psychiatric emergency service. Psychiatr Serv 58:1199–1204, 2007

Piechniczek-Buczek J: Psychiatric emergencies in the elderly: keys to diagnosis, assessment, and management. Psychiatric Times 27(7), July 9, 2010

Preston J, Johnson J: Clinical Psychopharmacology Made Ridiculously Simple, 7th Edition. Miami, FL, MedMaster, 2012

Ramadan MI: Managing psychiatric emergencies. The Internet Journal of Emergency Medicine 4(1), 2007

Sadock BJ, Sadock VA: Kaplan and Saddock's Synopsis of Psychiatry: Behavioral Sciences/Clinical Psychiatry, 10th Edition. Philadelphia, PA, Lippincott Williams & Wilkins, 2007

Schatzberg AF, Cole JO, DeBattista C: Manual of Clinical Psychopharmacology, 7th Edition. Washington, DC, American Psychiatric Publishing, 2010

Scott C (ed): Handbook of Correctional Mental Health, 2nd Edition. Washington, DC, American Psychiatric Publishing, 2010

Selverston S: Crisis: concepts and interventions, in Psychiatric Mental Health Nursing, 3rd Edition. Edited by Fortinash KM, Holoday-Worret PA. St. Louis, MO, Mosby, 2004, pp 507–518

Sernyak M, Rosenheck R: Experience of VA psychiatrists with pharmaceutical detailing of antipsychotic medications. Psychiatr Serv 58:1292–1296, 2007

Stahl SM: Stahl's Essential Psychopharmacology: Neuroscientific Basis and Practical Applications, 3rd Edition. New York, Cambridge University Press, 2008

Stahl S: The Prescriber's Guide: Stahl's Essential Psychopharmacology, 3rd Edition. New York, Cambridge University Press, 2009

Swartz MS, Perkins DO, Stroup TS, et al: Effects of antipsychotic medications on psychosocial functioning in patients with chronic schizophrenia: findings from the NIMH CATIE study. Am J Psychiatry 164:428–436, 2007

Townsend MC: Psychiatric Mental Health Nursing: Concepts of Care in Evidence-Based Practice, 5th Edition. Philadelphia, PA, FA Davis, 2005

Triebwasser J, Siever LJ: Pharmacotherapy of personality disorders. J Ment Health 16:5–50, 2007

Zeller S: Treatment of psychiatric patients in emergency settings. Prim Psychiatry 17:35–41, 2010

12

Management of Metabolic Side Effects of Psychotropic Medications

Barbara J. Limandri, Ph.D., A.P.R.N., P.M.H.-C.N.S., B.C.

He that wrestles with us strengthens our nerves
and sharpens our skills.
Our antagonist is our helper.

—Edmund Burke (1729–1797)

Overview of Medication-Associated Metabolic Side Effects

Since the 1920s, public health and nutrition scientists have studied metabolic syndrome, which is characterized by increased waist circumference, elevated fasting blood glucose and lipid levels, and hypertension, yet it has been only within the past decade that primary care providers have taken the phenomenon seriously. This confluence of risk factors for cardiovascular disease is an epidemic that has insidiously invaded the United States and the rest of the world and affects persons with severe mental illness disproportionately. In 1991, the *Healthy People 2000: National Health Promotion and Disease Prevention Objectives* targeted physical fitness and activity, diabetes, cardiovascular disease, and stroke as goals for improvement (U.S. Department of Health and Human Services 1991). However, the rate of obesity increased during that decade, contributing to an increase in diabetes, cardiovascular disease, and stroke and prompting *Healthy People 2010: Understanding and Improving Health* to make overweight and obesity second in the top 10 leading health indicators for improvement (U.S. Department of Health and Human Services 2000). Unfortunately, the rate of obesity increased even further, with *Healthy People 2020* citing that 34% of American adults are obese and 16.2% of American children and adolescents are obese (http://healthypeople.gov/2020). According to a large-scale survey of almost 9,000 men and women representative of the U.S. population (Ford et al. 2002), approximately 20% of the American public fulfills criteria for metabolic syndrome, and this figure increases to almost 50% for persons older than 60 years. The risk of metabolic syndrome is mainly based on increased morbidity of diabetes, hypertension, and musculoskeletal dysfunction and associated with increased mortality from cardiovascular disease, stroke, and other end-organ failure. The cost of treating metabolic syndrome and its consequences amounts to about 10% of our annual total health care expenditure. The human cost, however, is even greater in terms of loss of productivity and life as well as the burden of the disease on individuals, families, and society in general.

Individuals with severe mental illness are especially vulnerable to metabolic syndrome for reasons that are not completely clear. Common causes and general factors that contribute to the development of metabolic syndrome—such as genetic predisposition, lack of activity, and poor diet—may be more widely present in persons with psychiatric illness. In addition, many psychotropic medications potentially worsen glucose metabolism and, therefore, may contribute to the development and progression of metabolic syndrome.

Those with schizophrenia are three times more likely to develop metabolic syndrome, have a life expectancy 25–30 years less than those without schizophrenia, and have four to five times higher rates of type 2 diabetes (Batscha et al. 2010; Holt et al. 2010). Oddly, those having a first episode of schizophrenia and who are drug naïve still show higher rates of insulin resistance than do matched sample control subjects from the National Health and Nutrition Examination Survey (NHANES) (Raedler 2010; Ryan et al. 2003); therefore, the phenomenon is not totally related to the second-generation antipsychotics. In addition, glucose intolerance was described in schizophrenia before the advent of antipsychotics (e.g., Langfeldt 1952) and is also more common in unaffected family members (Mukherjee et al. 1989), which supports inherent susceptibility regardless of medications. Furthermore, premature death among those with schizophrenia is not limited to the United States; it seems to be a worldwide phenomenon. Similar studies in the United Kingdom, France, Finland, Canada, and Japan show a significant early mortality risk resulting from cardiovascular disease, with metabolic syndrome as the underlying precipitant (Raedler 2010).

Many clinicians believe that the metabolic syndrome is one of the consequences of the second-generation antipsychotic medications, but literature about the first-generation antipsychotics as well as literature related to other psychotropic medications and psychiatric disorders also describe this syndrome (Hermes et al. 2011; Jallon and Picard 2001; McIntyre et al. 2010). Therefore, all antipsychotic medications now carry a black box warning regarding increased mortality in elderly patients with dementia-related psychosis. Individuals with major depressive disorder show a high risk for insulin resistance, and conversely, those with diabetes show a higher risk for depression (Kloiber et al. 2010). Similarly, in the NHANES III study, those with diabetes had two to four times higher incidence of depression, and major depressive disorder was present in 48% of those with type 2 diabetes, suggesting some shared pathophysiology and causation (McIntyre et al. 2010). The serotonin reuptake inhibitors (with the exception of paroxetine) do not consistently affect blood glucose levels, nor do the serotonin-norepinephrine reuptake inhibitors. However, desvenlafaxine (Pristiq) shows a short-term elevation in blood glucose, and mirtazapine (Remeron) clearly shows a persistent increase in fasting blood glucose level and weight gain, especially noticeable at the lower dosages. Those with bipolar disorder also show a disproportionate prevalence for metabolic syndrome, with one study showing 51% meeting criteria (Jin et al. 2010). Certainly, combining the second-generation antipsychotics with mood stabilizers adds to this risk.

Metabolic syndrome remains a risk with several of the mood stabilizers, even without second-generation antipsychotics. Of those who take lithium (Eskalith, Lithobid), 25% gain weight, and if they develop hypothyroidism, this weight gain increases further. Weight gain is dose dependent, with the least amount of weight gain occurring at serum lithium levels of less than 0.8 mmol/L. Weight gain is also a problem with valproate (Depakene, Depakote): 3%–20% have between 3 and 10 kg increase in weight in 1 year of taking the medication. Of the persons taking gabapentin (Neurontin), 25% show a gain of 0.9–3.0 kg within 12 weeks of treatment. Lamotrigine (Lamictal) seems to have the lowest incidence of weight gain compared with lithium or gabapentin, with between −2.2 and +1.1 kg of change over 7 weeks of treatment (Torrent et al. 2008).

To provide high-quality care and safe prescribing for patients with psychiatric disorders, the advanced practice registered nurse (APRN) needs to understand the role of the metabolic syndrome in psychotropic medications, the possible mechanisms for this syndrome, and ways to prevent the syndrome as well as intervene as early as possible to prevent more serious consequences. A common problem is the failure to regularly screen for weight gain, hypertension, glucose tolerance, diabetes, and dyslipidemia in those with severe mental illness. In fact, a Medicaid study found that fewer than 20% of individuals receiving second-generation antipsychotics had baseline glucose testing, and fewer than 10% had baseline lipid panels (McIntyre et al. 2010).

Features of Metabolic Syndrome

The metabolic syndrome consists of five components that together raise the risk for cardiovascular disease (Table 12–1). Criteria for this syndrome (Grundy et al. 2005; Laaksonen et al. 2002; Taylor et al. 2010) require three of the five elements to be present.

These five core features are highly correlated with diabetes, coronary artery disease, and stroke; and some studies indicate that the earliest and most convenient measurement to consider is the waist circumference in conjunction with the body mass index (BMI). Abdominal fat cells produce a hormone, adiponectin, that contributes to insulin resistance, and the visceral fat located in the abdomen is also linked to higher total cholesterol, higher low-

Table 12–1.   Criteria for metabolic syndrome

Must have three of the following:

1. Fasting blood glucose >100 mg/dL

2. Triglycerides >150 mg/dL

3. High-density lipoprotein <40 mg/dL for men; <50 mg/dL for women

4. Systolic blood pressure >130 mm Hg; diastolic blood pressure >85 mm Hg

5. Waist circumference >102 cm (40 in) for men; >88 cm (35 in) for women

Source.   Adapted from Grundy et al. 2004.

density lipoprotein (LDL) cholesterol, and lower HDL cholesterol (Groth 2010; Hyman 2006; Mari et al. 1999).

Three systems affect appetite and metabolism: the nervous, endocrine, and immune systems. The hypothalamus controls feeding and expenditure of energy. Neuropeptides that increase feeding behavior include ghrelin, neuropeptide Y, and orexin; and neuropeptides that decrease feeding behavior include leptin, insulin, corticotropin-releasing hormone, and cholecystokinin. Leptin is produced by fat cells, with leptin receptors most dense in the medial hypothalamus. When these receptors are activated, it signals satiety and stops eating. Cells that line the stomach produce ghrelin. Several hours after eating, these cells increase the secretion of ghrelin, thereby stimulating the appetite for the next meal. The ventromedial hypothalamus and ventral tegmental area are the sites for ghrelin receptors. Bariatric surgery that removes or segregates the areas of the stomach with ghrelin cells may diminish appetite by decreasing the secretion of the neuropeptide. Neuropeptide Y receptors, found in the arcuate nucleus in the ventromedial hypothalamus, have a major role in energy expenditure and balance. When released, neuropeptide Y stimulates appetite and reduces energy expenditure. Leptin inhibits neuropeptide Y to counteract its effects and to restore balance of appetite and energy use, and ghrelin stimulates neuropeptide Y (Nogueiras et al. 2008).

The interlocking messengers that communicate between the three body systems regulate the process of food intake, metabolism, and energy use. The messengers from the nervous system are the neuropeptides and neurotransmitters already noted that influence appetite and food craving. The gastrointestinal tract, liver, and pancreas respond to the messages from the nervous systems with hormones such as leptin and insulin. The main endocrine system involved, however, is adipose tissue and specifically the adipocytes and adiponectin. Finally, the immune system responds with cytokines produced by adipose tissue. These cytokines, including interleukin-6, tumor necrosis factor α, and adiponectin, are mediators of an inflammatory response, resulting in insulin resistance (Arslan et al. 2010; Surendar et al. 2011).

Factors Associated With Metabolic Syndrome

The involvement of the immune system adds another layer to the metabolic syndrome that includes stress. Traditionally, we associate the hypothalamic-pituitary-adrenal (HPA) axis with stress; however, at least one study indicated that the autonomic nervous system has a more significant relation with stress and the metabolic syndrome. Specifically, what is apparent is dysregulation between the sympathetic system and the parasympathetic system. In those who had metabolic syndrome, Licht et al. (2010) found a decrease in parasympathetic activity and an increase in sympathetic activity in a large cohort sample of adults from primary care and mental health settings without an associated activation of the HPA axis. The inverse nature of the activity of the two branches of the autonomic nervous system was important; that is, metabolic syndrome was not associated with either the increase of both sympathetic and parasympathetic or the decrease of both sympathetic and parasympathetic systems. Although more research is needed to clarify the significance of these results, it appears that acute stress characterized by the HPA axis is less involved than the chronic stress associated with the autonomic system. The chronic stress of severe mental illness may contribute to metabolic syndrome regardless of medications, and the prescribed medications further compound the risk.

Under circumstances of acute stress, the adrenal cortex releases cortisol, and in chronic stress, the cortisol levels remain elevated over time. In both animal and human studies, chronic stress leads to excessive eating, especially of high-fat and high-carbohydrate foods. At this point, the elevated cortisol promotes overeating, gluconeogenesis, triglyceride production, catabolism of muscle protein, and deposition of fat stores in the visceral adipose (Dallman et al. 2003). Studies of military personnel with posttraumatic stress disorder showed an increased incidence of metabolic syndrome when compared with control subjects and nonmilitary participants (Heppner et al. 2009; Jakovljevi et al. 2006, 2008). Another perspective is that of loneliness as a measure of chronic stress that many people with severe and persistent mental disorders experience. In a British study of a large sample of men and women age 50 years and older who used a valid and reliable self-report tool to measure loneliness and controlled for smoking, loneliness was significantly associated with metabolic syndrome (Whisman 2010).

Two other significant factors in metabolic syndrome are smoking and alcohol consumption. Cigarette smokers have a 1.07–1.66 times greater risk for metabolic syndrome. Tobacco smoking is associated with decreased insulin sensitivity, insulin resistance, increased plasma lipid levels, and decreased HDL. Nicotine seems to contribute to a resistance to leptin, which suppresses appetite (Cena et al. 2011). However, smoking cessation by itself does not completely protect against metabolic syndrome unless the other factors such as BMI and waist circumference also decrease. In one large study in Japan, smoking cessation showed a 1.3 times risk for metabolic syndrome in those who also gained weight after quitting smoking (Hishida et al. 2009).

The effect of alcohol consumption on metabolic syndrome is less clear because of conflicting studies that used different definitions of high and low alcohol consumption and other methodological limitations such as diverse ethnicities, gender, age, and duration of drinking behavior. Controversy also exists about the effects of the types of alcohol consumed. Some studies suggest that wine has protective benefits because of its high phenolic composition that imparts antioxidant properties, which may reduce LDL oxidation (Rosell et al. 2003). However, a large cohort study in Switzerland that narrowly distinguished between high, medium, and low alcohol consumption as well as nondrinkers found that the type of beverage was not significantly related to metabolic syndrome (Clerc et al. 2010). In fact, this study showed a U-shaped relation between alcohol consumption and metabolic syndrome and diabetes, with a lower prevalence in low-risk drinkers, an increased prevalence in very-high-risk drinkers, but a nonsignificant prevalence in medium-risk and nondrinkers. Low-risk drinkers consumed between 1 and 13 drinks per week, medium-risk drinkers consumed between 14 and 34 drinks per week, and very-high-risk drinkers consumed 35 or more drinks per week. High alcohol consumption was associated with elevated triglyceride levels, blood pressure, fasting blood glucose levels, and fasting insulin levels, and with low HDL. Low-risk alcohol consumption was associated with smaller waist circumference and lower BMI, triglyceride levels, blood pressure, fasting blood glucose levels, and fasting insulin levels. Although this sample included men and women ages 35–75 years, all were white, thereby limiting the conclusions related to other ethnicities (Clerc et al. 2010). The Switzerland study results were similar to those of other studies that convincingly established that alcohol consumption and dependence are associated with metabolic syndrome with little evidence of a protective cardiovascular benefit, especially in those with alcohol dependence, even those in recovery (Fan et al. 2006; Hishida et al. 2009; Kahl et al. 2010).

Treatment Monitoring and Clinical Guidelines

APRNs, regardless of specialty, need to assess patients for metabolic syndrome and provide health promotion guidance in preventing and treating it (Tables 12–2 and 12–3). This begins with gathering baseline data that research shows to be risk factors: waist circumference, BMI, blood pressure, fasting blood glucose, triglycerides, and total and HDL cholesterol levels and their ratio. During the initial assessment, the APRN seeks information about the family health history for possible familial disorders and lifestyle practices, including activity level and duration, nutritional habits, and tobacco and alcohol use. Because a relation is found between schizophrenia, bipolar disorders, and depressive disorders, even with medication-naïve patients, these patients need to be monitored regardless of prescribing. Additionally, APRNs need to incorporate into their overall treatment planning motivational interviewing and nutritional and activity guidance.

When prescribing medication for psychiatric conditions, the clinician considers the appropriate medications for the symptomatology and discusses the pros and cons of these choices with the patient, including side effects and alternative choices. This discussion needs to include the probability of weight gain and how the patient and clinician will monitor this. Although the second-generation antipsychotics have a clear potential for metabolic syndrome, the clinician needs to use the same caution with the mood regulators. If the clinical situation warrants prescribing medication that may predispose to the metabolic syndrome, the APRN needs to monitor the basic markers at

Table 12–2. Recommended monitoring for metabolic syndrome

At baseline before adding medication:

- Anthropomorphic measures: height, weight, waist circumference, body mass index
- Lipid panel (including total cholesterol, low-density lipoprotein, high-density lipoprotein, triglycerides)
- Fasting blood glucose
- Blood pressure

At each follow-up visit:

- Blood pressure
- Weight

Every 3 months after initiation of medication until stable:

- Lipid panel
- Fasting blood glucose
- Anthropomorphic measures
- Blood pressure

Annually after stable:

- Lipid panel
- Fasting blood glucose
- Anthropometric measures
- Blood pressure

3-month intervals until a clear pattern emerges. If no significant changes occur in waist circumference, BMI, triglyceride levels, cholesterol ratio, and blood pressure, the patient can continue monitoring waist circumference and weight with annual clinical reevaluation. If changes occur, the APRN needs to review with the patient any dietary and activity changes as well as associated factors such as stress. At this point, the clinician uses counseling directed at the patient's level of motivation to improve these lifestyle behaviors and achieve evidence of change to prevent further development of metabolic syndrome. If necessary and possible, the nurse and patient may need to consider changing to another medication or adding medication such as metformin (Glucophage) to stabilize metabolism. Studies with olanzapine (Zyprexa) (Praharaj et al.

Table 12–3.   Treatment recommendations for metabolic syndrome

When initiating medication with the risk of metabolic syndrome

Select medication with lowest risk of weight gain relative to patient's symptoms.

Explain to the patient the risk of weight gain.

Discuss nutritional habits and recommend

- Portion sizes based on U.S. Department of Agriculture Choose My Plate Web site (www.choosemyplate.gov)

- Complex vs. simple carbohydrates

- Low-fat foods

- Antioxidant foods

Discuss activity level based on Choose My Plate, with minimum of 150 minutes per week for adults and 60 minutes per day for children and teenagers.

Encourage patient to stop smoking and avoid alcohol consumption.

When metabolic syndrome criteria are met

Consider changing medication to one with lower incidence of weight gain.

Consider adding metformin (Glucophage) 500 mg twice a day.

Assess motivational level.

Engage patient in agreement to increase activity level by 10%.

Engage patient in modifying diet in at least one way.

Help patient stop smoking and avoid alcohol consumption.

Assist patient in stress management.

2010) show that patients can lose weight and may even stabilize with metformin, although these data are based on short-term monitoring. Table 12–4 shows selected drugs commonly used in advanced practice mental health nursing, with the percentages of incidence of metabolic syndrome side effects (weight gain, blood pressure change, glycemic and lipid changes) based on available data from pre- and postmarketing pharmaceutical studies.

Some research with methodological limitations suggests various nutritional supplements for treatment of metabolic syndrome, including selenium (Bleys et al. 2008; Puchau et al. 2009) and magnesium (Ma et al. 1995;

McKeown et al. 2008). However, the most important intervention for APRNs is to have a serious discussion with patients about specifics of nutrition, including resources such as the U.S. Department of Agriculture Choose My Plate Web site (www.choosemyplate.gov). Nurses should explain the relation between the metabolic syndrome and diet and monitor with the patient dietary habits, including consumption of complex carbohydrates and high-fiber, low-fat, and deeply colored foods that are rich in antioxidants. Because children learn dietary habits primarily at home, clinicians need to remind parents to mindfully show these behaviors within the family.

The other side of food intake is caloric expenditure in the form of exercise and activity. Technology has advanced many areas of living, but it also has been a contributor to lower activity. Children prefer to play video and computer games rather than play tag, shoot baskets, or ride bicycles for fun. Similarly, adults focus on multitasking and conserving time so that they can work longer or participate in sedentary leisure. The APRN needs to inquire routinely about the amount of exercise or activity in which patients engage and to encourage adults to spend at least 150 minutes involved in vigorous activity every week. This can be as simple as walking and biking for short trips, parking as far away from destinations as reasonably safe, and walking during lunch and breaks at work; patients can also use more routinized plans such as fitness club membership, trainer-guided regular workouts, active sport activities, and partnered runs or walks. Engaging in activity is difficult even for the average individual, but the challenge for the patient with mental illness who is taking medications that may contribute to fatigue and metabolic syndrome is that much greater. Working with patients to develop a healthier, less sedentary lifestyle, as outlined in *The Surgeon General's Vision for a Healthy and Fit Nation* (U.S. Department of Health and Human Services 2010), is a responsibility of every APRN. Accountability holds humans responsible, and the nurse can help the patient find comfortable but assertive ways to develop and maintain activity habits.

Identifying the patient's readiness to change allows the APRN to motivate the patient appropriately with the Transtheoretical Model of Change. Although research on the effectiveness of this model in motivating patients to change has had inconsistent results, the consensus is that the model works as well as others and is more effective under certain conditions (Armitage and Arden 2008; Cahill et al. 2010). Collating the patient's behaviors that indicate

Table 12–4.   Percentage of metabolic side effects for selected psychotropic drugs

Drug	Weight changes	Blood pressure changes	Glycemic changes	Lipid changes
First-generation antipsychotics				
Chlorpromazine (Thorazine)	NDIA	Decrease	NDIA	NDIA
Fluphenazine (Prolixin)	Increase	Orthostasis	NDIA	NDIA
Haloperidol (Haldol)	NDIA	Increase and orthostasis	Increase and decrease	NDIA
Trifluoperazine (Stelazine)	Increase	Orthostasis	Increase and decrease	NDIA
Second-generation antipsychotics				
Aripiprazole (Abilify)	2%–30% increase; 5% decrease	<1% increase	<1% increase	<1% increase
Asenapine (Saphris)	2%–5% increase	2%–3% increase	5%–7% increase	13%–15% increased TRI; 8%–9% increased CHOL
Clozapine (Clozaril)	4%–31% increase	4% increase	<1% increase	Rare
Iloperidone (Fanapt)	1%–9% increase; ≥1% decrease	3%–5% orthostasis; 1%–3% decrease	NDIA	NDIA
Lurasidone (Latuda)	≥7% increase	<1% increase and decrease	10%–14% increase	NDIA

Table 12–4. Percentage of metabolic side effects for selected psychotropic drugs *(continued)*

Drug	Weight changes	Blood pressure changes	Glycemic changes	Lipid changes
Second-generation antipsychotics *(continued)*				
Olanzapine (Zyprexa)	5%–40% increase	1%–10% increase or decrease	<1% increase or decrease	<1% increase
Quetiapine (Seroquel)	3%–23% increase	15%–40% increase	2%–12% increase	8%–22% increase
Risperidone (Risperdal)	5% increase	4% increase (im only)	<1% increase	<1% increase
Ziprasidone (Geodon)	6%–10% increase	2%–3% increase	<1% increase	<1% increase
Antidepressants				
Bupropion (Wellbutrin)	14%–23% decrease	2%–4% increase; 3% decrease	<1% increase	NDIA
Citalopram (Celexa)	1%–10% increase or decrease	<1% increase	NDIA	NDIA
Escitalopram (Lexapro)	<1% increase	<1% increase	<1% increase	<1% increase
Clomipramine (Anafranil)	18% increase	6% decrease	<1% increase	<1% increase
Desvenlafaxine (Pristiq)	≤2% increase or decrease	≤1% increase (50–100 mg)	<1% increase	<1% increase
Venlafaxine (Effexor)	1%–6% decrease	3%–13% increase (dose related)	<1% increase	<1% increase

Table 12–4. Percentage of metabolic side effects for selected psychotropic drugs (*continued*)

Drug	Weight changes	Blood pressure changes	Glycemic changes	Lipid changes
Antidepressants (*continued*)				
Duloxetine (Cymbalta)	≥1% increase; 2% decrease	<1% increase	<1% increase	<1% increase
Fluoxetine (Prozac)	2% decrease; <1% increase	1%–10% increase	<1% decrease	<1% increase
Fluvoxamine (Luvox)	1%–2% decrease; 1%–10% increase	≤1% decrease	<1% increase or decrease	<1% increase
Milnacipran (Savella)	≥1% increase or decrease	5% increase	NDIA	≥1% increase
Mirtazapine (Remeron)	12%–49% increase	1%–10% increase	NDIA	>10% increase
Paroxetine (Paxil)	≥1% increase	≥1% increase	<1% increase	<1% increase
Sertraline (Zoloft)	1%–10% increase	NDIA	<1% increase	NDIA
Tricyclics in general	Increase or decrease	Increase or decrease	Increase or decrease	NDIA

Table 12–4. Percentage of metabolic side effects for selected psychotropic drugs *(continued)*

Drug	Weight changes	Blood pressure changes	Glycemic changes	Lipid changes
Mood stabilizers				
Gabapentin (Neurontin)	2%–3% increase	<1% increase or decrease	1% increase	<1% increase
Lamotrigine (Lamictal)	5% decrease; 1%–5% increase	<1% increase	<1% increase	NDIA
Lithium	Increase	NDIA	NDIA	NDIA
Topiramate (Topamax)	1% increase; 4%–9% decrease	1%–2% increase	1% increase	<1% increase
Valproic acid (Depakote)	6% decrease; 4%–9% increase	1%–5% increase or decrease	<1% increase	NDIA

Note.   Incidence rates are over variable time ranges (weeks to months). CHOL=cholesterol; im=intramuscular; NDIA=no definitive information available; TRI=triglycerides.

Source.   Turkoski BB: *Drug Information Handbook for Advanced Practice Nursing,* 13th Edition. Hudson, OH, Lexi-Comp, 2012.

readiness to change allows the clinician to tailor the change interventions to challenge the patient to achieve the stated goals and possibly move on to the next stage. Patients with severe mental illnesses have moved from preparation to action stage in increasing activity and decreasing smoking by targeting what they wanted personally and rewarding that achievement. The poorer the mental health of the patient, the less likely it is that the patient will make changes; however, change is still possible (Gorczynski et al. 2010; Schorr et al. 2009). This situation requires more creative strategies on the part of clinicians to identify what patients are willing to invest in making changes and what they need to do to assist the patient in taking those small steps.

The interventional strategy that psychiatric advanced practice registered nurses are most adept at and likely to incorporate into their practice is stress management (see Table 12–3). Because stress is one of the associated factors that contributes to metabolic syndrome, the clinician must assess patients' stressors and coping skills in an effort to assist them in lowering their stress response. Cognitive-behavioral therapy and dialectical behavior therapy have established track records in effectiveness in these areas. All patients deserve assistance and coaching in managing stress in their lives regardless of risk for metabolic syndrome. The risk only adds to the necessity of providing these strategies.

The lessons learned from the *Healthy People* initiative include the reality that obesity continues to increase each decade, even though it is a target of health promotion. As the obesity rate increases among the young, it is reasonable to project higher health care costs as they age. Nutritional and neurological science continues to provide greater understanding in how the metabolic syndrome occurs biologically, and pharmacological approaches are sure to follow. Clinicians need to have empathy for the difficulty in making lifestyle changes in the face of mental illness and disorder. At the same time, clinicians need to be encouraging and supportive of patients' self-efficacy in making internal changes without relying on medications to make changes. Clinicians need to assist patients by monitoring medications that are prescribed for their psychiatric symptoms and view patients holistically with health promotion needs and psychiatric intervention. At times, APRNs need to balance the benefits with the risks and choose the least harmful intervention but also help to mitigate possible harm. When patients need medication that is not covered by their insurance but provides benefits and less harm than other covered medications, the APRN must advocate for the patient with both insurance companies and pharmaceutical companies. As the U.S. Food and Drug Administration approves safer and more efficacious medications, the APRN needs to review the evidence of effect on other aspects of the person beyond their psychiatric symptoms and push for more effective strategies to manage the patient's medication needs.

Summary

When the APRN makes the clinical decision to use medications that may improve a patient's psychiatric symptoms at the risk of contributing to metabolic symptoms, it is critical to weigh the risks versus the benefits with the patient in a straightforward way. The mention of weight gain as a possible side effect frightens many patients to such an extent that they may refuse a promising medication because of the chance of gaining weight. It is helpful to discuss clinical data in simple terms to communicate not only the possibility of metabolic changes but also how the patient and the APRN will diligently monitor for these changes. Obtaining weight and blood pressure measurements at each visit demonstrates to the patient the importance of monitoring. Additionally, the APRN uses this opportunity to offer teaching and motivational counseling regarding basic health promotion, thereby building the patient's trust in the APRN's holistic concern. This is also a time to guide the patient to consider smoking cessation and exercise. The APRN would advise the patient about laboratory monitoring when initiating medication treatment and would discuss the laboratory results at baseline and at the 3-month, 6-month, and annual follow-up visits to monitor lipid levels and serum glucose. These conversations with the patient would occur with each contact as a gentle way of challenging him or her to make healthy lifestyle choices. If early indications of metabolic changes appear, the APRN can work with the patient to implement lifestyle adjustments (if the medication is providing significant mental health stability) or discuss possible changes in medication.

Changes in the Current Procedural Terminology (CPT) codes require the APRN to provide more specific documentation of Evaluation and Management (E/M) services. These changes may seem like an added burden and unnecessary paperwork; however, they also provide a mechanism for embedding general health promotion efforts within the clinical visit and a means of making the APRN's holistic concerns more visible. The psychiatric APRN is still a nurse, and this attention to the patient's body as well as mind is one of the defining characteristics of the nursing role. Incorporating fully transparent patient counseling and teaching into provision of care is what all nurses—regardless of specialty—are uniquely prepared and qualified to do.

Clinical Pearls

- While many psychotropic medications are associated with a potential for metabolic syndrome, the prevalence of metabolic syndrome has increased steadily in the general population, and persons with mental illness are at particular risk regardless of medications taken.

- Metabolic rates vary among different medications, and a risk-versus-benefit determination regarding medication choices is necessary before initiating treatment and in discussions with the patient.

- Psychoeducation about the potential metabolic effects of medications, monitoring of metabolic status, and counseling regarding healthy lifestyle behaviors need to occur before initiating treatment and at periodic intervals during treatment.

References

Armitage CJ, Arden MA: How useful are the stages of change for targeting interventions? Randomized test of a brief intervention to reduce smoking. Health Psychol 27:789–798, 2008

Arslan N, Erdur B, Aydin A: Hormones and cytokines in childhood obesity. Indian Pediatr 47:829–839, 2010

Batscha C, Schneiderhan ME, Kataria Y, et al: Treatment settings and metabolic monitoring for people experiencing first-episode psychosis. J Psychosoc Nurs Ment Health Serv 48:44–49, 2010

Bleys J, Navas-Acien A, Stranges S, et al: Serum selenium and serum lipids in US adults. Am J Clin Nutr 88:416–423, 2008

Cahill K, Lancaster T, Green N: Stage-based interventions for smoking cessation. Cochrane Database of Systematic Reviews 2010, Issue 11. Art. No.:CD004492. DOI: 10.1002/14651858.CD004492.pub4

Cena H, Fonte ML, Turconi G: Relationship between smoking and metabolic syndrome. Nutr Rev 69:745–753, 2011

Clerc O, Nanchen D, Cornuz J, et al: Alcohol drinking, the metabolic syndrome and diabetes in a population with high mean alcohol consumption. Diabet Med 27:1241–1249, 2010

Dallman MF, Pecoraro N, Akana SF, et al: Chronic stress and obesity: a new view of "comfort food." Proc Natl Acad Sci U S A 100:11696–11701, 2003

Fan AZ, Russell M, Dorn J, et al: Lifetime alcohol drinking pattern is related to the prevalence of metabolic syndrome: The Western New York Health Study (WNYHS). Eur J Epidemiol 21:129–138, 2006

Ford ES, Giles WH, Dietz WH: Prevalence of the metabolic syndrome among US adults: findings from the third National Health and Nutrition Examination Survey. JAMA 287:356–359, 2002

Gorczynski P, Faulkner G, Greening S, et al: Exploring the construct validity of the transtheoretical model to structure physical activity interventions for individuals with serious mental illness. Psychiatr Rehabil J 34:61–64, 2010

Groth SW: Adiponectin and polycystic ovarian syndrome. Biol Res Nurs 12:62–72, 2010

Grundy SM, Brewer HB, Cleeman JI, et al: Definition of metabolic syndrome: report of the National Heart, Lung, and Blood Institute/American Heart Association Conference on Scientific Issues Related to Definition. Circulation 109:433–438, 2004

Grundy SM, Cleeman JI, Daniels SR, et al: Diagnosis and management of the metabolic syndrome: an American Heart Association/National Heart, Lung, and Blood Institute Scientific Statement. Circulation 112:2735–2752, 2005

Heppner PS, Crawford EF, Haji UA, et al: The association of posttraumatic stress disorder and metabolic syndrome: a study of increased health risk in veterans. BMC Med 7:1–27, 2009

Hermes E, Nasrallah H, Davis V, et al: The association between weight change and symptom reduction in the CATIE schizophrenia trial. Schizophr Res 128:166–170, 2011

Hishida A, Koyama A, Tomota A, et al: Smoking cessation, alcohol intake and transient increase in the risk of metabolic syndrome among Japanese smokers at one health checkup institution. BMC Public Health 9:263–271, 2009

Holt R, Abdelrahman T, Hirsch M, et al: The prevalence of undiagnosed metabolic abnormalities in people with serious mental illness. J Psychopharmacol 24:867–873, 2010

Hyman MA: Diabetes—asking the right questions. Altern Ther Health Med 12:10–13, 2006

Jakovljevi M, Sari M, Nad S, et al: Metabolic syndrome, somatic and psychiatric comorbidity in war veterans with posttraumatic stress disorder: preliminary findings. Psychiatr Danub 18:169–176, 2006

Jakovljevi M, Babi, D, Cmcevi Z, et al: Metabolic syndrome and depression in war veterans with post-traumatic stress disorder. Psychiatr Danub 20:406–410, 2008

Jallon P, Picard F: Bodyweight gain and anticonvulsants: a comparative review. Drug Saf 24:969–978, 2001

Jin H, Meyer J, Mudaliar S, et al: Use of clinical markers to identify metabolic syndrome in antipsychotic-treated patients. J Clin Psychiatry 71:1273–1278, 2010

Kahl KG, Greggersen W, Schweiger U, et al: Prevalence of the metabolic syndrome in men and women with alcohol dependence: results from a cross-sectional study during behavioural treatment in a controlled environment. Addiction 105:1923–1927, 2010

Kloiber S, Kohli MA, Brueckl T, et al: Variations in tryptophan hydroxylase 2 linked to decreased serotonergic activity are associated with elevated risk for metabolic syndrome in depression [published erratum appears in Mol Psychiatry 15:1123, 2010]. Mol Psychiatry 15:736–747, 2010

Laaksonen DE, Lakka HM, Niskanen LK, et al: Metabolic syndrome and development of diabetes mellitus: application and validation of recently suggested definitions of the metabolic syndrome in a prospective cohort study. Am J Epidemiol 156:1070–1077, 2002

Langfeldt G: The insulin tolerance test in mental disorders. Acta Psychiatr Scand 80:189–200, 1952

Licht CMM, Vreeburg SA, van Reedt Dortland AKB, et al: Increased sympathetic and decreased parasympathetic activity rather than changes in hypothalamic-pituitary-adrenal axis activity is associated with metabolic abnormalities. J Clin Endocrinol Metab 95:2458–2466, 2010

Ma J, Folsom AR, Melnick SL, et al: Associations of serum and dietary magnesium with cardiovascular disease, hypertension, diabetes, insulin, and carotid arterial wall thickness: the ARIC study. Atherosclerosis Risk in Communities Study. J Clin Epidemiol 48:927–940, 1995

Mari O, Furuya R, Ohkawa S, et al: Altered abdominal fat distribution and its association with serum lipid profile in non-diabetic haemo-dialysis patients. Nephrol Dial Transplant 14:2427–2432, 1999

McIntyre RS, Danilewitz M, Liauw S, et al: Bipolar disorder and metabolic syndrome: an international perspective. J Affect Disord 126:366–387, 2010

McKeown NM, Jacques PF, Zhang XI, et al: Dietary intake is related to metabolic syndrome in older Americans. Euro J Nutr 47:210–216, 2008

Mukherjee S, Schnur DB, Reddy R: Family history of type 2 diabetes in schizophrenic patients (letter). Lancet 1(8636):495, 1989

Nogueiras R, Tschöp MH, Zigman JM: Central nervous system regulation of energy metabolism: ghrelin versus leptin. Ann N Y Acad Sci 1126:14–19, 2008

Praharaj K, Jana AK, Goyal N, et al: Metformin for olanzapine-induced weight gain: a systematic review and meta-analysis. Br J Clin Pharmacol 71:377–382, 2010

Puchau B, Zulet MA, de Echavarri AG, et al: Selenium intake reduces serum C3, an early marker of metabolic syndrome manifestations, in healthy young adults. Eur J Clin Nutr 63:858–864, 2009

Raedler TJ: Cardiovascular aspects of antipsychotics. Curr Opin Psychiatry 23:574–581, 2010

Rosell M, de Faire U, Hellenius M-L: Low prevalence of the metabolic syndrome in wine drinkers—is it the alcohol beverage or the lifestyle? Euro J Clin Nutr 57:227–234, 2003

Ryan MCM, Collins P, Thakore JH: Impaired fasting glucose tolerance in first-episode, drug-naïve patients with schizophrenia. Am J Psychiatry 160:284–289, 2003

Schorr G, Ulbricht S, Baumeister SE, et al: Mental health and readiness to change smoking behavior in daily smoking primary care patients. Int J Behav Med 16:347–354, 2009

Surendar J, Mohan V, Rao MM, et al: Increased levels of both Th1 and Th2 cytokines in subjects with metabolic syndrome (CURES-103). Diabetes Technol Ther 13:477–482, 2011

Taylor V, McKinnon MC, Macdonald K, et al: Adults with mood disorders have an increased risk profile for cardiovascular disease within the first 2 years of treatment. Can J Psychiatry 55:362–368, 2010

Torrent C, Amann B, Sanchez-Moreno J, et al: Weight gain in bipolar disorder: pharmacological treatment as a contributing factor. Acta Psychiatr Scand 118:4–18, 2008

U.S. Department of Agriculture: ChooseMyPlate.gov (available at: http://www.choosemyplate.gov). Accessed December 2011.

U.S. Department of Health and Human Services: Healthy People 2000: National Health Promotion and Disease Prevention Objectives (DHHS Publ PHS 91-50212). Washington, DC, U.S. Department of Health and Human Services, 1991

U.S. Department of Health and Human Services: Healthy People 2010: Understanding and Improving Health, 2nd Edition. Washington, DC, U.S. Government Printing Office, 2000

U.S. Department of Health and Human Services: The Surgeon General's Vision for a Healthy and Fit Nation. Rockville, MD, U.S. Department of Health and Human Services, Office of the Surgeon General, 2010

Whisman MA: Loneliness and the metabolic syndrome in a population-based sample of middle-aged and older adults. Health Psychol 29:550–554, 2010

13

Complementary and Alternative Pharmacotherapies

Bobbie Posmontier, Ph.D., C.N.M., A.P.R.N., P.M.H.-N.P., B.C.

> Every problem has in it the seeds of its own solutions.
> If you don't have any problems, you don't have any seeds.
>
> –Norman Vincent Peale (1898–1993)

Complementary and alternative medicine is practiced worldwide among patients in both Eastern and Western cultures to improve general health and well-being, treat a variety of both acute and chronic illnesses, cope with medication side effects, and achieve a measure of control over personal health (Barnes et al. 2008). According to a survey from the National Center for Health Statistics in 2007, approximately one in four adults and one in nine children have used complementary and alternative medicine to achieve these goals (Bercovitz et al. 2011). Use may be even more frequent among patients who have mental illness (Vermani et al. 2005). *Complementary medicine* refers to modalities that are used in concert with conventional medicine, whereas *alternative medicine* refers to those modalities that are used instead of conventional medicine (Barnes et al. 2008).

Complementary and alternative medicine encompasses many modalities, including herbs, vitamin and nutritional therapies, homeopathy, yoga, massage, chiropractic, acupuncture, energy therapies such as Reiki and therapeutic touch, music therapy, and horticultural therapy. Most patients use these modalities as an accompaniment to conventional medicine. For this reason, the potential exists for interactions—in particular, interactions between herbal remedies and psychotropic medications. The objective of this chapter is to introduce psychiatric clinicians to 10 herbal preparations commonly used for relief of mental illness symptoms by people in the United States that may have an effect on conventional psychopharmacological treatment: St. John's wort, valerian root, ginseng, kava, ginkgo biloba, schisandra, passionflower, black cohosh, gotu kola, and lemon balm (Table 13–1). There are many other herbal preparations not covered here; clinicians seeking a more in-depth understanding of this field should consult herbal texts within both the Eastern and Western traditions. Finally, although the focus of this chapter is on the psychiatric effects of herbs, readers should bear in mind that herbs may possess a wide range of medicinal qualities that affect many aspects of health.

Herbal Preparations Commonly Used to Treat Psychiatric Symptoms

St. John's Wort (*Hypericum perforatum*)

Description

St. John's wort, the most widely studied herb for depression and also known as goat weed and klamath weed, is an aromatic perennial that has been used for its antidepressant properties since the time of the ancient Greeks (Vermani et al. 2005). The leaves and flowers contain 0.1% hypericin and pseudohypericin, which are thought to be the active ingredients that promote its antidepressant effect (Butterweck and Schmidt 2007; Wong et al. 1998).

Mechanism of Action

The mechanism of action of St. John's wort may be attributed to monoamine oxidase (MAO) inhibition of MAO type A (MAO-A) or type B (MAO-B), inhibition of catechol O-methyltransferase (COMT), inhibition of serotonin reuptake, reduced serotonin receptor expression, inhibition of dopamine reuptake, N-methyl-D-aspartate (NMDA) antagonism, and inhibition of interleukin and cytokine release (Bladt and Wagner 1994; V. Kumar et al. 2006; Ruedeberg et al. 2010; Suzuki et al. 1984; Thiede and Walper 1994).

Efficacy

Three well-known meta-analyses have assessed the efficacy of St. John's wort. The first was a meta-analysis of 23 randomized controlled trials composed of 1,757 outpatients (Linde et al. 1996). Results suggested that St. John's wort was more effective than placebo in treating mild to moderate depressive symptoms and had efficacy comparable to that of conventional antidepressants, including sertraline. In the second meta-analysis, which reviewed 27 trials composed of 2,291 patients, St. John's wort was found to be more effective than placebo in mild to moderate depression; however, evidence was inadequate to conclude that it was as efficacious as conventional antidepressants (Linde and Mulrow 2000). Limitations of the studies included a short duration of only 4–8 weeks, varying diagnostic criteria, variable dosages of hypericin, and subtherapeutic dosages of antidepressants. In the third meta-analysis examining the efficacy of St. John's wort among 5,489 patients in 29 trials in major depression, St. John's wort was superior to placebo and was similar in efficacy to that of conventional antidepressants but had fewer side effects (Linde et al. 2008). In summary, the evidence suggests that St. John's wort is more effective than placebo for mild to moderate depression and has fewer side effects than conventional antidepressants.

Herbal and Medication Interactions

St. John's wort is both an inhibitor and an inducer of a variety of cytochrome P450 (CYP) enzymes, including 1A2, 3A4, 2B6, 2C19, and 2D6 (Hokkanen et al. 2011; Lei et al. 2010; Murphy et al. 2005; Van Strater and Bogers 2012). Given its action on serotonin, St. John's wort should be used with extreme caution in patients who are prescribed or who are taking other serotonergic agents. The risk of serotonin syndrome increases when St. John's wort is taken

Table 13–1.   Complementary and alternative pharmacotherapies commonly used for psychiatric symptoms

Agent	Potential indications	Dosing	Efficacy	Side effects
St. John's wort (*Hypericum perforatum*)	Mild to moderate depression	300 mg three times daily	+	+
Valerian (*Valeriana officinalis*)	Anxiety, mild insomnia	400–900 mg/day	+/–	+/– rare
Ginseng root (*Panax ginseng*)	Mood, anxiety, fatigue, endurance	1–2 g/day	+/–	+/– rare
Kava (*Piper methysticum*)	Anxiety	Total 140–210 mg/day in two to three divided doses	+	+
Ginkgo biloba *Ginkgo biloba*	Memory, mental acuity, fatigue, endurance	Total 120–160 mg/day in two to three divided doses (four to six are needed to determine effect)	+/–	+
Schisandra (*Schisandra chinensis*)	Mental clarity, endurance, cognitive impairment, fatigue/insomnia, alcohol abuse, depression, schizophrenia	500 mg–2 g of extract daily	–	+

Table 13–1. Complementary and alternative pharmacotherapies commonly used for psychiatric symptoms *(continued)*

Agent	Potential indications	Dosing	Efficacy	Side effects
Passionflower (*Passiflora incarnata*)	Insomnia, anxiety, opiate withdrawal, ADHD symptoms	2–5 g dried herb up to three times daily	+/–	+
Black cohosh (*Actaea racemosa* or *Cimicifuga racemosa*)	Irritability, mood swings, hot flashes, sleep disturbances related to menopause	20–40 mg twice daily	+/–	+
Gotu kola (*Centella asiatica*)	Fatigue, anxiety, depression, memory impairment, enhancement of intelligence	60–180 mg of extract daily	+/–	+
Lemon balm (*Melissa officinalis*)	Anxiety, sleep disorders, ADHD symptoms, agitation in dementia	2 g/day	+/–	+/–

Note.   ADHD=attention-deficit/hyperactivity disorder; – =no significant information known; +/– =possible; + =definite.

concomitantly with psychotropic medications such as the selective serotonin reuptake inhibitors and serotonin-norepinephrine reuptake inhibitors and the atypical antipsychotics. The risk of serotonin syndrome also increases when St. John's wort is taken with the triptan family of medications used to treat migraine headaches.

Adverse Effects

Possible adverse effects of St. John's wort include photosensitivity, stomach upset, dizziness, dry mouth, restlessness, constipation, and rare induction of mania or hypomania and psychosis (Joshi and Faubion 2005; Vermani et al. 2005). Caution is advised with the use of St. John's wort in pregnancy and lactation (Dugoua et al. 2006). Although no randomized clinical trials have been done among pregnant humans, in vitro animal studies suggested that St. John's wort does not cause long-term behavioral or cognitive effects in offspring but may result in low birth weight. In addition, animal studies suggested that St. John's wort has no effects on milk supply or infant weight but in a few cases may cause infant colic, lethargy, and drowsiness. St. John's wort is contraindicated in pheochromocytoma and in circumstances of intense exposure to sunlight (Wielgus et al. 2007). There are concerns about spontaneous bleeding (subarachnoid hemorrhage, subdural hematoma) in elderly individuals taking St. John's wort (Jacobs et al. 2007).

Valerian (*Valeriana officinalis*)

Description

Valerian root is an herbaceous perennial that was used in ancient Greece and Rome and currently is used to promote sleep and relieve anxiety. Its active ingredients, which promote its hypnotic and sedative effects, include valepotriates and sesquiterpenes.

Mechanism of Action

The mechanism of action of valerian is believed to be related to its γ-aminobutyric acid type B ($GABA_B$) receptor binding properties, GABA reuptake inhibition, and general GABA agonist actions (Benke et al. 2009). In addition, another study found that valerian is a partial agonist at the serotonin type 5A ($5\text{-}HT_{5A}$) receptor (Dietz et al. 2005).

Efficacy

Results of several studies confirmed the efficacy of valerian in improving measures of sleep quality, improving slow-wave sleep, and reducing time to onset of sleep but were limited by significant differences in design between studies (Bent et al. 2006; Salter and Brownie 2010). In a recent randomized triple-blind study of 100 postmenopausal women between 50 and 60 years old, findings suggested that valerian significantly improved sleep quality compared with placebo (Taavoni et al. 2011). In a meta-analysis of 18 randomized controlled trials evaluating the effectiveness of valerian for insomnia, findings suggested that although the studies indicated subjective improvement in sleep, further studies were needed to assess objective and quantitative measures of efficacy (Fernandez-San-Martin et al. 2010). Another meta-analysis of 29 randomized controlled trials found no significant effects of valerian on sleep (Taibi et al. 2007). Although an animal study found significant anxiolytic effects among mice (Benke et al. 2009), few studies have validated this effect in humans. One human study of 36 patients found a significant decrease in anxiety among valerian and diazepam (Valium) groups compared with placebo after 4 weeks of treatment, but results were limited by the small number of participants in each group, short duration of the study, and low dosages of active ingredients (Andreatini et al. 2002). In summary, preliminary studies suggested that valerian is effective in treating insomnia and anxiety, but more randomized controlled trials are needed to validate its efficacy.

Herbal and Medication Interactions

Some studies indicate adverse interactions between valerian and conventional psychotropics. One animal study reported an increase in hepatic delta-aminolevulinate dehydratase (delta-ALAD) activity, a marker for oxidative stress, and an increase in serum alanine aminotransferase (ALT) activity among rats given a combination of haloperidol (Haldol) and valerian (Dalla Corte et al. 2008). However, neither haloperidol nor valerian produced this effect alone. Findings from earlier studies suggested that valerian may act to potentiate the effects of barbiturates and the sedative effects of anesthetics and other central nervous system (CNS) depressants (Vermani et al. 2005). Another study suggested that valerian is unlikely to have any effects on the CYP enzymes (Gurley et al. 2005).

Adverse Effects

Findings from a meta-analysis of eight randomized controlled studies with sample sizes ranging from 20 to 830 suggested that adverse effects of valerian are rare but may include headaches, sweating, nausea, diarrhea, hangover effects, mental dullness, difficulty sleeping, depression, irritability, feeling detached, and an exaggerated feeling of well-being (Taibi et al. 2007).

Ginseng root (*Panax ginseng*)

Description

Ginseng is an ancient Asian folk remedy that has been used to treat mood and anxiety disorders, improve endurance, and relieve fatigue and stress (Vermani et al. 2005). Seven species of ginseng are found globally, and two, Siberian and Chinese ginseng, have distinctly different chemical structures (Attele et al. 1999; LaFrance et al. 2000). Active ingredients in the root are composed of at least 13 ginsenosides, which contain triterpenoid saponin glycosides. Ginseng preparations may be administered by mouth, intranasally, or via parenteral administration (Vermani et al. 2005).

Mechanism of Action

Studies from animal models suggest that the mechanism of action may involve an increase in acetylcholine release from the hippocampus, increased uptake of choline into cholinergic nerve endings, and promotion of nerve growth, which serves to facilitate learning and memory (Attele et al. 1999). In addition, ginseng inhibits the uptake of GABA, glutamate, dopamine, norepinephrine, and serotonin in animal models and competes with GABA agonists for binding at $GABA_A$ and $GABA_B$ receptors, which may promote CNS depression.

Efficacy

In a recent meta-analysis of eight studies that examined the effect of ginseng on psychomotor function among healthy volunteers and patients with Alzheimer's disease (sample sizes ranging from 15 to 97), findings suggested that ginseng significantly improved cognition and mood (Lee and Son 2011). However, studies were limited by small sample size, and most samples were composed of healthy volunteers.

Herbal and Medication Interactions

Although recent animal studies have found no evidence of ginseng's effect on CYP enzymes 2C9 or 2D6, it may affect medication serum levels through CYP1A2 induction and CYP3A4 inhibition (Bilgi et al. 2010; Liu et al. 2012).

Adverse Effects

According to a recent systematic review of 57 studies, ginseng appears to have a good safety profile with few adverse effects (Lee and Son 2011). Rare adverse effects that have been reported include insomnia, headache, chest discomfort, gastrointestinal upset, nausea, diarrhea, constipation, vomiting, hypoglycemia, hypertension, restlessness, anxiety, euphoria, mania, and psychosis (Joshi and Faubion 2005; Lee and Son 2011; Vermani et al. 2005).

Kava (*Piper methysticum*)

Description

Kava is a type of pepper grown in the South Pacific, whose root has been used to provide calming and mental clarity (LaFrance et al. 2000). The Latin meaning of *Piper* is "pepper," and *methysticum* means "intoxicating." The root contains psychoactive kava pyrones that have shown anticonvulsive properties through delayed inhibition of voltage-gated sodium channels as well as neuroprotection against focal cerebral ischemia in animal models. The main constituents are methysticin and dihydromethysticin. Use of kava has been restricted in Europe, Australia, Britain, and Canada over concerns of hepatotoxicity (Rychetnik and Madronio 2011; Sarris et al. 2009, 2011b). However, kava is still widely available in the United States and New Zealand and used for its anxiolytic effects.

Mechanism of Action

The mechanism of action of kava is believed to be related to selective binding to $GABA_A$ receptor complexes in the amygdala, hippocampus, and medulla and has similar effects to benzodiazepines, including muscle relaxation and anesthetic, anticonvulsant, and anxiolytic effects (LaFrance et al. 2000; Thompson et al. 2004). One of the kava pyrones, desmethoxyyangonin, may act as a reversible MAO-B inhibitor and boost the levels of dopamine, causing euphoric effects, whereas kavain may inhibit the reuptake of norepinephrine at the norepinephrine transporter and increase attention and arousal (Cairney et al. 2002, 2003; Uebelhack et al. 1998).

Efficacy

A comprehensive review found that kava was efficacious for the treatment of anxiety in four of six studies reviewed (Sarris et al. 2011a). In a 3-week double-blind, randomized controlled study of 60 adults with generalized anxiety, a significant decrease in depression and anxiety scores occurred after ingestion of aqueous kava without adverse effects (Sarris et al. 2009). An earlier meta-analysis evaluated six randomized controlled studies, which compared the effect of kava extract on nonpsychotic generalized anxiety disorder. Among 180 patients administered extract compared with 165 patients administered placebo, kava was significantly more effective than placebo (odds ratio = 3.30; 95% confidence interval = 2.09–5.22) in decreasing symptoms of anxiety (Witte et al. 2005).

Herbal and Medication Interactions

In a recent study, two constituents of kava, methysticin and 7,8-dihydromethysticin, were found to induce the CYP enzyme 1A1 (Li et al. 2011). In addition, kava may interact with CYP 2E1, 2D6, 2C9, 2C19, and 3A4 (Gurley et al. 2005; Mathews et al. 2005).

Adverse Effects

Adverse effects may include gastrointestinal upset, oral lingual dyskinesia, torticollis, vertigo, weight loss, loss of appetite, indigestion, and scaly rash (LaFrance et al. 2000; Rychetnik and Madronio 2011). Other adverse effects may include elevated liver enzymes (especially with heavy use of kava drink), elevated cholesterol levels, hepatotoxicity, elevated γ-glutamyltransferase, and decreased albumin and protein (Brown et al. 2007; LaFrance et al. 2000). In addition, use of kava may be associated with disorientation when taken with benzodiazepines. Finally, kava may result in rhabdomyolysis (Bodkin et al. 2012; LaFrance et al. 2000).

Ginkgo (*Ginkgo biloba*)

Description

Ginkgo leaf extract comes from a large and ancient species of tree, *Ginkgo biloba*, grown in China and used for its medicinal qualities for at least 5,000 years (Birks and Grimley Evans 2009). Ginkgo has been used for endurance, memory-enhancing effects in Alzheimer's disease and vascular dementia, mental alertness, and treatment of stress, fatigue, and cerebrovascular insufficiency. Active constituents in ginkgo biloba include flavonoids, terpenoids, and organic acids.

Mechanism of Action

Three major components, including ginkgo flavone glycosides, ginkgolides, and bilobalide, work in concert as free oxygen radical scavengers, which protect cell membrane integrity and inhibit platelet-activating factor (LaFrance et al. 2000). In animal models, ginkgo biloba has prevented choline release from the hippocampus when animals were subjected to hypoxia, increased GABA and glutamic acid decarboxylase activity, and increased muscarinic receptors in the hippocampus.

Efficacy

Findings from several studies have suggested that ginkgo biloba is efficacious in treating cerebrovascular insufficiency, erectile dysfunction, dementia, memory and concentration deficits, fatigue, anxiety, depressed mood, and tardive dyskinesia in schizophrenic patients administered antipsychotic medications and in improving glucose tolerance (LaFrance et al. 2000; Vermani et al. 2005; Zhang et al. 2011; Zhou et al. 2011). In addition, ginkgo biloba may have some efficacy in treating attention-deficit disorder (Niederhofer 2010). In a randomized controlled trial consisting of 3,069 subjects age 75 years or older, ginkgo biloba had no effects on the rate of dementia or Alzheimer's disease development and no effects on mild cognitive impairment compared with placebo (DeKosky et al. 2008). In a recent meta-analysis, however, consisting of nine randomized clinical trials and 2,372 patients, ginkgo biloba appeared more effective than placebo in treating cognitive deficits associated with Alzheimer's disease and vascular dementias (Weinmann et al. 2010).

Herbal and Medication Interactions

Ginkgo biloba may potentiate the effects of anticoagulants and increase the risk for spontaneous bleeding through its constituent ginkgolide because it inhibits platelet-activating factor (Vermani et al. 2005). Bilobalide, another major constituent of ginkgo extract, can induce the CYP enzyme S-warfarin hydroxylase and attenuate the anticoagulation effects of warfarin (Taki et al. 2012). Findings also suggest that ginkgo extract is an inducer of CYP3A4 (Robertson et al. 2008).

Adverse Effects

Few side effects are associated with ginkgo leaf extract use but may include headache, dizziness, palpitations, constipation, gastrointestinal upset, and allergic skin rash (Natural Medicines Comprehensive Database 2011). One case of Stevens-Johnson syndrome was reported when ginkgo leaf extract was taken with choline, vitamin B_6, and vitamin B_{12}. When used in large doses, ginkgo biloba may result in restlessness, diarrhea, nausea, vomiting, poor muscle tone, and weakness. One major concern with ginkgo biloba use is the potential for spontaneous bleeding, which has been cited in several case reports, especially after surgery. However, findings of large-scale trials do not support this effect. Ingestion of ginkgo biloba seed has been associated with abdominal pain, nausea, vomiting, diarrhea, restlessness, difficulty breathing, weak pulse, seizures, loss of consciousness, and shock. Ginkotoxin, which is found in small amounts in the leaves and larger amounts in the seeds, may cause seizures and death. However, causal evidence is insufficient to support the occurrence of seizures in patients ingesting only ginkgo leaf or ginkgo leaf extract.

Schisandra (*Schisandra chinensis*)

Description

The schisandra berry is an ancient herb native to Russia and China that has been used as a tonic in traditional Chinese medicine for a variety of effects, including cough suppression, immune enhancement, liver detoxification, mental clarity, and improved endurance, as well as to treat stress, cognitive impairment, fatigue, insomnia, weakness, schizophrenia, alcoholism, and depression (Pederson 2002; Yance and Valentine 1999). It has been widely used in Russia since the 1960s and is included in their *National Pharmacopoeia of the USSR* and *State Register of Drugs* (Panossian and Wikman 2008). Active ingredients include schizandrin, schizandrol, gomisins, schizanders, schisantherins, wuweizisus, citral, stigmasterol, other lignans, and vitamins C and E (Natural Medicines Comprehensive Database 2011).

Mechanism of Action

Animal studies of the effects of schizandrin, the main constituent affecting the CNS, suggest that it is a CNS stimulant and stabilizes bioelectric activity in the cerebral cortex (Panossian and Wikman 2008). In other animal studies, schizandrin and other constituents, including gomisin A, C, D, and G and schizandrol B, inhibit the activity of anticholinesterase, which may enhance cognition. Schisandra also may exert its anxiolytic, antidepressant, and memory-enhancing effects by reducing cortisol, nitric oxide, and phosphorylated stress-activated protein kinase; promoting antioxidant effects; and altering monoamine neurotransmitter levels (Chen et al. 2011; Panossian and Wikman 2008).

Efficacy

Although no human studies could be located, animal studies have found that schisandra is effective for reducing anxiety and depression and improving cognitive function (Chen et al. 2011; Giridharan et al. 2011; Panossian and Wikman 2008)

Herbal and Medication Interactions

Some findings suggest that schisandra strongly inhibits CYP3A4 and CYP2C9 (Panossian and Wikman 2008).

Adverse Effects

Use of schisandra extract may result in gastrointestinal upset, decreased appetite, skin rash, and itching (Natural Medicines Comprehensive Database 2011).

Passionflower (*Passiflora incarnata*)

Description

Passionflower, a climbing vine originating in the subtropical Americas, was recognized by early Spanish explorers as a sign of God's favor because the corona of the flower resembled the crown of thorns on Jesus, and the petals represented his 10 apostles (Natural Medicines Comprehensive Database 2011). It has been used by natural healers to treat insomnia, anxiety, opiate withdrawal, and attention-deficit/hyperactivity disorder. Active constituents include apigenin, luteolin, quercetin, kamferol, isovitexin, harmine, harmaline, harmalol, harman, harmin, maltol, and ethyl maltol.

Mechanism of Action

One of the constituents of passionflower, apigenin, is hypothesized to bind to CNS benzodiazepine receptors to exert its anxiolytic effects (Natural Medicines Comprehensive Database 2011). In animal studies, passionflower extracts also have been found to modulate levels of $GABA_A$ within hippocampal neurons (Elsas et al. 2010). In addition, evidence has been found that passionflower is an antagonist at the $GABA_B$ receptor (Appel et al. 2011).

Efficacy

Few human studies have examined the efficacy of passionflower. In a study of opiate withdrawal among 65 opiate-addicted persons, passionflower extract plus clonidine (Catapres) were more effective in reducing severe effects of opiate withdrawal than was clonidine alone (Akhondzadeh et al. 2001a). In a 4-week trial comparing the effects of oxazepam (Serax) and passionflower among 36 outpatients with generalized anxiety disorder, passionflower was equally effective but had less effect on job impairment than did oxazepam (Akhondzadeh et al. 2001b). A meta-analysis of passionflower that included two eligible studies and 198 patients concluded that there have been too few randomized clinical trials to draw conclusions about the efficacy of passionflower for anxiety (Miyasaka et al. 2007). A small randomized controlled trial comparing the hypnotic effects of passionflower tea with placebo among 45 patients found that passionflower was superior to placebo for improving sleep quality (Ngan and Conduit 2011). Further large-scale human clinical trials are warranted to fully assess the efficacy of passionflower for reducing symptoms of opiate withdrawal and anxiety and improving sleep.

Herbal and Medication Interactions

Because passionflower is sedating, it may potentiate the effects of CNS depressants such as pentobarbital (Nembutal), secobarbital (Seconal), clonazepam (Klonopin), lorazepam (Ativan), and zolpidem (Ambien) (Natural

Medicines Comprehensive Database 2011). In addition, passionflower may potentiate the effects of anticoagulants, anticonvulsants, tricyclic antidepressants, and MAO inhibitors (University of Maryland Medical Center 2011).

Adverse Effects

Reported adverse effects of passionflower include dizziness, confusion, sedation, and ataxia (Natural Medicines Comprehensive Database 2011). A case report of nausea, vomiting, prolonged QT interval, and ventricular tachycardia also was reported in the literature. One of the species of passionflower, *Passiflora edulis,* has been associated with liver and pancreatic toxicity.

Black Cohosh (*Actaea racemosa* or *Cimicifuga racemosa*)

Description

Black cohosh is a tall flowering plant in the buttercup family native to North America; the plant grows in rich, shady wooded areas (University of Maryland Medical Center 2011). It was discovered by Native Americans more than 200 years ago for its medicinal qualities, including decreasing irritability, mood swings, hot flashes, and sleep disturbances associated with menopause. Active constituents include phytosterin; isoferulic acid; fukinolic acid; caffeic acid; salicylic acid; sugars; tannins; long-chain fatty acids; and triterpene glycosides, including actein, cimicifugoside, and 27-deoxyacteine (Natural Medicines Comprehensive Database 2011).

Mechanism of Action

Fukinolic acid may inhibit neutrophil elastase, which may contribute to its anti-inflammatory effects (Natural Medicines Comprehensive Database 2011). Although black cohosh possesses estrogenic effects, the mechanism by which it accomplishes this is not fully understood. Findings from animal research suggest that it may suppress luteinizing hormone release from the pituitary gland. Results from preliminary research also suggest that black cohosh may act as a partial 5-HT agonist by binding to 5-HT_{1A}, 5-HT_{1D}, and 5-HT_7 receptors.

Efficacy

A meta-analysis of six double-blind, randomized controlled trials assessing the efficacy of black cohosh among 1,112 peri- and postmenopausal women did not find conclusive evidence supporting its efficacy (Borrelli and Ernst 2008). In addition, because the studies reviewed did not separate out the individual symptoms of menopause, it is difficult to ascertain whether black cohosh had an effect on psychiatric manifestations of menopause, including irritability, mood swings, and sleep disturbance. In contrast, another double-blind, randomized, placebo-controlled study evaluating the effects of black cohosh plus St. John's wort over a 16-week period among 301 women with menopausal symptoms found that women in the treatment group experienced significantly less depression and adverse menopausal symptoms than did those in the control group (Uebelhack et al. 2006). Further randomized controlled studies are warranted to fully ascertain the efficacy of black cohosh for psychiatric manifestations of menopause.

Herbal and Medication Interactions

Findings suggest that black cohosh is a modest inhibitor of CYP2D6, which may increase serum levels of medications metabolized by this route (Natural Medicines Comprehensive Database 2011). In addition, individual case reports have suggested that black cohosh also may elevate liver enzymes when taken with atorvastatin (Lipitor), as well as reduce the cytotoxic effects of the chemotherapeutic agent cisplatin in animal models. Risks of liver failure may increase when taken with hepatotoxic medications such as acetaminophen (Tylenol), carbamazepine (Tegretol), isoniazid (Tubizid), methotrexate (Rheumatrex, Trexall), and methyldopa (Aldoril).

Adverse Effects

Adverse effects of black cohosh may include gastrointestinal upset, rash, headache, dizziness, weight gain, cramping, breast tenderness, vaginal bleeding, liver toxicity, and a feeling of heaviness in the legs (Natural Medicines Comprehensive Database 2011). Other case reports have suggested that use of black cohosh may have a causal link to the onset of asthenia and muscle damage, cutaneous pseudolymphoma, venous thrombosis in protein S–deficient patients, and seizures. Because of its estrogenic effects, black cohosh could potentially increase the risk for metastasis in women with breast cancer.

Gotu Kola (*Centella asiatica*)

Description

Gotu kola is an herbaceous annual plant native to Asia (Natural Medicines Comprehensive Database 2011). It has been used in Ayurvedic and Chinese medicine to treat fatigue, anxiety, depression, and Alzheimer's disease, as well as to enhance memory and intelligence. Its active constituents include asiatic acid, madecassic acid, asiaticoside A (madecassoside), asiaticoside B, quercetin, kaempferol, sesquiterpenes, stigmasterol, sitosterol, and isothankuniside.

Mechanism of Action

The anxiolytic actions of gotu kola may be attributed to its binding with cholecystokinin and GABA receptors (Natural Medicines Comprehensive Database 2011). The efficacy of gotu kola in the treatment of Alzheimer's disease may be attributed to the asiaticoside derivatives, asiatic acid, asiaticoside 6, and SM2, which may play a role in neuroprotection from β-amyloid toxicity.

Efficacy

In a small recent pretest/posttest comparative study evaluating the effects of gotu kola on 33 patients with generalized anxiety disorder over a 60-day period, findings suggested that gotu kola significantly improved symptoms of anxiety, depression, and poor concentration (Jana et al. 2010). Another animal model study found that gotu kola decreased acetylcholinesterase activity and oxidative stress and reduced β-amyloid levels in the hippocampus, but no known studies have been performed to assess this effect in humans (Dhanasekaran et al. 2009; A. Kumar et al. 2009). Further double-blind, randomized controlled studies are warranted to fully evaluate the effects of gotu kola on psychiatric symptoms and Alzheimer's disease.

Herbal and Medication Interactions

Gotu kola may potentiate the effects of sedatives and hepatotoxic medications. A recent study found that gotu kola inhibits CYP 2C9, 2D6, and 3A4 (Pan et al. 2010).

Adverse Effects

Although generally well tolerated, gotu kola may cause gastrointestinal upset, nausea, drowsiness, dermatitis, and rare liver toxicity (Gomes et al. 2010; Natural Medicines Comprehensive Database 2011).

Lemon Balm (*Melissa officinalis*)

Description

Lemon balm, a perennial herb that is a member of the mint family and native to Europe, has been used since the Middle Ages to treat anxiety, sleep disorders, and attention-deficit/hyperactivity disorder and to reduce agitation in Alzheimer's disease patients (University of Maryland Medical Center 2011). It is often combined with other herbs such as valerian, hops, and chamomile to promote relaxation. It may be taken orally or used as aromatherapy. Active ingredients include citronellal, neral, and geranial monoterpenoid aldehydes; rosmarinic acid; and monoterpene glycosides (Natural Medicines Comprehensive Database 2011).

Mechanism of Action

The mechanism of action of lemon balm is related to its binding to nicotinic and muscarinic receptors and inhibition of GABA transaminase (Awad et al. 2009; Natural Medicines Comprehensive Database 2011).

Efficacy

In a small randomized controlled study evaluating the effects of lemon balm among 42 patients ages 65–80 years with mild to moderate Alzheimer's disease, findings suggested that the treatment group had higher levels of cognition and lower levels of agitation compared with the placebo group (Akhondzadeh et al. 2003). Another larger open multicenter study of 918 children younger than 12 years with restlessness and dyssomnias found that a combination of valerian and lemon balm decreased adverse symptoms from moderate or severe to mild or absent (Muller and Klement 2006).

Herbal and Medication Interactions

Lemon balm may potentiate the effects of CNS depressants and may interact with thyroid medications (Wong et al.1998).

Adverse Effects

Generally, lemon balm is very well tolerated but may cause nausea, vomiting, abdominal pain, dizziness, wheezing, and skin irritation (Natural Medicines Comprehensive Database 2011).

Summary

I have described 10 common herbal medications, including mechanisms of action, efficacy, herbal and medication interactions, and common adverse effects, that may be used by psychiatric patients. Psychiatric clinicians need to be aware of the pharmacological properties of these preparations to provide safe and effective care of their patients who use herbal remedies to relieve psychiatric symptoms.

Clinical Pearls

- Although many individuals consider complementary and alternative medicines to be "natural" and therefore safe, these agents are not without potential adverse effects and interactions. The psychiatric APRN should complete a thorough medication history when evaluating a patient and should provide education regarding the potential for interactions.

- St. John's wort is a rather popular alternative medication that can contribute to serotonin syndrome if taken with many of the psychotropic agents on the market.

- Black cohosh has been widely studied for its efficacy in reducing the symptoms associated with perimenopause and postmenopause in women. Although further studies are needed, caution is advised because of the potential for hepatotoxicity.

- Valerian has been used since ancient times to promote sleep and reduce anxiety. Although the studies have been small, reported outcomes have been positive with minimal adverse effects.

References

Akhondzadeh S, Kashani L, Mobaseri M, et al: Passionflower in the treatment of opiates withdrawal: a double-blind randomized controlled trial. J Clin Pharm Ther 26:369–373, 2001a

Akhondzadeh S, Naghavi HR, Vazirian M, et al: Passionflower in the treatment of generalized anxiety: a pilot double-blind randomized controlled trial with oxazepam. J Clin Pharm Ther 26:363–367, 2001b

Akhondzadeh S, Noroozian M, Mohammadi M, et al: Melissa officinalis extract in the treatment of patients with mild to moderate Alzheimer's disease: a double blind randomised placebo controlled trial. J Neurol Neurosurg Psychiatry 74:863–866, 2003

Andreatini R, Sartori VA, Seabra ML, et al: Effect of valepotriates (valerian extract) in generalized anxiety disorder: a randomized placebo-controlled pilot study. Phytother Res 16:650–654, 2002

Appel K, Rose T, Fiebich B, et al: Modulation of the gamma-aminobutyric acid (GABA) system by Passiflora incarnata L. Phytother Res 25:838–843, 2011

Attele AS, Wu JA, Yuan CS: Ginseng pharmacology: multiple constituents and multiple actions. Biochem Pharmacol 58:1685–1693, 1999

Awad R, Muhammad A, Durst T, et al: Bioassay-guided fractionation of lemon balm (Melissa officinalis L.) using an in vitro measure of GABA transaminase activity. Phytother Res 23:1075–1081, 2009

Barnes PM, Bloom B, Nahin RL: Complementary and alternative medicine use among adults and children: United States, 2007. Natl Health Stat Report 10(23):1–23, 2008

Benke D, Barberis A, Kopp S, et al: GABA A receptors as in vivo substrate for the anxiolytic action of valerenic acid a major constituent of Valerian root extracts. Neuropharmacology 56:174–181, 2009

Bent S, Padula A, Moore D, et al: Valerian for sleep: a systematic review and meta-analysis. Am J Med 119:1005–1012, 2006

Bercovitz A, Sengupta M, Jones A, et al: Complementary and Alternative Therapies in Hospice: The National Home and Hospice Care Survey: United States, 2007. Natl Health Stat Report 11(33):1–20, 2011

Bilgi N, Bell K, Ananthakrishnan AN, et al: Imatinib and Panax ginseng: a potential interaction resulting in liver toxicity. Ann Pharmacother 44:926–928, 2010

Birks J, Grimley Evans J: Ginkgo biloba for cognitive impairment and dementia. Cochrane Database of Systematic Reviews 2009, Issue 1. Art. No.: CD003120. DOI: 10.1002/14651858.CD003120.pub3

Bladt S, Wagner H: Inhibition of MAO by fractions and constituents of hypericum extract. J Geriatr Psychiatry Neurol 7 (suppl 1):S57–S59, 1994

Bodkin R, Schneider S, Rekkerth D, et al: Rhabdomyolysis associated with kava ingestion. Am J Emerg Med 30:635.e1–3, 2012

Borrelli F, Ernst E: Black cohosh (Cimicifuga racemosa) for menopausal symptoms: a systematic review of its efficacy. Pharmacol Res 58:8–14, 2008

Brown AC, Onopa J, Holck P, et al: Traditional kava beverage consumption and liver function tests in a predominantly Tongan population in Hawaii. Clin Toxicol 45:549–556, 2007

Butterweck V, Schmidt M: St. John's wort: role of active compounds for its mechanism of action and efficacy. Wien Med Wochenschr 157:356–361, 2007

Cairney S, Maruff P, Clough AR, et al: The neurobehavioural effects of kava. Aust N Z J Psychiatry 36:657–662, 2002

Cairney S, Clough AR, Maruff P, et al: Saccade and cognitive function in chronic kava users. Neuropsychopharmacology 28:389–396, 2003

Chen W, He R, Li YF, et al: Pharmacological studies on the anxiolytic effect of standardized Schisandra lignans extract on restraint-stressed mice. Phytomedicine 18:1144–1147, 2011

Natural Medicines Comprehensive Database. Stockton, CA, Therapeutic Research Faculty, 2011. Available at: http://naturaldatabase.therapeuticresearch.com. Accessed February 6, 2013.

Dalla Corte CL, Fachinetto R, Colle D, et al: Potentially adverse interactions between haloperidol and valerian. Food Chem Toxicol 46:2369–2375, 2008

DeKosky ST, Williamson JD, Fitzpatrick AL, et al: Ginkgo biloba for prevention of dementia: a randomized controlled trial. JAMA 300:2253–2262, 2008

Dhanasekaran M, Holcomb LA, Hitt AR, et al: Centella asiatica extract selectively decreases amyloid beta levels in hippocampus of Alzheimer's disease animal model. Phytother Res 23:14–19, 2009

Dietz BM, Mahady GB, Pauli GF, et al: Valerian extract and valerenic acid are partial agonists of the 5-HT5a receptor in vitro. Brain Res Mol Brain Res 138:191–197, 2005

Dugoua JJ, Mills E, Perri D, et al: Safety and efficacy of St. John's wort (hypericum) during pregnancy and lactation. Can J Clin Pharmacol 13:e268–276, 2006

Elsas SM, Rossi DJ, Raber J, et al: Passiflora incarnata L (Passionflower) extracts elicit GABA currents in hippocampal neurons in vitro and show anxiogenic and anticonvulsant effects in vivo varying with extraction method. Phytomedicine 17:940–949, 2010

Fernandez-San-Martin MI, Masa-Font R, Palacios-Soler L, et al: Effectiveness of Valerian on insomnia: a meta-analysis of randomized placebo-controlled trials. Sleep Med 11:505–511, 2010

Giridharan VV, Thandavarayan RA, Sato S, et al: Prevention of scopolamine-induced memory deficits by schisandrin B, an antioxidant lignan from Schisandra chinensis in mice. Free Radic Res 45:950–958, 2011

Gomes J, Pereira T, Vilarinho C, et al: Contact dermatitis due to Centella asiatica. Contact Dermatitis 62:54–55, 2010

Gurley BJ, Gardner SF, Hubbard MA, et al: In vivo effects of goldenseal, kava kava, black cohosh, and valerian on human cytochrome P450 1A2, 2D6, 2E1, and 3A4/5 phenotypes. Clin Pharmacol Ther 77:415–426, 2005

Hokkanen J, Tolonen A, Mattila S, et al: Metabolism of hyperforin, the active constituent of St. John's wort, in human liver microsomes. Eur J Pharm Sci 42:273–284, 2011

Jacobs S, Pies R, Katz I: Clinical Manual of Geriatric Psychopharmacology. Washington, DC, American Psychiatric Publishing, 2007, p 254

Jana U, Sur TK, Maity LN, et al: A clinical study on the management of generalized anxiety disorder with Centella asiatica. Nepal Med Coll J 12:8–11, 2010

Joshi KG, Faubion MD: Mania and psychosis associated with St. John's wort and ginseng. Psychiatry 2:56–61, 2005

Kumar A, Dogra S, Prakash A: Neuroprotective effects of Centella asiatica against intracerebroventricular colchicine-induced cognitive impairment and oxidative stress. Int J Alzheimers Dis 2009:pii, 2009

Kumar V, Mdzinarishvili A, Kiewert C, et al: NMDA receptor-antagonistic properties of hyperforin, a constituent of St. John's wort. J Pharmacol Sci 102:47–54, 2006

LaFrance W, Lauterbach EC, Coffey CE, et al: The use of herbal alternative medicines in neuropsychiatry: a report of the ANPA Committee on Research. J Neuropsychiatry Clin Neurosci 12:177–192, 2000

Lee NH, Son CG: Systematic review of randomized controlled trials evaluating the efficacy and safety of ginseng. J Acupunct Meridian Stud 4:85–97, 2011

Lei HP, Yu XY, Xie HT, et al: Effect of St. John's wort supplementation on the pharmacokinetics of bupropion in healthy male Chinese volunteers. Xebiotica 40:275–281, 2010

Li Y, Mei H, Wu Q, et al: Methysticin and 78-dihydromethysticin are two major kavalactones in kava extract to induce CYP1A1. Toxicol Sci 124:388–399, 2011

Linde K, Ramirez G, Mulrow CD, et al: St. John's wort for depression—an overview and meta-analysis of randomised clinical trials. BMJ 313:253–258, 1996

Linde K, Berner MM, Kriston L: St. John's wort for major depression. Cochrane Database of Systematic Reviews 2008, Issue 4. Art. No.: CD000448. DOI: 10.1002/14651858.CD000448.pub3.

Liu R, Qin M, Hang P, et al: Effects of Panax notoginseng saponins on the activities of CYP1A2, CYP2C9, CYP2D6 and CYP3A4 in rats in vivo. Phytother Res 26:1113–1118, 2012

Mathews JM, Etheridge AS, Valentine JL, et al: Pharmacokinetics and disposition of the kavalactone kawain: interaction with kava extract and kavalactones in vivo and in vitro. Drug Metab Dispos 33:1555–1563, 2005

Miyasaka LS, Atallah ÁN, Soares BG: Passiflora for anxiety disorder. Cochrane Database of Systematic Reviews 2007, Issue 1. Art. No.: CD004518. DOI: 10.1002/14651858.CD004518.pub2.

Muller SF, Klement S: A combination of valerian and lemon balm is effective in the treatment of restlessness and dyssomnia in children. Phytomedicine 13:383–387, 2006

Murphy PA, Kern SE, Stanczyk FZ, et al: Interaction of St. John's wort with oral contraceptives: effects on the pharmacokinetics of rethindrone and ethinyl estradiol ovarian activity and breakthrough bleeding. Contraception 71:402–408, 2005

Ngan A, Conduit R: A double-blind placebo-controlled investigation of the effects of Passiflora incarnata (passionflower) herbal tea on subjective sleep quality. Phytother Res 25:1153–1159, 2011

Niederhofer H: Ginkgo biloba treating patients with attention-deficit disorder. Phytother Res 24:26–27, 2010

Pan YB, Abd-Rashid BA, Ismail Z, et al: In vitro modulatory effects on three major human cytochrome P450 enzymes by multiple active constituents and extracts of Centella asiatica. J Ethnopharmacol 130:275–283, 2010

Panossian A, Wikman G: Pharmacology of Schisandra chinensis Bail.: an overview of Russian research and uses in medicine. J Ethnopharmacol 118:183–212, 2008

Pederson M: Nutritional Herbology: A Reference Guide to Herbs. Warsaw, IN, Wendell W Whitman, 2002

Robertson SM, Davey RT, Voell J, et al: Effect of Ginkgo biloba extract on lopinavir, midazolam and fexofenadine pharmacokinetics in healthy subjects. Curr Med Res Opin 24:591–599, 2008

Ruedeberg C, Wiesmann UN, Brattstroem A, et al: Hypericum perforatum L. (St. John's wort) extract Ze 117 inhibits dopamine re-uptake in rat striatal brain slices: an implication for use in smoking cessation treatment? Phytother Res 24:249–251, 2010

Rychetnik L, Madronio CM: The health and social effects of drinking water-based infusions of kava: a review of the evidence. Drug Alcohol Rev 30:74–83, 2011

Salter S, Brownie S: Treating primary insomnia—the efficacy of valerian and hops. Aust Fam Physician 39:433–437, 2010

Sarris JD, Kavanagh J, Byrne G, et al: The Kava Anxiety Depression Spectrum Study (KADSS): a randomized placebo-controlled crossover trial using an aqueous extract of Piper methysticum. Psychopharmacology 205:399–407, 2009

Sarris J, LaPorte E, Schweitzer I: Kava: a comprehensive review of efficacy safety and psychopharmacology. Aust N Z J Psychiatry 45:27–35, 2011a

Sarris J, Teschke R, Stough C, et al: Re-introduction of kava (Piper methysticum) to the EU: is there a way forward? Planta Med 77:107–110, 2011b

Suzuki O, Katsumata Y, Oya M, et al: Inhibition of monoamine oxidase by hypericin. Planta Med 50:272–274, 1984

Taavoni S, Ekbatani N, Kashaniyan M, et al: Effect of valerian on sleep quality in postmenopausal women: a randomized placebo-controlled clinical trial. Menopause 18:951–955, 2011

Taibi DM, Landis CA, Petry H, et al: A systematic review of valerian as a sleep aid: safe but not effective. Sleep Med Rev 11:209–230, 2007

Taki Y, Yokotani K, Yamada S, et al: Ginkgo biloba extract attenuates warfarin-mediated anticoagulation through induction of hepatic cytochrome P450 enzymes by bilobalide in mice. Phytomedicine 19:177–182, 2012

Thiede HM, Walper A: Inhibition of MAO and COMT by hypericum extracts and hypericin. J Geriatr Psychiatry Neurol 7 (suppl 1):S54–S56, 1994

Thompson R, Ruch W, Hasehrl RU: Enhanced cognitive performance and cheerful mood by standardized extracts of Piper methysticum (kava-kava). Hum Psychopharmacol 19:243–250, 2004

Uebelhack R, Franke L, Schewe HJ: Inhibition of platelet MAO-B by kava pyrone-enriched extract from Piper methysticum Forster (kava-kava). Pharmacopsychiatry 31:187–192, 1998

Uebelhack R, Blohmer JU, Graubaum HJ, et al: Black cohosh and St. John's wort for climacteric complaints: a randomized trial. Obstet Gynecol 107:247–255, 2006

University of Maryland Medical Center: Medical Alternative Medicine Index. 2011. Available at: http://www.umm.edu/altmed. Accessed December 24, 2011.

Van Strater AC, Bogers JP: Interaction of St. John's wort (Hypericum perforatum) with clozapine. Int Clin Psychopharmacol 27:121–124, 2012

Vermani M, Milosevic I, Smith F, et al: Herbs for mental illness: effectiveness and interaction with conventional medicines. J Fam Pract 54:789–800, 2005

Weinmann S, Roll S, Schwarzbach C, et al: Effects of Ginkgo biloba in dementia: systematic review and meta-analysis. BMC Geriatr 10:14, 2010

Wielgus AR, Chignell CF, Miller DS, et al: Phototoxicity in human retinal pigment epithelial cells promoted by hypericin a component of St. John's wort. Photochem Photobiol 83:706–713, 2007

Witte S, Loew D, Gaus W: Meta-analysis of the efficacy of the acetonic kava-kava extract WS1490 in patients with non-psychotic anxiety disorders. Phytother Res 19:183–188, 2005

Wong A, Smith HM, Boon HS: Herbal remedies in psychiatric practice. Arch Gen Psychiatry 55:1033–1044, 1998

Yance D, Valentine A: Herbal Medicine Healing and Cancer: A Comprehensive Program for Prevention and Treatment. Lincolnwood, IL, Keats Publishing, 1999

Zhang WF, Tan YL, Zhang XY, et al: Extract of Ginkgo biloba treatment for tardive dyskinesia in schizophrenia: a randomized double-blind placebo-controlled trial. J Clin Psychiatry 72:615–621, 2011

Zhou L, Meng Q, Qian T, et al: Ginkgo biloba extract enhances glucose tolerance in hyperinsulinism-induced hepatic cells. J Nat Med 65:50–56, 2011

14

Culturally Sensitive Psychopharmacology

Barbara Jones Warren, Ph.D., A.P.R.N., P.M.H.-C.N.S., B.C., F.A.A.N.

Culture is a matrix of infinite possibilities and choices.

—Wole Soyinka, Nigerian Nobel Laureate

The need to address cultural issues within mental health care settings has been systematically investigated for more than 20 years. However, this information was not compiled until the late 1990s and early 2000s when the Office of the Surgeon General formulated two hallmark research and practice-based reports that emphasized the importance of mental health as a basis for overall health (U.S. Department of Health and Human Services 1999, 2001). Findings of the reports also indicated that persons from culturally and ethnically diverse populations incur stigma and health care disparities at a higher rate

379

than do persons who are not from these populations. The presence of mental health care stigma and health care disparities contributes to patient dissatisfaction, patient nonadherence, and ineffective treatment outcomes. The Surgeon General reports also emphasized the need for the ongoing examination of the role of culture in development of evidence-based treatments, including psychotherapeutic and psychopharmacological interventions (U.S. Department of Health and Human Services 1999, 2001).

Psychiatric mental health nursing's scope of practice and holistic paradigm are well suited to facilitate the development of culturally sensitive strategies and interventions for patients and their families who are affected by mental illness. The previous chapters in this manual provide information on the psychopharmacological management of patients' symptoms within the context of their mental health disorders. The purpose of this chapter is to provide information on culturally sensitive psychopharmacological mental health care strategies that psychiatric mental health nurses (PMHNs) can use within their practice settings. PMHNs can incorporate this information into development of treatment strategies aimed at the holistic management of their patients. More specifically, I discuss 1) the role of culture in relation to mental health, wellness, and illness; 2) culturally sensitive assessment techniques; and 3) implications for psychiatric mental health practice when culturally sensitive psychotherapeutic and psychopharmacological strategies are integrated into practice settings.

Role of Culture in Relation to Mental Health, Wellness, and Illness

> The relation(ship) between the body and the mind is so intimate that, if either of them got out of order, the whole system would suffer. (Mohandas K. Gandhi, *Guide to Health*, 1930)

Culture is one of the most important aspects of people's lives because it guides and shapes how they think, function, and interact with others (Leininger 2006). More specifically, culture imparts value and meaning to everyday existence because it is the foundation for how a person, group, or community internally and externally expresses and practices its beliefs, values, and norms (Warren 2011). A person's culture may be self-defined or defined by society. Cultural layers also exist within the life of every person. Individuals are born into a culture of origin and then add cultural layers as they grow and develop throughout life (Warren 2009). Furthermore, these layers are influenced by individuals' genetic makeup (Consensus Panel on Genetic/Genomic Nursing Competencies 2008; Spector 2004; Warren 2008). To prepare themselves to meet the challenge of providing quality care for racially and ethnically diverse patient populations, PMHNs and other mental health care practitioners need to examine their own beliefs, assumptions, and perceptions about culture.

It is important that PMHNs, as holistic mental health providers, acknowledge and understand the role and complexity of culture in the lives of their patients from racially and ethnically diverse backgrounds. Patients feel a sense of comfort when they are able to speak freely about their cultural beliefs and practices. Being unable to express these beliefs and values often creates or intensifies stress, creates illness, and exacerbates symptoms. Reports from the Surgeon General (U.S. Department of Health and Human Services 1999, 2001) and the Institute of Medicine (Smedley et al. 2004) emphasized that patients are more adherent to treatment plans when their cultural perspectives and needs are incorporated into screening, assessment, and health care procedures. Patient adherence increases the likelihood of successful mental health outcomes and improvement of health.

Health Care Disparities

The literature and research on health care disparities indicate that persons from racially and ethnically diverse populations incur a greater disability burden from mental illness because of unmet mental health needs (Munoz et al. 2007; U.S. Department of Health and Human Services 2001). Persons from these populations often have access to fewer monetary and health care resources because they are devalued and stigmatized within society. Thus, the lack of health care access and availability are contributing factors to disparate health care, poor overall health, and less productivity in life. The cost of not treating mental illness is high for the persons who are left untreated and for society as a whole. Untreated mental illness is exacerbated and negatively affects the everyday quality of life for persons with the illness. Persons have lost workdays because of a lack of productivity, and illness-related absences affect the work environments and society (Noonan et al. 2007).

Cultural Issues in Mental Health Care and Psychopharmacology: Terminology

A number of specialized terms are used in discussions about cultural issues in mental health care and strategies for reducing communication barriers based on racial, ethnic, cultural, or linguistic differences.

Cultural competence is an ongoing, dynamic skill process whereby a PMHN or other health care provider develops expertise regarding knowledge about patients' cultural perspectives and needs and then immerses this expertise into the development of treatment plans with culturally and ethnically diverse patients (Campinha-Bacote 2007; Warren and Broome 2011). Many health care providers prefer and interchangeably use the terms *cultural appropriateness, cultural humility, cultural sensitivity,* and *cultural relevance* instead of *cultural competence* because they see competence as an endpoint of learning. However, many cultural experts think that *cultural competence* is a more inclusive term than the other terms that may be used. Moreover, the other terms are viewed as being a point-in-time learning skill. From the standpoint of certain health care providers, the interchangeable terms have the following meanings:

- *Cultural appropriateness* indicates that a treatment strategy is the correct one to use.
- *Cultural humility* indicates that the provider feels the need to honor and respect a patient's cultural perspectives and needs.
- *Cultural sensitivity* and *cultural relevance* are the same in that they indicate that a provider understands the importance and significance of matching the treatment strategy with a patient's cultural perspectives and needs (Warren 2009).

Two basic terms—*race* and *ethnicity*—are also often used interchangeably, but they are different. *Race* classifies a person or group based on a set of socially determined genetic factors and biological traits, whereas *ethnicity* represents the common set of beliefs that a group shares and practices (U.S. Department of Health and Human Services 2001). In a simplistic sense and narrow view, some health care providers define the term *race* on the basis of what a patient looks and sounds like (e.g., color of skin, texture of hair, use of language).

However, it is important that the PMHN not stereotype a person based on what the nurse perceives or observes the person's race to be.

Genotype refers to an individual's genetic makeup; it has nothing to do with the person's physical appearance. The genotype is a person's unique and individual set of genes. It is expressed when encoded deoxyribonucleic acid (DNA) translates to ribonucleic acid (RNA) molecules and proteins, and this expression of the genotype plays a part in a person's observable traits (e.g., phenotype) (Patwardham 2005). Hence, prescribing and monitoring a medication based on personal impressions or visual observations is a dangerous and culturally incompetent approach. Incorrect identification of a person's race can lead to choice of an inappropriate medication and prescription of an improper dosage (Lawson 1999). These mistakes may potentially result in serious and even lethal physical consequences for patients, depending on the side-effect profile of the medication (Keltner and Vance 2011). Undesirable side effects often contribute to patient nonadherence. Thus, the choice of a medication and the monitoring of its effects need to be based on accurate information about a patient's genetic profile, including genetic factors that influence drug metabolism (Warren 2008).

Polymorphism refers to genetic variations in the human population that give rise to distinct subgroups who differ in their response to medications. Genetic polymorphisms have implications for the effect of a person's body on a medication and the effect of the medication on the person's body (Stahl 2009); these variations determine the individual's capacity to metabolize various medications used in treatment. It is not feasible to conduct a genetic panel on every patient because it is expensive and not covered by insurance, and patients may object to it being done because they have concerns about how information from the panel may be used by or shared with other individuals. In any case, the state of knowledge does not, as of yet, inform prescribing of psychiatric medications.

Individuals from racially and ethnically diverse backgrounds often do not trust providers and the health care system. This mistrust is grounded in past persecution, past abuse of research participants, negative experiences with providers, and current discriminatory practices within society (U.S. Department of Health and Human Services 2001). Stigma around mental illness adds to the concerns that these persons may have about accessing and receiving mental health care. The use of psychiatric medications remains a concern to individuals from diverse backgrounds because they often have cultural beliefs that affect their perception of medication use (Campinha-Bacote 2007; Spector 2004). Thus, knowledge about culture and medication issues is an important consideration when treatment plans are developed for patients from racially and ethnically diverse backgrounds (Rodriquez 2007).

Ethnic pharmacology or *ethnopharmacology* is the scientific study of how biological traits and cultural perspectives influence pharmacological response in persons from culturally and ethnically diverse backgrounds (Scott and Hewett 2008; Stepp and Moerman 2001; Warren 2007). *Ethnic psychopharmacology* refers to the study of the effect of psychotropic drugs on persons from racially and ethnically diverse populations (Lawson 1999). The study of these pharmacological responses encompasses prescribed agents, herbal agents, and folk remedies.

The genome and epigenetics have become important areas of study over the last 10 years. The *genome* is the essential component within persons that contains all of the biological information needed to build and sustain them. The biological data are encoded in DNA, which is further divided into genes. The genes code proteins that attach at specific positions to switch off and on a series of chemical reactions (gene expression) (Consensus Panel on Genetic/Genomic Nursing Competencies 2008). Thus, the growth and development of a person is coordinated by chemical reactions that switch the genome off and on at specific times and sites. *Epigenetics* is the study of these reactions and the factors that influence them. The genome is dynamic in its response to environment, and biopsychosocial variables such as stress, diet, behavior, and toxins can activate and alter the chemical reactions that regulate gene expression. Furthermore, culture, the genome, and epigenetics affect brain functioning and behavior in a synergistic manner.

Genetic factors also determine a person's response to pharmacological agents, including *pharmacodynamics* (mechanism of action and effect on the target site) and *pharmacokinetics* (absorption, metabolism, distribution, and elimination) (Muñoz and Hilgenberg 2006). Thus, patients' perceptions about mental health, wellness, and illness not only are grounded in their cultural beliefs, values, and norms but also may be affected by their physical response to medications because of genetic polymorphisms. Factors that should guide decision making surrounding the choice of a medication include the drug's overall profile, availability, and monitoring in connection with the patient's cultural belief systems and language/communication patterns; the provider's cultural belief systems and language/communication patterns; and the provider's prescribing philosophy and practices (Okpaku 1999; K. Y. Wang et al. 2010; X. Wang et al. 2011). A provider's understanding and acknowledgment of the importance of a patient's cultural belief system contribute to the establishment and maintenance of the therapeutic relationship. This relationship enhances patient adherence and promotes successful mental health outcomes. Thus, it is important that PMHNs understand the biopsychosocial connection regarding the role of culture and the influence of genetic factors within the lives of their patients so that they can provide culturally sensitive, competent, high-quality care for patients (Ward-Smith 2010). This is the formula for culturally competent care.

Drug Metabolism and the Cytochrome P450 System

As already noted, individuals differ in their metabolic responses to pharmacological agents depending on their genetic profile (i.e., polymorphisms). When medications enter the body, they are converted into active metabolites via enzymes and isoenzymes in the liver. It is important to note that because of genetic variations in the population, some individuals have a reduced capacity to metabolize certain medications. This decreased efficiency can potentially lead to toxic response to medications. For example, someone with an inefficient metabolism (i.e., a "poor metabolizer") will have reduced drug clearance in the body, resulting in medication buildup and possible toxicity. Conversely, someone with a normal, well-functioning metabolism (i.e., an "extensive metabolizer") will have efficient drug clearance without risk of buildup or toxicity (Al Koudsi et al. 2010; Consensus Panel on Genetic/Genomic Nursing Competencies 2008; Keltner and Folks 2005; Munoz et al. 2007).

The primary enzyme system about which PMHNs need to be knowledgeable is the cytochrome P450 (CYP) system. The enzymes of the CYP system, located in the liver, are involved in metabolism of most drugs. Enzymes such as CYP2D6 and CYP2C19 collectively are responsible for almost one-third of all drug metabolism, including the metabolism of 36 antidepressants and 38 antipsychotics (Aulinskas 2010). Therefore, they are also involved in many drug-drug interactions, the clinical effect of the drug, and manifestation of potential adverse events. Medications are broken down and excreted by the liver and kidney through the action of these enzymes. Certain herbal and folk remedies may inhibit the functioning of the CYP system, thereby changing or inactivating the metabolism of medications. The use of tobacco and dietary practices also can alter or inactivate the functioning within these enzyme systems (Frackiewicz et al. 1999).

Ethnopharmacological research has found biological variations among different race and population groups in the ability to produce enzymes within these systems (Keltner and Vance 2011; Muñoz and Hilgenberg 2006). The genetic polymorphisms of the CYP system are important because different ethnic groups may have greater or lesser ability to metabolize drugs influenced by a specific metabolic enzyme. For instance, 15%–20% of Asian populations are poor metabolizers of CYP2C19, whereas only 3%–5% of Caucasian (white) populations are poor metabolizers (Bertilsson 1995; Desta et al. 2002). As another example, Asians, Pacific Islanders, Africans, and African Americans have a much higher percentage of reduced or nonfunctional CYP2D6 alleles (40%–50%) than do their counterparts of European (white) origin (26%) (Aulinskas 2010). These ethnic genetic polymorphisms may contribute to drug intolerance, elevated risk of side effects, and poorer health outcomes, especially in regard to psychotropic medications. Please refer to Appendix 2, "Psychotropic and Other Medications Influenced by the Cytochrome P450 (CYP) System," for a table outlining commonly prescribed psychotropic and other agents metabolized by various CYP enzymes.

Stereotyping or Culturally Competent Care?

The study of ethnopharmacology creates some challenges because of the variations that exist within racial and ethnic groups. Scientific information about the enzyme systems, metabolic processes, and polymorphisms can help educate nurses. However, it is important to note that the commonly used terms and defined categories such as Caucasian, white, European American, Asian American, African American, Native American, and Hispanic American are imprecise because of the intraracial, ethnic, and genotype differences within these categories (Muñoz and Hilgenberg 2006; U.S. Department of Health and Human Services 2001). Individuals from racially and ethnically diverse populations can respond as a poor metabolizer for one classification or medication and as an extensive metabolizer for another classification (AlAmeri et al. 2010; Muñoz and Hilgenberg 2006) because of the genotype variations. The ability of the PMHN to understand these variations is a component of cultural competence. Such understanding also protects against stereotyping of patients based on their race or ethnic origins.

Some important metabolic variations are worth noting. Persons from Native American and Asian cultural groups may be more sensitive to the effects of alcohol compared with persons who are not from these groups. This sensitivity is a result of the relative deficiency of aldehyde dehydrogenase, and this deficiency creates a slower-than-usual metabolism of the intermediate product acetylaldehyde. This produces a toxic reaction (known as the *flushing syndrome*) that leads to increased pulse and heart rates. A growing body of literature exists regarding the enzymatic processes of the CYP system and their effect on the use of psychotropic medications. Medications that are substrates of 2D6 and 2C19 enzymes are linked to slow metabolic processing in persons from African and Native American as well as Eastern Asian cultures. This slow metabolism leads to cell buildup of medication as a result of ineffective breakdown and distribution of drugs within body systems (de Almeida et al. 2011; Muñoz and Hilgenberg 2006; Warren 2008).

The Culturally Competent Therapeutic Relationship

The PMHN's ability to understand and interpret the role and significance of his or her culture and that of patients is the key in developing a therapeutic nurse-patient relationship. The therapeutic relationship forms the foundation of the process by which patient and nurse come to consensus about patient needs and treatment plan development and implementation. Shared decision making in the relationship is part of the establishment of recovery processes for patients and their families and significant others. Also not to be forgotten is that standards for *cultural competence in nursing* exist that define the discipline's cultural and educational perspectives, delineate how the discipline establishes nurse-patient relationships, and help nurses enact their specialty roles within health care environments and systems (Muñoz and Luckmann 2005; Warren 2011).

According to Peplau (1956), successful development and progression of the nurse-patient relationship is facilitated by the nurse. Recovery and resilience are important components within the relationship. *Recovery* is a cultural process by which a person who is affected by mental illness reestablishes his or her sense of hope and self-worth to develop successful life opportunities (Anthony 1993; Warren 2011). The person develops knowledge about the illness and available treatment options. *Resilience* is a cultural concept embedded within the recovery process: it is the protective and strength aspect that helps a patient to recover by appropriately coping with the stress and issues associated with mental illness. Thus, the therapeutic PMHN-patient relationship continues to evolve through the nurse's application of culturally competent knowledge about patient recovery and resilience processes.

Stop, Think, and Respond Box
How might your feelings and attitudes about the behavior of a patient from a different culture or ethnic group affect your ability to assess the patient? Would you possibly misinterpret the patient's needs or communication style?

Psychiatric nurses are often the initial health care provider that patients encounter when they attempt to access the mental health care system. Thus, the nurse's use of culturally competent strategies may be the single most important factor in helping patients to feel comfortable and embrace treatment suggestions by the nurse. Nurses' beliefs about patients whose racial and ethnic backgrounds differ from their own evolve out of several sources. Among these are the nurses' own cultural inheritance (e.g., culture of origin) perspectives, their face-to-face experiences with individuals from other cultures or races, and societal influences of stigma and bias toward racially and ethnically diverse individuals. Table 14–1 presents a list of questions for nurses to use in the cultural assessment.

Table 14–1. Nursing cultural assessment questions

1. How would you describe your cultural inheritance?

2. Do you have a specific culture or ethnic group that you consider yourself part of? How would you describe your group?

3. Have you had any personal or professional experience with persons who are racially, ethnically, or culturally different from you? How would you describe these experiences? Is there knowledge about these experiences that might help or not help you in developing a therapeutic relationship with someone who is culturally different from you?

Cultural Language and Patterns of Communication

Language and communication patterns influence how nurses and patients interact with and assess each other. Moreover, nurses' and patients' health care beliefs and practices are grounded in their perceptions of the way illness occurs and their worldviews. Language serves as the primary way for persons to communicate; it is the most salient component in development of the therapeutic nurse-patient relationship. Interpersonal conflicts appear and intensify when language barriers occur between the nurse and the patient. For example, patients may use communication approaches that are culturally alien to their health care providers. These approaches may include the use of a different spoken language, signing, gesturing, and written communication practices. Nurses need to address the issue of different spoken or sign languages. Having a list of available interpreters is advised. However, it may be more prudent and culturally competent for the nurse to become adept at using the necessary spoken or sign language that most potential patients are comfortable with or use (Muñoz and Luckmann 2005).

Language also includes nonverbal communication. In fact, patients are often more sensitive to and aware of nurses' nonverbal patterns, particularly when the nurse says one thing but uses a tone or facial expression that clearly indicates another feeling or attitude.

Cultural Language and Concepts About Illness and Disease

When describing their symptoms, patients may use unique terms and phrases that reflect specific concepts and viewpoints from their culture. It is important for PMHNs to be familiar with these terms so that they may better understand the way that patients perceive and define themselves through cultural lenses. This understanding is critical not only to facilitating communication between nurses and their patients but also to developing culturally appropriate treatment strategies and protocols. Table 14–2 lists selected cultural terms for emotional symptoms and their psychiatric language equivalents.

Most psychiatric nurses accept the scientific model as the primary explanation for illness and disease occurrences. However, patients from diverse cultural or ethnic backgrounds may hold other ideas or beliefs about the causes of illness and disease, including natural and outside forces (Campinha-Bacote 2007; Warren 2011). See Table 14–3 for the explanations offered by different models.

Worldviews

Nurses' and patients' worldviews affect how they perceive and value relationships. The four worldviews are *analytical, relational, community,* and *ecological.* It is important that PMHNs understand patients' worldviews as well as their own because these views form the foundation of what patients and nurses value in communication patterns and relationships. For example, a patient or nurse with an *analytical* view values an individual decision-making process and prefers a learning approach that uses written and visual media. Information about medications can be provided through the use of pamphlets, books, and videos that facilitate self-instruction as opposed to interactive learning with the nurse. Direct eye contact and questioning are also valued (Warren 2007).

The *relational* view values development of relationships and interactions. The patient or nurse with this view prefers a verbal and interactive communication style to elicit information and present health-related information. The nurse also may need to incorporate enough time within visits to be able to meet the needs of a patient with this view. The inclusion of family, friends, and significant others such as community cultural health care providers is an important concept in this view.

Table 14–2.   Cultural and psychiatric language descriptions of emotional symptoms

Cultural language	Psychiatric language
Amok: used by some persons from Polynesian and Malaysian cultures. Symptoms include confusion, anger, aggression, amnesia, and exhaustion.	Dissociative event symptoms
Ataque de nervios: used by some persons from Latino and Mediterranean culture to describe their moderate to severe levels of anxiety.	Panic attack–like symptoms
Brain fag: used by some persons from West African cultures. Symptoms include concentration, memory, and thinking problems.	Anxiety, depressive, or somatoform symptoms
Falling-out or *blacking out:* used by some persons from the American South or Caribbean cultures. Symptoms include dizziness, fainting, or an inability to move or respond to others.	Conversion or dissociative event symptoms
Heart pain or *broken heart:* used by some persons from Native American cultures. Symptoms include depressive and anxious behaviors.	Anxiety and depressive symptoms
Hwa-byung (anger syndrome): used by some persons from Korean cultures. Symptoms can be attributed to suppressing one's anger and include sleeping and eating problems, panic, fear, pains and aches, and dyspnea.	Anxiety and depressive symptoms

Source.   Adapted from Appendix I, "Outline for Cultural Formulation and Glossary of Culture-Bound Syndromes," of DSM-IV-TR (American Psychiatric Association 2000).

Table 14–3.   Models of illness and disease

Model	Explanation of cause of illness and disease
Scientific model	Entry of bacteria, viruses, and germs; failure of the immune system; body stressors
Natural model	Natural breaks within interrelated environments within the world (e.g., flood, earthquakes) that create an imbalance within nature and thus persons
Outside Forces model	A supernatural being uses spells and hexes to produce illness in persons who have wronged another individual, group, or community.

A patient or nurse with the *community* view values polite, respectful communication. He or she also values the opinions of family, friends, and community members and makes decisions on the basis of their input. The inclusion of family, friends, and significant others such as community cultural health care providers is also an important concept in this view.

The *ecological* view promotes a quiet, parsimonious community style. Eye contact may not be part of communication, especially when persons are speaking to others whom they consider to be important and powerful. The concept of balance between the mind, body, and spirit is also part of this view. PMHNs need to incorporate this holistic concept and discuss information in a quiet, respectful manner. Ongoing direct eye contact also needs to be minimized or avoided (Warren and Broome 2011).

Stop, Think, and Respond Box

Take a minute to assess and think about your culture. Are you made up of only one culture? Do you express one viewpoint, value, and belief? The answer to these questions relies on your ability, as a PMHN, to begin to assess your cultural beliefs, values, norms, and worldviews. Remember that understanding your own cultural beliefs will facilitate your ability to understand your patient's cultural perspectives.

Inclusion of Family, Friends, and Significant Others

PMHNs need to be aware of and sensitive to the roles that family, friends, and significant others play within the lives of patients. Many persons within American society value the individual decision-making process. The opinions of health care providers of family members may or may not be an important consideration within a patient's decision-making process. Yet persons from many cultural groups often value the opinions of family, friends, and other community members over the advice of "traditional health care experts." Neither approach is wrong or better than the other. However, the nurse needs to be able to collect data and develop a nursing plan that is culturally meaningful to the patient and others whom the patient deems important. Nurses' failure to adhere to this assessment approach generally erodes the therapeutic nurse-patient relationship and creates an atmosphere of cultural incompetence.

For example, the use of family surnames, accompanied by a person's official title, is a cultural preference when addressing others for many persons from racially and ethnically diverse groups. This approach indicates a level of respect and self-esteem that one has for another person. Nurses' failure to use this approach might indicate to patients that nurses do not respect them or their cultural preferences (Leininger 2006; Spector 2004).

Similarly, persons from many cultures may initially consult with their culturally based physicians, elders, healers, and shamans before consulting with a physician or nurse who uses a more Western-based medicine treatment approach. Cultural health care providers also may use complementary and alternative therapies in the care of their patients because these therapies are viewed as more holistic and natural and less invasive than Western-based ones. Moreover, patients, their families, friends, and significant others often have more trust in health care practitioners who acknowledge the cultural importance of their health care beliefs and practices. It is important that the perspectives of these individuals be included in the treatment planning process. All of these factors increase patient adherence to medication treatment (U.S. Department of Health and Human Services 2001).

Culturally Competent Psychiatric Assessment: Implications for Practice

Now it is time to focus on how all the information in this chapter fits together. PMHNs' culturally competent psychopharmacological management of patients requires an assessment of the biopsychosocial components that have been discussed within this chapter. The assessment of these holistic components includes PMHNs' understanding of the role of culture, definition of cultural terms, health care disparities, and the use of the process of cultural competence within all aspects of psychiatric mental health nursing practice. It is also critical that PMHNs be aware that some ethnic groups carry genetic variants of drug-metabolizing enzymes that may affect their response to medications. Central to all management is the nurse's development and maintenance of a culturally competent therapeutic nurse-patient relationship. PMHNs need to understand not only their patients' cultural perspectives but also their own cultural perspectives. "Stop, Think, and Respond" boxes and Table 14–1 presented some questions for a PMHN's consideration about these perspectives. Cultural patterns of language and communication and cultural perspectives on the causes of illness and disease were discussed within the chapter. Tables 14–2 and 14–3 provided information about assessment of these perspectives.

Finally, PMHNs can incorporate four areas of assessment in their culturally competent care of patients: 1) an overall cultural assessment collection of questions that are used to assess patients, 2) cause of illnesses and disease, 3) cultural medication assessment areas, and 4) areas for discussion with patients about their medication management.

Table 14–4 shows the overall assessment questions that PMHNs must use as the basis for their initial assessment of patients. This assessment provides a clear picture of what the patient believes and how he or she maintains health and wellness and treats illnesses or disease processes.

Table 14–5 presents questions to ask patients regarding their perceptions about the cause of illnesses and disease. For example, some patients may believe that illness is caused by imbalances in nature, divine interventions, or outside magical forces. This understanding then is incorporated into the collaborative patient and PMHN care planning.

Table 14–6 presents cultural assessment questions on medication treatment. These questions assess the patient's feelings and perceptions about taking medications. These are important areas for consideration in PMHNs' provision of culturally competent patient care.

Table 14–7 presents areas for discussion with patients regarding their medication adherence and management. This is the final component of the initial discussion and shared decision-making process between the patient and the nurse. This component evolves from the other assessment areas.

Table 14–8 provides a list of helpful Internet resources containing information relevant to the ethnopsychopharmacological management of psychiatric mental health patients.

Table 14–4.   Overall assessment questions

Cultural pattern	Assessment prompts
Communication styles	What language does the patient fluently use? What is the patient's first language? Does the patient want or prefer an interpreter? What is the patient's preferences related to personal touch and space parameters?
Environmental orientation	How long has the patient lived where he or she is currently living? Where was the patient born and raised? Is there a specific cultural group that the patient identifies with? Are there traditional beliefs and values that are important to the patient? What is the patient's worldview?
Nutritional practices	Does the patient have favorite foods? Are there foods that the patient eats or avoids to stay healthy or get well? Does the patient avoid foods based on spiritual or religious bases?
Role of family and significant others	Does the patient have someone he or she wants called, contacted, and consulted or not regarding development of the treatment plan and implementation processes? Who are the important persons within the patient's life? How does the patient make decisions? Does he or she make decisions alone or with input from others?
Health care influences	Ask the patient what he or she needs from you, as a nurse, today. What do you fear most about treatment?
Educational preferences	How does the patient like to learn new tasks and develop new ideas? What formal and informal education does the patient have?

Table 14–4. Overall assessment questions *(continued)*

Cultural pattern	Assessment prompts
Spirituality and religious practices	Does the patient consider himself or herself to be spiritual or religious? If so, what does it mean to him or her?
	Are there persons to whom the patient wants to talk about spiritual or religious ideas?
Biological and physical status	Are there specific emotional or physical illnesses within the patient's family history?
	Are there medications, vitamins, or herbal remedies that the patient uses or avoids?
	Does the patient have specific health care, grooming, or hair care needs?
	Does the patient do any of the following, and if so, how often and how much: smoke anything; drink wine, hard liquor, spirits, energy drinks, colas or other sodas, coffee, milk, or tea; or eat chocolate or energy bars?

Table 14–5. Questions to assess patient perceptions regarding causes of illness and disease

1. What do you call the problem?
2. What do you think caused the problem?
3. Why do you think it started when it did?
4. What do you think the illness does? How does it work?
5. How severe is the illness?
6. What kind of treatment do you think you should receive?
7. What are the most important results you hope to receive from the treatment?
8. What are the chief problems the illness has caused?
9. What do you fear most about the treatment?

Source. Warren 2008; Warren and Broome 2011.

Table 14–6. Cultural assessment questions on medication treatment

1. Explore the patient's feelings about taking potential treatment and medications. Does the patient think they are necessary or required?

2. Explore the meaning of taking medication. Does the patient believe medications are even needed for what illness he or she now has?

3. Do the patient's family, friends, or significant others have opinions or feelings about taking medications? What are these opinions and feelings? Do these opinions and feelings affect what the patient wants or needs to do?

4. Does the patient have spiritual or religious beliefs about taking medications? If so, what are they?

5. Does the patient think there are benefits or no benefits to taking medication?

6. Are there any special meanings connected to taking a medication (e.g., size, shape, color, connections to balancing types of medications)?

7. Does the patient have any concerns about losing control when taking medications?

Table 14–7. Cultural discussion areas for patient instructions

1. Level of symptomatology as culturally perceived and discussed by the patient

2. Level of symptomatology as culturally perceived and discussed by the nurse

3. Actions and side effects for any medication regimen and therapies, including any complementary and alternative therapies used by the patient

4. Role of the patient's daily schedule and the connection of this to medication regimens, including dietary, work, and sleep practices

5. Role and use of support systems (e.g., family; significant others; spiritual or religious advisers; culturally specific health care providers: shaman, medicine woman or man, curandera/o, faith healers; and other non–culturally specific health care providers)

Table 14–8.   Internet resources

- National Standards on Culturally and Linguistically Appropriate Services: http://minorityhealth.hhs.gov/templates/browse.aspx?lvl=2&lvlID=15

- Culture, Language, and Health Literacy (Health Resources and Services Administration): www.hrsa.gov/culturalcompetence

- EthnoMed: http://ethnomed.org

- National Center for Cultural Competence: http://nccc.georgetown.edu

Summary

This chapter has presented information about culturally competent psychotherapeutic and psychopharmacological management within psychiatric mental health nursing practice settings. The role of culture and biopsychosocial connections in the context of assessment and implementation strategy development was discussed. The process of developing cultural competence is particularly salient to psychiatric mental health nursing practice because this specialty focuses on the holistic interface of mind, body, and spirit within the therapeutic nurse-patient relationship. An understanding of the higher load of genetic metabolic polymorphisms carried by some racial and ethnic groups is critical to nurses' ability to manage medication regimens for these individuals. This chapter provided an overview of how PMHNs can deliver culturally competent psychopharmacological care for their racially and ethnically diverse patients. The provision of culturally competent psychopharmacological care minimizes the reticence on the part of the patient to engage in treatment, while helping the patient to develop recovery- and resiliency-based competencies. Psychiatric mental health practice "specializes in the promotion of mental health through assessment, diagnosis, and treatment of human responses to mental health problems and psychiatric disorders…It employs a purposeful use of self as its art…and neurobiological theories and research evidence as its science" (American Psychiatric Nurses Association et al. 2007, p. 1).

Clinical Pearls

- How do nurses' cultural perspectives and experiences affect patient care?
  - Essential for quality culturally inclusive care and effective outcomes.
  - Facilitate development of the therapeutic relationship.
- What does ethnopharmacology have to do with nurses' evidence-based care of patients?
  - A thorough understanding of metabolism and polymorphisms should inform prescribing and administrative practices for all nurses.
  - Knowledge about ethnopharmacology helps nurses provide evidence-based care for their patients.
- Describe your nursing philosophy for providing quality care for racially and ethnically diverse patients: How you will incorporate culturally sensitive psychopharmacology into your practice, academic, and/or research settings?
  - Worldviews and cultural experiences affect relationships between nurses and their patients.
  - Cultural inclusiveness is a key component in all aspects of nursing (e.g., education, practice, research environment).

References

AlAmeri M, Epstein M, Johnston A: Generic and therapeutic substitutions: are they always ethical in their own terms? Pharm World Sci 32:691–695, 2010

Al Koudsi N, Hoffmann EB, Assadzadeh A, et al: Hepatic C CYP2A6 levels and nicotine metabolism: impact of genetic, physiological, environmental, and epigenetic factors. Eur J Clin Pharmacol 66:239–251, 2010

American Psychiatric Association: Diagnostic and Statistical Manual of Mental Disorders, 4th Edition, Text Revision. Washington, DC, American Psychiatric Association, 2000

American Psychiatric Nurses Association (APNA), International Society of Psychiatric Mental Health Nurses (ISPN), American Nurses Association (ANA): Psychiatric-Mental Health Nursing: Scope and Standards of Practice. Silver Spring, MD, American Nurses Association, 2007

Anthony WA: Recovery from mental illness: the guiding vision of the mental health services in the 1990s. Psychiatric Rehabilitation Journal 2(3):17–24, 1993

Aulinskas T: Genelex New York informed consent: DNA drug sensitivity testing, version 10/11. Seattle, WA, Genelex Corporation, March 2010. Available at: http://genelex.com/NYconsent.pdf. Accessed May 7, 2012.

Bertilsson L: Geographical/interracial differences in polymorphic drug oxidation: current state of knowledge of cytochromes P450 (CYP) 2D6 and 2C19. Clin Pharmacokinet 29:192–209, 1995

Campinha-Bacote J: The Process of Cultural Competence in the Delivery of Healthcare Services: The Journey Continues. Cincinnati, OH, Transcultural CARE Associates, 2007

Consensus Panel on Genetic/Genomic Nursing Competencies: Essentials of Genetic and Genomic Nursing: Competencies, Curricula Guidelines, and Outcome Indicators, 2nd Edition. Silver Spring, MD, American Nurses Association, 2008

de Almeida Cde F, de Amorim EL, de Albuquerque UP: Insights into the search for new drugs from traditional knowledge: an ethnobotanical and chemical-ecological perspective. Pharm Biol 49:864–873, 2011

Desta Z, Zhao X, Shin JG, et al: Clinical significance of the cytochrome P450 2C19 genetic polymorphism. Clin Pharmacokinet 41:913–958, 2002

Frackiewicz EJ, Sramek JJ, Herrera JM, et al: Review of neuroleptic dosage in different ethnic groups, in Cross-Cultural Psychiatry. Edited by Herrera JM, Lawson WB, Sramek JJ. New York, Wiley, 1999, pp 107–130

Keltner NL, Folks DG: Psychotropic Drugs, 4th Edition. St. Louis, MO, Elsevier Mosby, 2005

Keltner NL, Vance DE: Introduction to psychotropic drugs, in Psychiatric Nursing, 6th Edition. Edited by Keltner NL, Bostrom CE, McGuinness T. St. Louis, MO, Elsevier Mosby, 2011, pp 142–154

Lawson WB: The art and science of ethnopharmacology, in Cross-Cultural Psychiatry. Edited by Herrera JM, Lawson WB, Sramek JJ. New York, Wiley, 1999, pp 67–74

Leininger MM: Culture care diversity and universality theory and evolution of the ethnonursing method, in Culture Care and Universality: A Worldwide Nursing Theory. Edited by Leininger MM, McFarland MR. Boston, MA, Jones & Bartlett, 2006, pp 1–41

Muñoz C, Hilgenberg C: Ethnopharmacology: understanding how ethnicity can affect drug response is essential to providing culturally competent care. Holist Nurs Pract 20:227–234, 2006

Muñoz C, Luckmann J: Transcultural Communication in Nursing, 2nd Edition. Clifton Park, NJ, Thomson Delmar, 2005

Munoz R, Primm A, Ananth J, et al: Life in Color: Culture in American Psychiatry. Munster, IN, Hilton Publishing, 2007

Noonan P, Warren BJ, White D: Psychiatric nurse: diagnosis and pharmacologic treatment of bipolar disorder: a roundtable discussion. Counseling Points: Enhancing Patient Communication for the Psychiatric Nurse 1(4):1–12, 2007

Okpaku SM: Prescribing for Africans: some transcultural guidelines, in Cross-Cultural Psychiatry. Edited by Herrera JM, Lawson WB, Sramek JJ. New York, Wiley, 1999, pp 53–62

Patwardham B: Ethnopharmacology and drug discovery. J Ethnopharmacol 100:50–52, 2005

Peplau H: Interpersonal Relations in Nursing. New York, Putnam, 1956

Rodriquez E: Plants of restricted use indicated by three cultures in Brazil (Caboclo-river dweller, Indian and Quilombola). J Ethnopharmacol 111:295–302, 2007

Scott G, Hewett ML: Pioneers in ethnopharmacology: the Dutch East India company (VOC) at the Cape from 1650–1800. J Ethnopharmacol 115:339–360, 2008

Smedley BD, Butler AS, Bristow LR: In the Nation's Compelling Interest: Ensuring Diversity in the Health-Care Workforce. Washington, DC, National Academies Press, 2004

Spector RE: Cultural Diversity in Health and Illness, 6th Edition. Upper Saddle River, NJ, Pearson Prentice Hall, 2004

Stahl SM: The Prescriber's Guide: Stahl's Essential Psychopharmacology, 3rd Edition. New York, Cambridge University Press, 2009

Stepp JR, Moerman DE: The importance of weeds in ethnopharmacology. J Ethnopharmacol 75:19–23, 2001

U.S. Department of Health and Human Services: Mental Health: A Report of the Surgeon General. Washington, DC, U.S. Department of Health and Human Services, 1999

U.S. Department of Health and Human Services: Mental Health: Culture, Race, and Ethnicity: A Supplement to Mental Health: A Report of the Surgeon General. Washington, DC, U.S. Department of Health and Human Services, 2001

Wang KY, Chian CF, Lai HR, et al: Clinical pharmacist counseling improves outcomes for Taiwanese asthma patients. Pharm World Sci 32:721–729, 2010

Wang X, Sun H, Zhang A, et al: Potential role of metabolomics approaches in the area of traditional Chinese medicine: as pillars of the bridge between Chinese and Western medicine. J Pharm Biomed Anal 55:859–868, 2011

Ward-Smith P: Individual variations in drug responses. Urol Nurs 30:22–27, 2010

Warren BJ: Cultural aspects of bipolar disorder: interpersonal meaning for clients and psychiatric nurses. J Psychos Nurs 45:1–5, 2007

Warren BJ: Ethnopharmacology: the effect on patients, health care professionals, and systems. Urol Nurs 28:292–295, 2008

Warren BJ: Teaching the fluid process of cultural competence at the graduate level: a constructionist approach, in Transforming Nursing Education: The Culturally Inclusive Environment. Edited by Bosher SD, Pharris MD. New York, Springer, 2009, pp 179–206

Warren BJ: Cultural competence in psychiatric nursing, in Psychiatric Nursing, 6th Edition. Edited by Keltner NL, Bostrom CE, McGuinness T. St. Louis, MO, Elsevier Mosby, 2011, pp 128–134

Warren BJ, Broome B: The culture of mental illness in adolescents with urologic problems. Urol Nurs 31:95–104, 2011

PART III

Appendixes

Approximate Psychotropic Drug Dose Equivalencies

The information contained in this appendix is offered to provide the prescriber with approximate dose equivalencies within classes of psychotropic medications. These equivalency guidelines can assist the practitioner in managing a patient's medication to avoid side effects and maximize symptom response. Below, two example scenarios are offered to illustrate how a psychiatric advanced practice registered nurse (APRN) might use these data to switch a patient from one psychotropic agent to another utilizing a cross-tapering approach (i.e., gradually introducing the new agent while tapering the dosage of the old one).

Example 1

Patient is prescribed alprazolam (Xanax) 1 mg bid but is experiencing breakthrough anxiety during the mid-afternoon. The psychiatric APRN decides to switch the patient to a different medication, diazepam (Valium), which has a longer half-life.

- Week 1: Reduce alprazolam to 0.5 mg bid and start diazepam 5 mg bid.
- Week 2: Discontinue alprazolam and increase diazepam to 10 mg bid.

With this plan, the patient should not experience withdrawal symptoms or any significant discomfort, given that the dosing of the two agents is approximately equivalent.

Example 2

Patient is prescribed sertraline (Zoloft) 200 mg/day but it no longer seems to be working. The psychiatric APRN decides to cross-taper the patient to duloxetine (Cymbalta).

- Week 1: Reduce sertraline to 150 mg daily and start duloxetine 30 mg daily.
- Week 2: Reduce sertraline to 100 mg daily and increase duloxetine to 60 mg daily.
- Week 3: Reduce sertraline to 50 mg daily and increase duloxetine to 90 mg daily.
- Week 4: Discontinue sertraline and continue duloxetine 90 mg daily.

While theoretically the duloxetine should be increased to 120 mg/day in week 4, the two agents differ in their mechanism of action, with sertraline solely targeting serotonin and duloxetine targeting both serotonin and norepinephrine. As this example explores the cross-taper of two different classes of antidepressant, it may not be necessary to maximize the hypothetical dose equivalency for the duloxetine, given its reuptake inhibition of both serotonin and norepinephrine.

Of course, in all situations, the patient's symptoms, comorbid medical conditions, other medications, and life circumstances should ultimately guide the decision-making process. This table is offered as a potential guideline.

Drug	Dosage*
Benzodiazepines (for anxiety/panic disorder)	
Ativan (lorazepam)	1.0 mg
Klonopin (clonazepam)	0.5 mg
Librium (chlordiazepoxide)	10 mg
Serax (oxazepam)	15 mg
Tranxene (clorazepate)	7.5 mg
Valium (diazepam)	5.0 mg
Xanax (alprazolam)	0.5 mg
Xanax XR (alprazolam)	0.5 mg
Selective serotonin reuptake inhibitors (for depression and anxiety)	
Celexa (citalopram)	20 mg
Lexapro (escitalopram)	10 mg
Luvox (fluvoxamine)	50 mg bid
Luvox CR (fluvoxamine ER)	100 mg
Paxil (paroxetine)	20 mg
Paxil CR (paroxetine ER)	25 mg
Prozac/Sarafem (fluoxetine)	20 mg
Prozac Weekly (fluoxetine weekly)	90 mg/week
Viibryd (vilazodone)	20 mg
Zoloft (sertraline)	50 mg
Serotonin-norepinephrine reuptake inhibitors (for depression and anxiety)	
Effexor XR (venlafaxine ER)	75 mg
Pristiq (desvenlafaxine)	50 mg
Cymbalta (duloxetine)	30 mg

Drug	Dosage*
Psychostimulants (for attention-deficit/hyperactivity disorder)	
Adderall (amphetamine salts)	7.5 mg bid
Adderall XR (amphetamine salts ER)	15 mg
Concerta (methylphenidate ER)	18 mg
Daytrana (methylphenidate transdermal)	20 mg
Dexedrine (dextroamphetamine)	15 mg
Focalin (dexmethylphenidate)	5 mg bid
Focalin XR (dexmethylphenidate ER)	10 mg
Metadate ER/Metadate CD (methylphenidate ER)	15 mg
Ritalin (methylphenidate)	5 mg tid
Ritalin LA/Ritalin-SR (methylphenidate ER)	15 mg
Vyvanse (lisdexamfetamine)	20–30 mg
First-generation (typical) antipsychotics	
Haldol (haloperidol)	2 mg
Loxitane (loxapine)	10 mg
Navane (thiothixene)	5 mg
Prolixin (fluphenazine)	2 mg
Thorazine (chlorpromazine)	100 mg
Trilafon (perphenazine)	16 mg
Second- and third-generation (atypical) antipsychotics	
Abilify/Abilify Discmelt (aripiprazole)	15 mg
Fanapt (iloperidone)	8 mg bid
Geodon (ziprasidone)	40 mg bid
Invega (paliperidone)	6 mg
Invega Sustenna (paliperidone LAI)	156 mg im q 4 weeks
Latuda (lurasidone)	60 mg
Risperdal/Risperdal M-Tab (risperidone)	1 mg bid

Drug	Dosage*
Second- and third-generation (atypical) antipsychotics (continued)	
Risperdal Consta (risperidone LAI)	25 mg im q 2 weeks
Saphris (asenapine)	5–10 mg bid
Seroquel (quetiapine)	100 mg bid
Seroquel XR (quetiapine ER)	200 mg
Zyprexa/Zyprexa Zydis (olanzapine)	10 mg
Zyprexa Relprevv (olanzapine LAI)	210 mg im q 2 weeks or 405 mg im q 4 weeks
Nonbenzodiazepine hypnotics (for insomnia/sleep disorders)	
Ambien (zolpidem)	10 mg
Ambien CR (zolpidem ER)	12.5 mg
Benadryl (diphenhydramine)	25–50 mg
Desyrel (trazodone)	50–100 mg
Lunesta (eszopiclone)	3 mg
Rozerem (ramelteon)	8 mg
Silenor (doxepin)	6 mg
Sonata (zaleplon)	10 mg
Vistaril (hydroxyzine)	50 mg
Benzodiazepine hypnotics (for insomnia)	
Dalmane (flurazepam)	15–30 mg
Halcion (triazolam)	0.5 mg
Restoril (temazepam)	15 mg

Note.   These approximate dose equivalencies are intended solely as guidelines. bid = twice a day; im = intramuscularly; q = every; tid = three times a day. ER = extended release; LAI = long-acting injectable.
*Dosages are per day unless otherwise noted.

Psychotropic and Other Medications Influenced by the Cytochrome P450 (CYP) System

This appendix presents an overview of the psychotropic and other medications influenced by the cytochrome P450 (CYP) system. The CYPs are the major enzymes involved in drug metabolism in the liver. Psychiatric advanced practice registered nurses (APRNs) need to be aware of which psychotropic medications are inducers and which are inhibitors of specific CYP enzymes. It is those actions that will impact adverse events of the medications, drug-drug interactions, and overall efficacy of the agent.

Caution should be exercised when the agent being prescribed is known to be a CYP inducer or inhibitor, as the target drug dosage may need to be adjusted to account for the potential increase or decrease in metabolism. Additionally, when patients are prescribed medications that are metabolized by the same CYP enzyme, there may be a cumulative effect and exacerbation of adverse events, which may lead to toxicity and potentially harmful effects for the patient.

This table offers an overview of the most common CYP enzymes and their impact on various psychotropic medications.

Substrates

1A2	2B6	2C8	2C9
acetaminophen, amitriptyline, caffeine, clomipramine, clozapine, cyclobenzaprine, estradiol, fluvoxamine, haloperidol, imipramine, mexilletine, naproxen, olanzapine, ondansetron, phenacetin, propranolol, riluzole, ropivacaine, tacrine, theophylline, tizanidine, verapamil, R-warfarin, zileuton, zolmitriptan	bupropion, cyclophosphamide, efavirenz, ifosfamide, methadone	amodiaquine, cerivastatin, paclitaxel, repaglinide, torsemide	amitriptyline, celecoxib, diclofenac, fluoxetine, fluvastatin, glibenclamide, glimepiride, glipizide, glyburide, ibuprofen, irbesartan, lornoxicam, losartan, meloxicam, S-naproxen, nateglinide, phenytoin, piroxicam, rosiglitazone, suprofen, tamoxifen, tolbutamide, torsemide, S-warfarin

2C19	2D6	2E1	3A4/5/7
amitriptyline, carisoprodol, chloramphenicol, citalopram, clomipramine, cyclophosphamide, diazepam, hexobarbital, imipramine, indomethacin, lansoprazole, S-mephenytoin, R-mephobarbital, moclobemide, nelfinavir, nilutamide, omeprazole,	alprenolol, amitriptyline, amphetamine, aripiprazole, atomoxetine, bufuralol, carvedilol, chlorpheniramine, chlorpromazine, clomipramine, codeine, debrisoquine, desipramine, dexfenfluramine, dextromethorphan, duloxetine, encainide, flecainide, fluoxetine, fluvoxamine,	acetaminophen, aniline, benzene, chlorzoxazone, N,N-dimethyl formamide, enflurane, ethanol, halothane, isoflurane, methoxyflurane, sevoflurane, theophylline	alfentanyl, alprazolam, amlodipine, aprepitant, aripiprazole, astemizole, atorvastatin, buspirone, cafergot, caffeine, cerivastatin, chlorpheniramine, cilostazol, cisapride, clarithromycin, cocaine, codeine, cyclosporine, dapsone, dexamethasone, dextromethorphan, diazepam, diltiazem,

Substrates *(continued)*

2C19 *(cont'd)*	2D6 *(cont'd)*	2E1	3A4/5/7 *(cont'd)*
pantoprazole, phenobarbitone, phenytoin, primidone, progesterone, proguanil, propranolol, rabeprazole, teniposide, R-warfarin	haloperidol, imipramine, lidocaine, methoxyamphetamine, metoclopramide, S-metoprolol, mexilletine, minaprine, nebivolol, nortriptyline, ondansetron, oxycodone, paroxetine, perhexiline, perphenazine, phenacetin, phenformin, promethazine, propafenone, propranolol, risperidone, sparteine, tamoxifen, thioridazine, timolol, tramadol, venlafaxine, zuclopenthixol		docetaxel, domperidone, eplerenone, erythromycin, estradiol, felodipine, fentanyl, finasteride, gleevec, haloperidol, hydrocortisone, indinavir, irinotecan, LAAM, lercanidipine, lidocaine, lovastatin, methadone, midazolam, nateglinide, nelfinavir, nifedipine, nisoldipine, nitrendipine, ondansetron, pimozide, progesterone, propranolol, quetiapine, quinidine, quinine, risperidone, ritonavir, salmeterol, saquinavir, sildenafil, simvastatin, sirolimus, tacrolimus (FK506), tamoxifen, taxol, telithromycin, terfenadine, testosterone, trazodone, triazolam, verapamil, vincristine, zaleplon, ziprasidone

Inhibitors

1A2	2B6	2C8	2C9
amiodarone, cimetidine, ciprofloxacin, fluoroquinolones, fluvoxamine, furafylline, interferon, methoxsalen, mibefradil	thiotepa, ticlopidine	gemfibrozil, glitazones, montelukast, quercetin, trimethoprim	amiodarone, fenofibrate, fluconazole, fluvastatin, fluvoxamine, isoniazid, lovastatin, phenylbutazone, probenicid, sertraline, sulfamethoxazole, sulfaphenazole, teniposide, voriconazole, zafirlukast

2C19	2D6	2E1	3A4/5/7
chloramphenicol, cimetidine, felbamate, fluoxetine, fluvoxamine, indomethacin, ketoconazole, lansoprazole, modafinil, omeprazole, oxcarbazepine, pantoprazole, probenicid, rabeprazole, ticlopidine, topiramate	amiodarone, bupropion, celecoxib, chlorpheniramine, chlorpromazine, cimetidine, citalopram, clemastine, clomipramine, cocaine, diphenhydramine, doxepin, doxorubicin, duloxetine, escitalopram, fluoxetine, halofantrine, haloperidol_red, hydroxyzine, levomepromazine, methadone, metoclopramide, mibefradil, midodrine, moclobemide, paroxetine, perphenazine, quinidine, ranitidine, ritonavir, sertraline, terbinafine, ticlopidine, tripelennamine	diethyldithio-carbamate, disulfiram	amiodarone, aprepitant, chloramphenicol, cimetidine, ciprofloxacin, clarithromycin, delaviridine, diethyldithiocarbamate, diltiazem, erythromycin, fluconazole, fluvoxamine, gestodene, grapefruit juice, imatinib, indinavir, itraconazole, ketoconazole, mibefradil, mifepristone, nefazodone, nelfinavir, norfloxacin, norfluoxetine, ritonavir, saquinavir, star fruit, telithromycin, verapamil, voriconazole

Inducers

1A2	2B6	2C8	2C9
broccoli, brussels sprouts, char-grilled meat, insulin, methylcholanthrene, modafinil, nafcillin, beta-naphthoflavone, omeprazole, tobacco	phenobarbital, rifampin	rifampin	rifampin, secobarbital

2C19	2D6	2E1	3A4/5/7
carbamazepine, norethindrone, prednisone, rifampin	dexamethasone, rifampin	ethanol, isoniazid	barbiturates, carbamazepine, efavirenz, glucocorticoids, modafinil, nevirapine, oxcarbazepine, phenobarbital, phenytoin, pioglitazone, rifabutin, rifampin, St. John's wort, troglitazone

Note.   CYP = cytochrome P450.
Source.   Adapted from data from Flockhart DA: Drug interactions: cytochrome P450 drug interaction table. Indianapolis, IN, Indiana University School of Medicine, 2007. Available at: http://medicine.iupui.edu/clinpharm/ddis/table.aspx. Accessed January 15, 2013.

Psychopharmacogenetic Variations

Implications for Practice

Over 25% of ALL common medications have genetic information that can be tested and used to personalize medical treatment.

—Frueh et al. 2008

*P*ersonalized *medicine* has recently become a "buzz term" in psychiatry. Given the lack of definitive diagnostic testing available, pharmacogenetic testing has offered a means of reducing the "trial and error" prescribing that often occurs in the field of psychiatry. Through identifying the various genotypes and their impact on symptom expression and hypothetical impact on the psychotropic medications, practitioners now have a new tool to augment their clinical assessment.

This table offers an overview of the psychopharmacogenetic variations exerted by the patient's genetic profile. These genes and genotypes impact the expression of psychiatric symptoms and the potential for adverse effects of psychotropic medications. Using the information provided in this chart, coupled with the clinical assessment, and the results of pharmacogenetic testing, the psychiatric advanced practice registered nurse (APRN) can narrow down the prescribing options to "personalize" medication therapy for the patient.

Gene	Purpose	Genotype	Hypothetical implications	Personalized medicine options
Serotonin transporter (*SLC6A4*)—serotonin pathway (Weizman et al. 2012)	Presynaptic serotonin reuptake	S/S, S/LG, or LG/LG: short allele variant (S) or (LG)	↑ Cortisol burden secondary to ↑ negative feedback on HPA axis; ↓ Response to SSRIs; ↑ Risk for TRD, PTSD	Consider use of non-SSRI antidepressants; Use caution when initiating or discontinuing SSRI or SNRI treatment
		LA/LA: long allele variant (LA)	↑ Transcription activity; "Normal" genotype; may be protective for adverse events	Consider use of SSRI antidepressants
Serotonin receptor (*5HT2C*)—serotonin pathway (Zhang and Malhotra 2011)	Satiety signaling activity	C/C: "C" allele antagonism	↑ Risk for weight gain, metabolic syndrome with psychotropics	Monitor for metabolic syndrome, weight gain; Use caution with atypical antipsychotics
		C/T or T/T: "T" allele variant	"Normal" genotype; may be protective for adverse events	Consider use of SSRI antidepressants
Gated calcium channel (*CACNA1C*)—glutamate pathway (Ferreira et al. 2008)	Regulation of calcium influx along cell membrane	G/A: "A" allele variant (A)	↑ Excitatory neurotransmission; ↑ Risk for mood disorder recurrence; ↑ Risk for bipolar disorder, schizophrenia, MDD; ↑ Response to mood-stabilizing anticonvulsants, atypical antipsychotics	Consider use of anticonvulsant mood stabilizers, atypical antipsychotic mood stabilizers, lithium

Gene	Purpose	Genotype	Hypothetical implications	Personalized medicine options
Gated calcium channel (*CACNA1C*) (*continued*)		G/G: no variant	No clinical implications	Patient assessment of symptoms should guide clinical decision making regarding medications
Ankyrin 3 (*ANK3*)— cell membrane maintenance (Ferreira et al. 2008)	Stabilization of sodium channels and excitatory neurotransmission	T/T: "T" allele variant	↑ Risk for bipolar disorder, schizophrenia, cyclothymic mood disorder ↑ Risk for decreased sustained attention	Consider use of anticonvulsant mood stabilizers, stimulants, wake-promoting agents
Methylenetetrahydro-folate reductase (*MTHFR*)— metabolism (Robinson 2009)	Conversion of folic acid to its most usable/active form— methylfolate	T/T: "T" allele variant	Inefficient production of methylfolate ↓ Ability to regulate flow of monoamines across synapse ↑ Risk for depression, autism, bipolar disorder, schizophrenia	Consider use of L-methylfolate, the most usable form of folic acid, which is able to cross the blood-brain barrier

Gene	Purpose	Genotype	Hypothetical implications	Personalized medicine options
Catechol-O-methyltransferase (*COMT*)—dopamine pathway (Zhang and Malhotra 2011)	Regulation of dopamine and norepinephrine levels in PFC, which impacts memory, attention, judgment, and other executive functions	Val/Val: "Val" allele variant	↓ Dopamine in PFC ↓ Executive functioning	Consider use of psychostimulants, bupropion, atomoxetine, wake-promoting agents
		Met/Met: "Met" allele variant	↓ Dopamine in PFC ↑ Sensitivity to euphoric effects of substances of abuse	Consider use of bupropion to enhance dopamine in PFC
Dopamine receptor (*DRD2*)—dopamine pathway (Zhang and Malhotra 2011)	Movement and perception	Ins/Del or Del/Del: deletion variant (Del)	↑ Risk for adverse effects ↓ Response to atypical antipsychotics	Consider use of non-antipsychotic mood stabilizers such as anticonvulsants
		Ins/Ins: insertion allele (Ins)	"Normal" genotype; may be protective for adverse events	Consider use of atypical antipsychotic mood stabilizers
Cytochrome P450 enzymes—metabolism CYP2D6 (Zhang and Malhotra 2011) CYP2C19 (Weizman et al. 2012)	Enzymes responsible for metabolism of medications in the liver	EM: extensive metabolizer	"Normal" drug metabolism	EMs usually respond as clinically indicated for medications; typically no dosing adjustments necessary
		IM: intermediate metabolizer	Variation in one allele	Dosage adjustments may be required for medications that are substrates of these systems
		PM: poor metabolizer	Variation in two alleles	

Gene	Purpose	Genotype	Hypothetical implications	Personalized medicine options
CYP3A4/5+ (Plesnicar 2010)			Both IMs and PMs may be at increased risk for drug-induced side effects, unpredictable treatment response	
		UM: ultrarapid metabolizer	Higher-than-average rate of drug metabolism ↑ Risk of therapeutic failure ↑ Risk of drug-induced side effects secondary to ↑ exposure to drug metabolites	Dosage adjustments may be required for medications that are substrates of these systems

Note. ↑ = increased; ↓ = decreased; HPA = hypothalamic-pituitary-adrenal; MDD = major depressive disorder; PTSD = posttraumatic stress disorder; PFC = prefrontal cortex; SSRI = selective serotonin reuptake inhibitor; SNRI = serotonin-norepinephrine reuptake inhibitor; TRD = treatment-resistant depression.

References

Ferreira MA, O'Donovan MC, Meng YA, et al: Collaborative genome-wide association analysis supports a role for ANK3 and CACNA1C in bipolar disorder. Nat Genet 40:1056–1058, 2008

Frueh FW, Amur S, Mummaneni P, et al: Pharmacogenomic biomarker information in drug labels approved by the United States food and drug administration: prevalence of related drug use. Pharmacotherapy 28:992–998, 2008

Plesnicar BK: Personalized antipsychotic treatment: the adverse effects perspectives. Psychiatr Danub 22:329–334, 2010

Robinson DS: Vitamins, monoamines, and depression. Primary Psychiatry 16:19–21, 2009

Weizman S, Gonda X, Dome P, et al: Pharmacogenetics of antidepressive drugs: a way towards personalized treatment of major depressive disorder. Neuropsychopharmacol Hung 14:87–101, 2012

Zhang JP, Malhotra AK: Pharmacogenetics and antipsychotics: therapeutic efficacy and side effects prediction. Expert Opin Drug Metab Toxicol 7:9–37, 2011

Psychiatric Rating Scales

Clinical rating scales provide assistance in identifying a patient's initial symptoms as well as monitoring symptoms over time. For the prescribing psychiatric advanced practice registered nurse (APRN), the various psychiatric rating scales can also serve as tools for tracking the effectiveness of a patient's medication based on reduction of symptoms over time.

This appendix offers a sampling of the most widely used psychiatric rating scales across symptom clusters and diagnostic categories of mental disorders (see table below for a listing of the relevant chapter[s] for each scale). The prescribing APRN will find these instruments to be a valuable resource.

	Relevant chapter(s) in manual
Patient Health Questionnaire: Somatic, Anxiety, and Depressive Symptoms (PHQ-SADS)	2, 3

The PHQ-SADS is a universal screening tool for identifying patients at risk for depression and anxiety associated with somatic complaints. It is useful for both primary care practitioners and psychiatric clinicians.

Hamilton Anxiety Scale (Ham-A)	2

The Ham-A is one of the most popular anxiety rating scales utilized in both clinical and research settings. Clinicians will find this instrument helpful in assessing a patient's progress and in adjusting medication dosages.

17-Item Hamilton Rating Scale for Depression (Ham-D-17)	3

Like the Ham-A, the Ham-D-17 is one of the most widely utilized rating scales. The psychiatric advanced practice nurse will find this tool helpful in tracking a patient's progress over time as well as making medication dosage adjustments.

Edinburgh Postnatal Depression Scale (EPDS)	3

The EPDS is a tool used to screen women at risk for postpartum depression. To obtain the most accurate glimpse of the woman's current mental state, it is important that she complete the scale based on her mood, thoughts, and feelings over the past month.

Parent Version of the Young Mania Rating Scale (P-YMRS)	4

The Young Mania Rating Scale (YMRS) is an excellent tool for identifying the severity of manic symptoms in patients diagnosed with bipolar disorder. The Parent Version of the YMRS is modified for use in the pediatric population. This scale allows the practitioner to interview parents or guardians about a child's symptoms in order to determine whether the child should be referred for further evaluation by a mental health professional and also to help assess whether a child's symptoms are responding to treatment.

	Relevant chapter(s) in manual
Abnormal Involuntary Movement Scale (AIMS)	4, 5, 10

The AIMS is the gold standard for evaluating extrapyramidal and tardive dyskinesia symptoms in patients prescribed antipsychotic medications. This rating scale aids in the early detection of movement disorders and allows the clinician and patient to determine the best course of action to minimize further adverse events.

Vanderbilt ADHD Diagnostic Parent Rating Scale (VADPRS) **Vanderbilt ADHD Diagnostic Teacher Rating Scale (VADTRS)**	6

The VADPRS and VADTRS are customized to evaluate a child's symptoms in the home or school environment. Scores from these scales can aid the practitioner in identifying the various subtypes of ADHD as well as common comorbidities such as oppositional defiant disorder, depression, anxiety, and conduct disorder. The VADPRS and VADTRS can also be used to evaluate the child's improvement over time and the need for medication adjustment.

Adult ADHD Self-Report Scale—Version 1.1 (Adult ASRS-v1.1) **Symptom Checklist**	6

The ASRS-v1.1 Symptom Checklist is a self-report rating scale to assist with evaluating the symptoms of ADHD in adults. It has been useful in prompting conversation between the patient and practitioner.

Clinical Institute Withdrawal Assessment of Alcohol Scale, Revised (CIWA-Ar)	7

The CIWA-Ar is commonly utilized in inpatient settings to evaluate the severity of a patient's withdrawal symptoms during detoxification from alcohol. It is particularly helpful in identifying the risk of disorientation and potential for seizures.

	Relevant chapter(s) in manual
Sleep Disorder Scales: Pittsburgh Insomnia Rating Scale (PIRS) Epworth Sleepiness Scale (ESS)	8

Because insomnia is one of the most prominent symptoms across the psychiatric disorders, it is important that the practitioner ascertain whether the patient's insomnia is part of the primary psychiatric presentation or a comorbid condition requiring its own treatment.

- The PIRS is a 7-day rating scale to track patterns of insomnia.
- The ESS is a brief rating scale to assess a patient's risk for idiopathic hypersomnolence, narcolepsy, and sleep apnea by evaluating patterns of dozing behavior and their impact on quality of life.

PTSD Checklist—Civilian Version (PCL-C)	9

The PCL-C is a self-report rating scale used in screening for symptoms of posttraumatic stress disorder in the general (civilian) population. This scale can be applied to most traumatic events and is useful for prompting dialogue between the patient and practitioner.

Patient Health Questionnaire: Somatic, Anxiety, and Depressive Symptoms (PHQ-SADS)

The PHQ-SADS consists of the Patient Health Questionnaire somatic symptom items (PHQ-15), the generalized anxiety disorder items (GAD-7), and the depression items (PHQ-9), plus the panic items from the original Patient Health Questionnaire. Copies of the PHQ family of measures, including the GAD-7, are available at the PHQ Screeners Web site (www.phqscreeners.com). Translations, a bibliography, an instruction manual, and other information are also provided on this Web site.

	Score range	Severity	Proposed treatment
PHQ-15	0–4	Minimal	Monitor symptoms, repeat PHQ-15 at follow-up
	5–9	Mild	Therapy; coping skills; consider medications; refer for additional testing
	10–14	Moderate	Ongoing therapy; psychotropic medications; collaborate with other providers
	15–30	Severe	Consider hospitalization; ongoing therapy; medications and collaboration
GAD-7	0–5	Mild	Monitor symptoms; stress management/relaxation techniques; repeat GAD-7 at follow-up
	6–10	Moderate	Therapy; continue stress management/relaxation; consider medications
	11–15	Moderately severe	Ongoing therapies and medications
	16–21	Severe	Possible partial program or hospitalization; ongoing therapy and psychotropic medications
PHQ-9	0–4	None—minimal	None
	5–9	Mild	Monitor symptoms; repeat PHQ-9 at follow-up
	10–14	Moderate	Therapy; coping skills; consider medications
	15–19	Moderately severe	Ongoing therapy and medications
	20–27	Severe anxiety	Consider partial program or hospitalization; ongoing therapy and psychotropic medications

Source Reference. Kroenke K, Spitzer RL, Williams JB, Löwe B: "The Patient Health Questionnaire Somatic, Anxiety, and Depressive Symptom Scales: A Systematic Review." *General Hospital Psychiatry* 32:345–359, 2010.

Web Source. Psychiatric Times "Clinically Useful Psychiatric Scales" Web site (www.psychiatrictimes.com/clinical-scales).

Patient Health Questionnaire (PHQ-SADS)

This questionnaire is an important part of providing you with the best health care possible. Your answers will help in understanding problems that you may have. Please answer every question to the best of your ability.

Patient Health Questionnaire somatic symptom items (PHQ-15)

A. During the <u>last 4 weeks</u>, how much have you been bothered by any of the following problems?	Not bothered (0)	Bothered a little (1)	Bothered a lot (2)
1. Stomach pain			
2. Back pain			
3. Pain in your arms, legs, or joints (knees, hips, etc.)			
4. Feeling tired or having little energy			
5. Trouble falling or staying asleep, or sleeping too much			
6. Menstrual cramps or other problems with your periods			
7. Pain or problems during sexual intercourse			
8. Headaches			
9. Chest pain			
10. Dizziness			
11. Fainting spells			
12. Feeling your heart pound or race			
13. Shortness of breath			
14. Constipation, loose bowels, or diarrhea			
15. Nausea, gas, or indigestion			

PHQ-15 Score   =   ___ + ___

Generalized Anxiety Disorder items (GAD-7)

B. Over the last 2 weeks, how often have you been bothered by any of the following problems?	Not at all (0)	Several days (1)	More than half the days (2)	Nearly every day (3)
1. Feeling nervous anxiety or on edge				
2. Not being able to stop or control worrying				
3. Worrying too much about different things				
4. Trouble relaxing				
5. Being so restless that it is hard to sit still				
6. Becoming easily annoyed or irritable				
7. Feeling afraid as if something awful might happen				

GAD-7 Score   =   ___ + ___ + ___

C. Questions about anxiety attacks	No (1)	Yes (2)
a. In the last 4 weeks, have you had an anxiety attack? suddenly feeling fear or panic?		
If you checked "NO", go to question E.		
b. Has this ever happened before?		
c. Do some of these attacks come suddenly out of the blue—that is, in situations where you don't expect to be nervous or uncomfortable?		
d. Do these attacks bother you a lot or are you worried about having another attack?		
e. During your last bad anxiety attack, did you have symptoms like shortness of breath, sweating, or your heart racing, pounding, or skipping?		

Patient Health Questionnaire depression items (PHQ-9)

D. Over the last 2 weeks, how often have you been bothered by any of the following problems?	Not at all (0)	Several days (1)	More than half the days (2)	Nearly every day (3)
1. Little interest or pleasure in doing things				
2. Feeling down, depressed, or hopeless				
3. Trouble falling or staying asleep, or sleeping too much				
4. Feeling tired or having little energy				
5. Poor appetite or overeating				
6. Feeling bad about yourself—or that you are a failure or have let yourself or your family down				
7. Trouble concentrating on things, such as reading the newspaper or watching television				
8. Moving or speaking so slowly that other people could have noticed; or the opposite—being so fidgety or restless that you have been moving around a lot more than usual				
9. Thoughts that you would be better off dead of or hurting yourself in some way				

PHQ-9 Score   =   ___ + ___ + ___

E. If you checked off any problems on this questionnaire, how difficult have these problems made it for you to do your work, take care of things at home, or get along with other people?

Not difficult at all	Somewhat difficult	Very difficult	Extremely difficult
☐	☐	☐	☐

The PHQ and GAD screeners were developed by Drs. Robert L. Spitzer, Janet B.W. Williams, Kurt Kroenke, and colleagues, with an educational grant from Pfizer Inc. No permission is required to reproduce, translate, display, or distribute them.

Hamilton Anxiety Scale (Ham-A)

Instructions for the Clinician

The Hamilton Anxiety Scale (Ham-A) is a widely used and well-validated tool for measuring the severity of a patient's anxiety. It should be administered by an experienced clinician.

The Ham-A probes 14 parameters and takes 15–20 minutes to complete the interview and score the results. Each item is scored on a 5-point scale, ranging from 0 = not present to 4 = severe.

The major value of Ham-A is to assess the patient's response to a course of treatment, rather than as a diagnostic or screening tool. By administering the scale serially, a clinician can document the results of drug treatment or psychotherapy.

Developed in 1959 by Dr. Max Hamilton, the scale has proven useful not only in following individual patients but also in research involving many patients.

Ham-A Scoring Instructions

Sum the scores from all 14 parameters.
14–17 = Mild Anxiety
18–24 = Moderate Anxiety
25–30 = Severe Anxiety

Source.   Hamilton M: "The Assessment of Anxiety States by Rating." *British Journal of Medical Psychology* 32:50–55, 1959.

Web Source.   Psychiatric Times "Clinically Useful Psychiatric Scales" Web site (www.psychiatrictimes.com/clinical-scales).

Hamilton Anxiety Scale (Ham-A)

The Hamilton Anxiety Scale (Ham-A) is a rating scale developed to quantify the severity of anxiety symptomatology, often used in psychotropic drug evaluation. It consists of 14 items, each defined by a series of symptoms. Each item is rated on a 5-point scale, ranging from 0 (not present) to 4 (severe).

1. ANXIOUS MOOD
   - Worries
   - Anticipates worst

2. TENSION
   - Startles
   - Cries easily
   - Restless
   - Trembling

3. FEARS
   - Fear of the dark
   - Fear of strangers
   - Fear of being alone
   - Fear of animal

4. INSOMNIA
   - Difficulty falling asleep or staying asleep
   - Difficulty with nightmares

5. INTELLECTUAL
   - Poor concentration
   - Memory impairment

6. DEPRESSED MOOD
   - Decreased interest in activities
   - Anhedonia
   - Insomnia

7. SOMATIC COMPLAINTS: MUSCULAR
   - Muscle aches or pains
   - Bruxism

8. SOMATIC COMPLAINTS: SENSORY
   - Tinnitus
   - Blurred vision

9. CARDIOVASCULAR SYMPTOMS
   - Tachycardia
   - Palpitations
   - Chest pain
   - Sensation of feeling faint

10. RESPIRATORY SYMPTOMS
    - Chest pressure
    - Choking sensation
    - Shortness of breath

11. GASTROINTESTINAL SYMPTOMS
    - Dysphagia
    - Nausea or vomiting
    - Constipation
    - Weight loss
    - Abdominal fullness

12. GENITOURINARY SYMPTOMS
    - Urinary frequency or urgency
    - Dysmenorrhea
    - Impotence

13. AUTONOMIC SYMPTOMS
    - Dry mouth
    - Flushing
    - Pallor
    - Sweating

14. BEHAVIOR AT INTERVIEW
    - Fidgets
    - Tremor
    - Paces

The HAM-A is in the public domain.

17-Item Hamilton Rating Scale for Depression (Ham-D-17)

Instructions for the Clinician

The Hamilton Depression Rating Scale (Ham-D) has proven useful for many years as a way of determining a patient's level of depression before, during, and after treatment. It should be administered by a clinician experienced in working with psychiatric patients.

Although the Ham-D form lists 21 items, the scoring is based on the first 17. It generally takes 15–20 minutes to complete the interview and score the results. Eight items are scored on a 5-point scale, ranging from 0 = not present to 4 = severe. Nine are scored from 0 to 2.

Since its development in 1960 by Dr. Max Hamilton of the University of Leeds, England, the scale has been widely used in clinical practice and become a standard in pharmaceutical trials.

Ham-D Scoring Instructions

Sum the scores from the first 17 items.

0–7	=	Normal
8–13	=	Mild Depression
14–18	=	Moderate Depression
19–22	=	Severe Depression
≥23	=	Very Severe Depression

Source Reference.   Hamilton M: "A Rating Scale for Depression." *Journal of Neurology, Neurosurgery, and Psychiatry* 23:56–62, 1960.

Web Source.   University of Massachusetts Medical School "e-Mental Health in Central Massachusetts" Web site (http://library.umassmed.edu/ementalhealth/clinical/index.cfm).

17-Item Hamilton Depression Rating Scale (Ham-D-17)

The HAM-D is designed to rate the severity of depression in patients. Although it contains 21 areas, the patient's score should be calculated on the first 17 answers.

1. DEPRESSED MOOD
   (Gloomy attitude, pessimism about the future, feeling of sadness, tendency to weep)
   0 Absent
   1 Sadness, etc.
   2 Occasional weeping
   3 Frequent weeping
   4 Extreme symptoms

2. FEELINGS OF GUILT
   0 Absent
   1 Self-reproach, feels he/she has let people down
   2 Ideas of guilt
   3 Present illness is a punishment; delusions of guilt
   4 Hallucinations of guilt

3. SUICIDE
   0 Absent
   1 Feels life is not worth living
   2 Wishes he/she were dead
   3 Suicidal ideas or gestures
   4 Attempts at suicide

4. INSOMNIA—Initial
   (Difficulty in falling asleep)
   0 Absent
   1 Occasional
   2 Frequent

5. INSOMNIA—Middle
   (Complains of being restless and disturbed during the night; waking during the night)
   0 Absent
   1 Occasional
   2 Frequent

6. INSOMNIA—Delayed
   (Waking in early hours of the morning and unable to fall asleep again)
   0 Absent
   1 Occasional
   2 Frequent

7. WORK AND INTERESTS
   0 No difficulty
   1 Feelings of incapacity, listlessness, indecision, and vacillation
   2 Loss of interest in hobbies, decreased social activities
   3 Productivity decreased
   4 Unable to work. Stopped working because of present illness only. (Absence from work after treatment or recovery may rate a lower score.)

8. RETARDATION
   (Slowness of thought, speech, and activity; apathy; stupor)
   0 Absent
   1 Slight retardation at interview
   2 Obvious retardation at interview
   3 Interview difficult
   4 Complete stupor

9. AGITATION
   (Restlessness associated with anxiety)
   0 Absent
   1 Occasional
   2 Frequent

10. ANXIETY—PSYCHIC
    0 No difficulty
    1 Tension and irritability
    2 Worrying about minor matters
    3 Apprehensive attitude
    4 Fears

17-Item Hamilton Depression Rating Scale (Ham-D-17) *(continued)*

11. ANXIETY—SOMATIC
(Gastrointestinal, indigestion;
Cardiovascular, palpitation; Headaches;
Respiratory; Genitourinary, etc.)

0   Absent
1   Mild
2   Moderate
3   Severe
4   Incapacitating

12. SOMATIC SYMPTOMS—
GASTROINTESTINAL
(Loss of appetite, heavy feeling in
abdomen; constipation)

0   Absent
1   Mild
2   Severe

13. SOMATIC SYMPTOMS—GENERAL
(Heaviness in limbs, back, or head; diffuse
backache; loss of energy and fatigability)

0   Absent
1   Mild
2   Severe

14. GENITAL SYMPTOMS
(Loss of libido, menstrual disturbances)

0   Absent
1   Mild
2   Severe

15. HYPOCHONDRIASIS

0   Not present
1   Self-absorption (bodily)
2   Preoccupation with health
3   Querulous attitude
4   Hypochondriacal delusions

16. WEIGHT LOSS

0   No weight loss
1   Slight
2   Obvious or severe

17. INSIGHT
(Must be interpreted in terms of patient's
understanding and background)

0   No loss
1   Partial or doubtful loss
2   Loss of insight

TOTAL ITEMS 1–17: _____

0–7	=	Normal
8–13	=	Mild Depression
14–18	=	Moderate Depression
19–22	=	Severe Depression
≥23	=	Very Severe Depression

The HAM-D-17 is in the public domain.

Edinburgh Postnatal Depression Scale (EPDS) for Postpartum Depression

Background

The Edinburgh Postnatal Depression Scale (EPDS) was developed in 1987 for screening postpartum women in outpatient, home visiting settings, or at the 6–8 week postpartum examination. It has been utilized among numerous populations, including U.S. women and Spanish-speaking women in other countries. The scale has since been validated, and evidence from a number of research studies has confirmed the tool to be both reliable and sensitive in detecting depression.

The EPDS consists of 10 questions and can usually be completed in less than 5 minutes. Validation studies have utilized various threshold scores in determining which women were positive and in need of referral. Cut-off scores range from 9 to 13 points. A woman scoring 9 or more points or indicating any suicidal ideation—that is, she scores 1 or higher on question 10—should be referred immediately for follow-up.

The EPDS score should not override clinical judgment. A careful clinical assessment should be carried out to confirm the diagnosis. The scale indicates how the mother has felt during the previous week. In doubtful cases it may be useful to repeat the tool after 2 weeks. The scale will not detect mothers with anxiety neuroses, phobias, or personality disorders.

Scoring

- Questions 1, 2, and 4 (without an *) are scored 0, 1, 2, or 3, with the top box scored as a 0 and the bottom box scored as a 3.
- Questions 3 and 5–10 (marked with an *) are reverse-scored, with the top box scored as a 3 and the bottom box scored as 0.
- Maximum score: 30
- Possible depression: 10 or higher
- Always look at Question 10, which indicates suicidal thoughts.

Instructions

- The mother is asked to check one of four possible responses that comes the closest to how she has been feeling the previous 7 days.
- All 10 items must be completed.
- Care should be taken to avoid the possibility of the mother discussing her answers with others.
- The mother should complete the scale herself, unless she has limited English or has difficulty with reading.

Source Reference. Cox JL, Holden JM, Sagovsky R: "Detection of Postnatal Depression: Development of the 10-Item Edinburgh Postnatal Depression Scale." *British Journal of Psychiatry* 150:782–786, 1987.

Web Source. Psychiatric Times "Clinically Useful Psychiatric Scales" Web site (www.psychiatrictimes.com/clinical-scales).

Edinburgh Postnatal Depression Scale Form

INSTRUCTIONS AND SAMPLE QUESTION:

Because you are pregnant or have recently had a baby, we would like to know how you are feeling. Please CHECK the answer that comes closest to how you have felt IN THE PAST 7 DAYS, not just how you feel today. Below is an example, already completed:

I have felt happy
- ❑ Yes, all the time
- ■ Yes, most of the time
- ❑ No, not very often
- ❑ No, not at all

This would mean "I have felt happy most of the time" during the past week. Please complete the other questions in the same way.

In the past 7 days:

1. I have been able to laugh and see the funny side of things.
   - ❑ As much as I always could
   - ❑ Not quite so much now
   - ❑ Definitely not so much now
   - ❑ Not at all

2. I have looked forward with enjoyment to things.
   - ❑ As much as I ever did
   - ❑ Rather less than I used to
   - ❑ Definitely less than I used to
   - ❑ Hardly at all

*3. I have blamed myself unnecessarily when things went wrong.
   - ❑ Yes, most of the time
   - ❑ Yes, some of the time
   - ❑ Not very often
   - ❑ No, never

4. I have been anxious or worried for no good reason.
   - ❑ No, not at all
   - ❑ Hardly ever
   - ❑ Yes, sometimes
   - ❑ Yes, very often

*5. I have felt scared or panicky for no very good reason.
   - ❑ Yes, quite a lot
   - ❑ Yes, sometimes
   - ❑ No, not much
   - ❑ No, not at all

*6. Things have been getting on top of me.
   - ❑ Yes, most of the time I haven't been able to cope at all
   - ❑ Yes, sometimes I haven't been coping as well as usual
   - ❑ No, most of the time I have coped quite well
   - ❑ No, I have been coping as well as ever

*7. I have been so unhappy that I have had difficulty sleeping.
   - ❑ Yes, most of the time
   - ❑ Yes, sometimes
   - ❑ Not very often
   - ❑ No, not at all

*8. I have felt sad or miserable.
   - ❑ Yes, most of the time
   - ❑ Yes, quite often
   - ❑ Not very often
   - ❑ No, not at all

*9. I have been so unhappy that I have been crying.
   - ❑ Yes, most of the time
   - ❑ Yes, quite often
   - ❑ Only occasionally
   - ❑ No, never

*10. The thought of harming myself has occurred to me.
   - ❑ Yes, quite often
   - ❑ Sometimes
   - ❑ Hardly ever
   - ❑ Never

Parent Version of the Young Mania Rating Scale (P-YMRS)

The P-YMRS consists of 11 questions that parents are asked about their child's present state. The original rating scale (Young Mania Rating Scale; see below) was developed to assess severity of symptoms in adults hospitalized for mania. This revision was developed in an effort to help clinicians such as pediatricians determine when children should be referred for further evaluation by a mental health professional (such as a child psychiatrist) and also to help assess whether a child's symptoms are responding to treatment. The scale is NOT intended to diagnose bipolar disorder in children; such a diagnosis requires a thorough evaluation by an experienced mental health professional, preferably a board-certified child psychiatrist.

The average scores in children studied were approximately 25 for mania (a syndrome found in patients with bipolar I disorder) and 20 for hypomania (a syndrome found in patients with bipolar II disorder, bipolar disorder not otherwise specified, and cyclothymic disorder). Anything above 13 indicated a potential case of mania or hypomania for the group that was studied, while anything above 21 was a probable case. In situations where the odds of bipolar diagnosis are high to begin with (a child with mood symptoms with 2 parents having bipolar disorder), the P-YMRS can be extremely helpful. But for most groups of people, the base rate of bipolar disorder is unknown but low. Then, the most that a high score can do is raise a red flag (similar to having a family history of bipolar disorder).

Even a high score is unlikely to indicate a bipolar diagnosis. The P-YMRS performs similarly to the screening test for prostate cancer, in that it will identify most cases of bipolar disorder, but with an extremely high false-positive rate. The P-YMRS is presently being studied in a community pediatrics practice to determine its validity in that setting. The P-YMRS is provided here for educational purposes only, and should not be used as a substitute for evaluation by mental health professionals.

Source References.   The P-YMRS was revised from the Young Mania Rating Scale (YMRS):

Young RC, Biggs JT, Ziegler VE, Meyer DA: "A Rating Scale for Mania: Reliability, Validity and Sensitivity." *British Journal of Psychiatry* 133:429–435, 1978)

and was presented at the First Annual International Conference on Bipolar Disorders, Pittsburgh, PA, June 1996 (Gracious BL et al.). Its statistical properties are outlined in the following source:

Gracious BL, Youngstrom EA, Findling RL, Calabrese JR, et al: "Discriminative Validity of a Parent Version of the Young Mania Rating Scale." *Journal of the American Academy of Child and Adolescent Psychiatry* 41: 1350–1359, 2002.

Web Source.   Tennessee Department of Mental Health and Substance Abuse Services Web site (www.tn.gov/mental/policy/best_pract_children.shtml).

Parent Version of the Young Mania Rating Scale (P-YMRS)

Instructions: Please read each question below and circle the answer number that most closely describes your child.

1. **Mood—Is your child's mood higher (better) than usual?**
   0   No
   1   Mildly or possibly increased
   2   Definite elevation—more optimistic, self-confident; cheerful; appropriate to their conversation
   3   Elevated but inappropriate to content; joking, mildly silly
   4   Euphoric; inappropriate laughter; singing/making noises; very silly

2. **Motor Activity/Energy—Does your child's energy level or motor activity appear to be greater than usual?**
   0   No
   1   Mildly or possibly increased
   2   More animated; increased gesturing
   3   Energy is excessive; hyperactive at times; restless but can be calmed
   4   Very excited; continuous hyperactivity; cannot be calmed

3. **Sexual Interest—Is your child showing more than usual interest in sexual matters?**
   0   No
   1   Mildly or possibly increased
   2   Definite increase when the topic arises
   3   Talks spontaneously about sexual matters; gives more detail than usual; more interested in girls/boys than usual
   4   Has shown open sexual behavior—touching others or self inappropriately

4. **Sleep—Has your child's sleep decreased lately?**
   0   No
   1   Sleeping less than normal amount by up to 1 hour
   2   Sleeping less than normal amount by more than 1 hour
   3   Need for sleep appears decreased; less than 4 hours
   4   Denies need for sleep; has stayed up 1 night or more

5. **Irritability—Has your child appeared irritable?**
   0   No more than usual
   2   More grouchy or crabby
   4   Irritable openly several times throughout the day; recent episodes of anger with family, at school, or with friends
   6   Frequently irritable to point of being rude or withdrawn
   8   Hostile and uncooperative about all the time

6. **Speech (Rate and Amount)—Is your child talking more quickly or more than usual?**
   0   No change
   2   Seems more talkative
   4   Talking faster or more to say at times
   6   Talking more or faster to point he/she is difficult to interrupt
   8   Continuous speech; unable to interrupt

Parent Version of the Young Mania Rating Scale (P-YMRS) *(continued)*

7. Thoughts—Has your child shown changes in his/her thought patterns?
   0   No
   1   Thinking faster; some decrease in concentration; talking "around the issue"
   2   Distractible; loses track of the point; changes topics frequently; thoughts racing
   3   Difficult to follow; goes from one idea to the next; topics do not relate; makes rhymes or repeats words
   4   Not understandable; he/she doesn't seem to make any sense

8. Content—Is your child talking about different things than usual?
   0   No
   2   He/she has new interests and is making more plans
   4   Making special projects; more religious or interested in God
   6   Thinks more of him/herself; believes he/she has special powers; believes he/she is receiving special messages
   8   Is hearing unreal noises/voices; detects odors no one else smells; feels unusual sensations; has unreal beliefs

9. Disruptive/Aggressive Behavior—Has your child been more disruptive or aggressive?
   0   No; he/she is cooperative
   2   Sarcastic; loud; defensive
   4   More demanding; making threats
   6   Has threatened a family member or teacher; shouting; knocking over possessions/ furniture or hitting a wall
   8   Has attacked family member, teacher, or peer; destroyed property; cannot be spoken to without violence

10. Appearance—Has your child's interest in his/her appearance changed recently?
    0   No
    1   A little less or more interest in grooming than usual
    2   Doesn't care about washing or changing clothes, or is changing clothes more than three times a day
    3   Very messy; needs to be supervised to finish dressing; applying makeup in overly-done or poor fashion
    4   Refuses to dress appropriately; wearing bizarre styles

11. Insight—Does your child think he/she needs help (for his/her behavior) at this time?
    0   Yes; admits difficulties and wants treatment
    1   Believes there might be something wrong (but has not asked for help)
    2   Admits to change in behavior but denies he/she needs help
    3   Admits behavior might have changed but denies need for help
    4   Denies there have been any changes in his/her behavior/thinking

Source.   Reprinted from Gracious BL, Youngstrom EA, Findling RL, Calabrese JR: "Discriminative Validity of a Parent Version of the Young Mania Rating Scale." *Journal of the American Academy of Child and Adolescent Psychiatry* 41(11):1350–1359, 2002, with permission from Elsevier.

Abnormal Involuntary Movement Scale (AIMS)

AIMS Examination Procedure

> Should be completed before entering the ratings on the AIMS form.
>
> Either before or after completing the Examination Procedure, observe the patient unobtrusively at rest (e.g., in waiting room).
>
> The chair to be used in this examination should be a hard, firm one without arms.

1. Ask patient whether there is anything in his/her mouth (gum, candy, etc.) and if there is, to remove it.

2. Ask patient about the current condition of his/her teeth. Ask patient if he/she wears dentures. Do teeth or dentures bother patient now?

3. Ask patient whether he/she notices any movements in mouth, face, hands, or feet. If yes, ask to describe and to what extent they currently bother patient or interfere with his/her activities.

4. Have patient sit in chair with hands on knees, legs slightly apart, and feet flat on floor. (Look at entire body for movements while in this position).

5. Ask patient to sit with hands hanging unsupported. If male, between legs, if female, and wearing a dress, hanging over knees. (Observe hands and other body areas.)

6. Ask patient to open mouth. (Observe tongue at rest within mouth.) Do this twice.

7. Ask patient to protrude tongue. (Observe abnormalities of tongue movement.)

*8. Ask patient to tap thumb, with each finger, as rapidly as possible for 10–15 seconds: separately with right hand, then with left hand. (Observe facial and leg movements.)

9. Flex and extend patient's left and right arms, one at a time. (Note any rigidity and rate it.)

10. Ask patient to stand up. (Observe in profile. Observe all body areas again, hips included.)

*11. Ask patient to extend both arms outstretched in front with palms down. (Observe trunk, legs, and mouth.)

*12. Have patient walk a few paces, turn, and walk back to chair. (Observe hands and gait.) Do this twice.

---

*Activated movements.

Source Reference. Guy W (ed): ECDEU Assessment Manual for Psychopharmacology, Revised (DHEW Publ No ADM 76-388). Rockville, MD, U.S. Department of Health, Education and Welfare, 1976.

Web Source. Psychiatric Times "Clinically Useful Psychiatric Scales" Web site (www.psychiatrictimes.com/clinical-scales).

Abnormal Involuntary Movement Scale (AIMS)

Patient's name (please print): _____ Patient's ID information: _____

Examiner's name: _____

Current medications and total mg/day

Medication #1: _____ Total mg/day: ___ Medication #2: _____ Total mg/day: ___

Instructions: Complete the examination procedure before entering these ratings.

	None, normal (0)	Minimal (may be extreme normal) (1)	Mild (2)	Moderate (3)	Severe (4)
Facial and Oral Movements					
1. Muscles of facial expression (e.g., movements of forehead, eyebrows, periorbital area, cheeks; include frowning, blinking, smiling, grimacing)	❑	❑	❑	❑	❑
2. Lips and perioral area (e.g., puckering, pouting, smacking)	❑	❑	❑	❑	❑
3. Jaw (e.g., biting, clenching, chewing, mouth opening, lateral movement)	❑	❑	❑	❑	❑
4. Tongue (Rate only increases in movement both in and out of mouth, NOT inability to sustain movement)	❑	❑	❑	❑	❑
Extremity Movements					
5. Upper (arms, wrists, hands, fingers)—Include choreic movements (i.e., rapid, objectively purposeless, irregular, spontaneous); athetoid movements (i.e., slow, irregular, complex, serpentine); DO NOT include tremor (i.e., repetitive, regular, rhythmic)	❑	❑	❑	❑	❑
6. Lower (legs, knees, ankles, toes) (e.g., lateral knee movement, foot tapping, heel dropping, foot squirming, inversion and eversion of foot)	❑	❑	❑	❑	❑
Trunk Movements					
7. Neck, shoulders, hips (e.g., rocking, twisting, squirming, pelvic gyrations)	❑	❑	❑	❑	❑

Abnormal Involuntary Movement Scale (AIMS) *(continued)*

SCORING:
- Score the highest amplitude or frequency in a movement on the 0–4 scale, not the average.
- Score activated movements the same way; do not lower those numbers.
- A positive AIMS examination is a score of 2 in two or more movements or a score of 3 or 4 in a single movement.
- Do not sum the scores (e.g., a patient who scores 1 in four movements DOES NOT have a positive AIMS score of 4).

	None, normal	Minimal (may be extreme normal)	Mild	Moderate	Severe
	(0)	(1)	(2)	(3)	(4)
Overall Severity					
8. Severity of abnormal movements	❑	❑	❑	❑	❑
9. Incapacitation due to abnormal movements	❑	❑	❑	❑	❑

	No awareness	Aware, no distress	Aware, mild distress	Aware, moderate distress	Aware, severe distress
	(0)	(1)	(2)	(3)	(4)
10. Patient's awareness of abnormal movements (rate only patient's report)	❑	❑	❑	❑	❑

	Yes	No
Dental Status		
11. Current problems with teeth and/or dentures?	❑	❑
12. Does patient usually wear dentures?	❑	❑

Comments: _____

Examiner's signature: _____ Next exam date: _____

The AIMS is in the public domain.

Vanderbilt ADHD Diagnostic Parent Rating Scale (VADPRS)

Scoring Instructions for the VADPRS

Behaviors are counted if they are scored 2 (often) or 3 (very often).

Predominantly inattentive subtype	Requires 6 or more counted behaviors on items 1–9 and a performance problem (score of 1 or 2) in any of the items on the performance section.
Predominantly hyperactive/ impulsive subtype	Requires 6 or more counted behaviors on items 10–18 and a performance problem (score of 1 or 2) in any of the items on the performance section.
Combined subtype	Requires 6 or more counted behaviors each on both the inattention and hyperactivity/impulsivity dimensions.
Oppositional defiant disorder	Requires 4 or more counted behaviors on items 19–26.
Conduct disorder	Requires 3 or more counted behaviors on items 27–40.
Anxiety or depression	Requires 3 or more counted behaviors on items 41–47.

The **performance section** is scored as indicating some impairment if a child scores 1 or 2 on at least 1 item.

Source Reference.   Wolraich ML, Lambert W, Doffing MA, et al: "Psychometric Properties of the Vanderbilt ADHD Diagnostic Parent Rating Scale in a Referred Population." *Journal of Pediatric Psychology* 28:559–567, 2003.

Web Source.   "Developmental Behavioral Tools" page of the University of Oklahoma Health Sciences Center (UOHSC) Child Study Center Consultation Services Web site (http://dbp2doc.org/online-resources/developmental-behavioral-tools).

Vanderbilt ADHD Diagnostic Parent Rating Scale (VADPRS)

Patient Name: _____ Date of Birth:_____

Today's Date: _____ Age:_____

Grade:_____

Each rating should be considered in the context of what is appropriate for the age of your child.

Frequency Code: 0 = Never; 1 = Occasionally; 2 = Often; 3 = Very Often

1. Does not pay attention to details or makes careless mistakes, such as in homework	1	2	3	4
2. Has difficulty sustaining attention to tasks or activities	1	2	3	4
3. Does not seem to listen when spoken to directly	1	2	3	4
4. Does not follow through on instruction and fails to finish schoolwork (not due to oppositional behavior or failure to understand)	1	2	3	4
5. Has difficulty organizing tasks and activities	1	2	3	4
6. Avoids, dislikes, or is reluctant to engage in tasks that require sustained mental effort	1	2	3	4
7. Loses things necessary for tasks or activities (school assignments, pencils, or books)	1	2	3	4
8. Is easily distracted by extraneous stimuli	1	2	3	4
9. Is forgetful in daily activities	1	2	3	4
10. Fidgets with hands or feet or squirms in seat	1	2	3	4
11. Leaves seat when remaining seated is expected	1	2	3	4
12. Runs about or climbs excessively in situations when remaining seated is expected	1	2	3	4
13. Has difficulty playing or engaging in leisure activities quietly	1	2	3	4
14. Is "on the go" or often acts as if "driven by a motor"	1	2	3	4
15. Talks too much	1	2	3	4
16. Blurts out answers before questions have been completed	1	2	3	4
17. Has difficulty waiting his or her turn	1	2	3	4
18. Interrupts or intrudes on others (butts into conversations or games)	1	2	3	4
19. Argues with adults	1	2	3	4
20. Loses temper	1	2	3	4

Vanderbilt ADHD Diagnostic Parent Rating Scale (VADPRS) *(continued)*

21.	Actively defies or refuses to comply with adults' requests or rules	1	2	3	4
22.	Deliberately annoys people	1	2	3	4
23.	Blames others for his or her mistakes or misbehaviors	1	2	3	4
24.	Is touchy or easily annoyed by others	1	2	3	4
25.	Is angry or resentful	1	2	3	4
26.	Is spiteful and vindictive	1	2	3	4
27.	Bullies, threatens, or intimidates others	1	2	3	4
28.	Initiates physical fights	1	2	3	4
29.	Lies to obtain goods for favors or to avoid obligations ("cons" others)	1	2	3	4
30.	Is truant from school (skips school) without permission	1	2	3	4
31.	Is physically cruel to people	1	2	3	4
32.	Has stolen items of nontrivial value	1	2	3	4
33.	Deliberately destroys others' property	1	2	3	4
34.	Has used a weapon that can cause serious harm (bat, knife, brick, gun)	1	2	3	4
35.	Is physically cruel to animals	1	2	3	4
36.	Has deliberately set fires to cause damage	1	2	3	4
37.	Has broken into someone else's home, business, or car	1	2	3	4
38.	Has stayed out at night without permission	1	2	3	4
39.	Has run away from home overnight	1	2	3	4
40.	Has forced someone into sexual activity	1	2	3	4
41.	Is fearful, anxious, or worried	1	2	3	4
42.	Is afraid to try new things for fear of making mistakes	1	2	3	4
43.	Feels worthless or inferior	1	2	3	4
44.	Blames self for problems, feels guilty	1	2	3	4
45.	Feels lonely, unwanted, or unloved; complains that "no one loves" him or her	1	2	3	4
46.	Is sad, unhappy, or depressed	1	2	3	4
47.	Is self-conscious or easily embarrassed	1	2	3	4

Vanderbilt ADHD Diagnostic Parent Rating Scale (VADPRS) *(continued)*

Performance

	Problematic		Average	Above average	
Academic Performance					
1. Reading	1	2	3	4	5
2. Mathematics	1	2	3	4	5
3. Written expression	1	2	3	4	5
Classroom Behavior					
1. Relationships with peers	1	2	3	4	5
2. Following directions/rules	1	2	3	4	5
3. Disrupting class	1	2	3	4	5
4. Assignment completion	1	2	3	4	5
5. Organizational skills	1	2	3	4	5

The Vanderbilt scales were developed by Mark L. Wolraich, M.D., and colleagues at the University of Oklahoma Health Science Center in Oklahoma City. They are in the public domain.

Vanderbilt ADHD Diagnostic Teacher Rating Scale (VADTRS)

Scoring Instructions for the VADTRS

Behaviors are counted if they are scored 2 (often) or 3 (very often).

Inattentive subtype	Requires 6 or more counted behaviors from questions 1– 9.
Hyperactive/ impulsive subtype	Requires 6 or more counted behaviors from questions 10–18.
Combined subtype	Requires 6 or more counted behaviors each on both the inattention and the hyperactivity/impulsivity dimensions.
Oppositional defiant and conduct disorders	Requires 3 or more counted behaviors from questions 19–28.
Anxiety or depression	Requires 3 or more counted behaviors from questions 29–35.

The **performance section** is scored as indicating some impairment if a child scores 1 or 2 on at least 1 item.

Source Reference. Wolraich ML, Feurer I, Hannah JN, et al: "Obtaining Systematic Teacher Reports of Disruptive Behavior Disorders Utilizing DSM-IV." *Journal of Abnormal Child Psychology* 26:141–152, 1998.

Web Source. "Developmental Behavioral Tools" page of the University of Oklahoma Health Sciences Center (UOHSC) Child Study Center Consultation Services Web site (http://dbp2doc.org/online-resources/developmental-behavioral-tools).

Vanderbilt ADHD Diagnostic Teacher Rating Scale (VADTRS)

Patient Name: _____ Date of Birth:_____

Today's Date: _____ Age:_____

Grade:_____

Each rating should be considered in the context of what is appropriate for the age of the children you are rating.

Frequency Code: 0 = Never; 1 = Occasionally; 2 = Often; 3 = Very Often

1. Fails to give attention to details or makes careless mistakes in schoolwork	1	2	3	4
2. Has difficulty sustaining attention to tasks or activities	1	2	3	4
3. Does not seem to listen when spoken to directly	1	2	3	4
4. Does not follow through on instruction and fails to finish schoolwork (not due to oppositional behavior or failure to understand)	1	2	3	4
5. Has difficulty organizing tasks and activities	1	2	3	4
6. Avoids, dislikes, or is reluctant to engage in tasks that require sustained mental effort	1	2	3	4
7. Loses things necessary for tasks or activities (school assignments, pencils, or books)	1	2	3	4
8. Is easily distracted by extraneous stimuli	1	2	3	4
9. Is forgetful in daily activities	1	2	3	4
10. Fidgets with hands or feet or squirms in seat	1	2	3	4
11. Leaves seat in classroom or in other situations in which remaining seated is expected	1	2	3	4
12. Runs about or climbs excessively in situations in which remaining seated is expected	1	2	3	4
13. Has difficulty playing or engaging in leisure activities quietly	1	2	3	4
14. Is "on the go" or often acts as if "driven by a motor"	1	2	3	4
15. Talks excessively	1	2	3	4
16. Blurts out answers before questions have been completed	1	2	3	4
17. Has difficulty waiting in line	1	2	3	4
18. Interrupts or intrudes on others (e.g., butts into conversations or games)	1	2	3	4

Vanderbilt ADHD Diagnostic Teacher Rating Scale (VADTRS) *(continued)*

19. Loses temper	1	2	3	4
20. Actively defies or refuses to comply with adults' requests or rules	1	2	3	4
21. Is angry or resentful	1	2	3	4
22. Is spiteful and vindictive	1	2	3	4
23. Bullies, threatens, or intimidates others	1	2	3	4
24. Initiates physical fights	1	2	3	4
25. Lies to obtain goods for favors or to avoid obligations ("cons" others)	1	2	3	4
26. Is physically cruel to people	1	2	3	4
27. Has stolen items of nontrivial value	1	2	3	4
28. Deliberately destroys others' property	1	2	3	4
29. Is fearful, anxious, or worried	1	2	3	4
30. Is self-conscious or easily embarrassed	1	2	3	4
31. Is afraid to try new things for fear of making mistakes	1	2	3	4
32. Feels worthless or inferior	1	2	3	4
33. Blames self for problems, feels guilty	1	2	3	4
34. Feels lonely, unwanted, or unloved; complains that "no one loves" him or her	1	2	3	4
35. Is sad, unhappy, or depressed	1	2	3	4

Vanderbilt ADHD Diagnostic Teacher Rating Scale (VADTRS) *(continued)*

Performance		Problematic		Average		Above average
Academic Performance						
1. Reading		1	2	3	4	5
2. Mathematics		1	2	3	4	5
3. Written expression		1	2	3	4	5
Classroom Behavioral Performance						
1. Relationships with peers		1	2	3	4	5
2. Following directions/rules		1	2	3	4	5
3. Disrupting class		1	2	3	4	5
4. Assignment completion		1	2	3	4	5
5. Organizational skills		1	2	3	4	5

The Vanderbilt scales were developed by Mark L. Wolraich, M.D., and colleagues at the University of Oklahoma Health Science Center in Oklahoma City. They are in the public domain.

Adult ADHD Self-Report Scale—Version 1.1 (Adult ASRS-v1.1) Symptom Checklist

Instructions

The Symptom Checklist is an instrument consisting of the 18 DSM-IV-TR criteria. Six of the 18 questions were found to be the most predictive of symptoms consistent with ADHD. These 6 questions are Part A of the Symptom Checklist. Part B of the Symptom Checklist contains the remaining 12 questions.

Symptoms

1. Ask the patient to complete both Part A and Part B of the Symptom Checklist by marking an X in the box that most closely represents the frequency of occurrence of each of the symptoms.
2. Score Part A. If four or more marks appear in the darkly shaded boxes within Part A then the patient has symptoms highly consistent with ADHD in adults and further investigation is warranted.
3. The frequency scores on Part B provide additional cues and can serve as further probes into the patient's symptoms. Pay particular attention to marks appearing in the dark shaded boxes. The frequency-based response is more sensitive with certain questions. No total score or diagnostic likelihood is utilized for the 12 questions. It has been found that the 6 questions in Part A are the most predictive of the disorder and are best for use as a screening instrument.

Impairments

1. Review the entire Symptom Checklist with your patients and evaluate the level of impairment associated with the symptom.
2. Consider work/school, social and family settings.
3. Symptom frequency is often associated with symptom severity, therefore the Symptom Checklist may also aid in the assessment of impairments. If your patients have frequent symptoms, you may want to ask them to describe how these problems have affected the ability to work, take care of things at home, or get along with other people such as their spouse/significant other.

History

Assess the presence of these symptoms or similar symptoms in childhood. Adults who have ADHD need not have been formally diagnosed in childhood. In evaluating a patient's history, look for evidence of early-appearing and long-standing problems with attention or self-control. Some significant symptoms should have been present in childhood, but full symptomatology is not necessary.

Source Statement

The Adult ADHD Self-Report Scale—Version 1.1 (ASRS-V1.1) Symptom Checklist was developed in conjunction with the World Health Organization and the Workgroup on Adult ADHD (Lenard Adler, M.D.; Ronald Kessler, Ph.D.; and Thomas Spencer, M.D.). The Adult ASRS-v1.1 is downloadable from Harvard School of Medicine's National Comorbidity Survey Web site (www.hcp.med.harvard.edu/ncs/asrs.php), from which methodological data are also available.

No approval is required to use the ASRS so long as the user acknowledges in all print materials that it is copyrighted by the World Health Organization. In addition, we also request citation of the key methodological paper on these instruments as follows: Kessler RC, Adler L, Ames M, et al: "The World Health Organization Adult ADHD Self-Report Scale (ASRS): A Short Screening Scale for Use in the General Population." *Psychological Medicine* 35:245–256, 2005.

Adult ADHD Self-Report Scale (Adult ASRS-v1.1) Symptom Checklist

Patient Name: _____ Today's Date: _____

Please answer the questions below, rating yourself on each of the criteria shown using the scale on the right side of the page. As you answer each question, place an X in the box that best describes how you have felt and conducted yourself over the past 6 months. Please give this completed checklist to your health care professional to discuss during today's appointment.

	Never	Rarely	Sometimes	Often	Very often
Part A					
1. How often do you have trouble wrapping up the final details of a project, once the challenging parts have been done?					
2. How often do you have difficulty getting things in order when you have to do a task that requires organization?					
3. How often do you have problems remembering appointments or obligations?					
4. When you have a task that requires a lot of thought, how often do you avoid or delay getting started?					
5. How often do you fidget or squirm with your hands or feet when you have to sit down for a long time?					
6. How often do you feel overly active and compelled to do things, like you were driven by a motor?					

Adult ASRS-v1.1 Symptom Checklist *(continued)*

	Never	Rarely	Sometimes	Often	Very often
Part B					
7. How often do you make careless mistakes when you have to work on a boring or difficult project?					
8. How often do you have difficulty keeping your attention when you are doing boring or repetitive work?					
9. How often do you have difficulty concentrating on what people say to you, even when they are speaking to you directly?					
10. How often do you misplace or have difficulty finding things at home or at work?					
11. How often are you distracted by activity or noise around you?					
12. How often do you leave your seat in meetings or other situations in which you are expected to remain seated?					
13. How often do you feel restless or fidgety?					
14. How often do you have difficulty unwinding and relaxing when you have time to yourself?					
15. How often do you find yourself talking too much when you are in social situations?					
16. When you're in a conversation, how often do you find yourself finishing the sentences of the people you are talking to, before they can finish them themselves?					
17. How often do you have difficulty waiting your turn in situations when turn taking is required?					
18. How often do you interrupt others when they are busy?					

No approval is required to use the ASRS so long as the user acknowledges in all print materials that it is copyrighted by the World Health Organization.

Clinical Institute Withdrawal Assessment of Alcohol Scale, Revised (CIWA-Ar)

Procedure

This assessment for monitoring withdrawal symptoms requires approximately 5 minutes to administer. The maximum score is 67 (see instrument). Patients scoring less than 10 do not usually need additional medication for withdrawal.

CIWA-Ar Scoring

   0–9   = absent or minimal withdrawal (only prn medications)

 10–19 = mild to moderate withdrawal (scheduled medications + prn medications)

  ≥20   = severe withdrawal (assess hourly; maximize scheduled medications + prn medications; transfer to intensive care unit if needed)

Source Reference.   Sullivan JT, Sykora K, Schneiderman J, Naranjo CA, Sellers EM: "Assessment of Alcohol Withdrawal: The Revised Clinical Institute Withdrawal Assessment for Alcohol Scale (CIWA-Ar)." *British Journal of Addiction* 84:1353–1357, 1989.

Web Source.   U.S. Department of Veterans Affairs Center for Health Care Evaluation (CHCE) Web Site (www.chce.research.va.gov/apps/PAWS/content/downloads.htm).

Clinical Institute Withdrawal Assessment of Alcohol Scale—Revised (CIWA-Ar)

Patient:_____   Date:_____   Time:_____
VITAL SIGNS: Pulse:_____ Respiratory Rate:_____ Blood pressure:_____ Temperature:_____

NAUSEA AND VOMITING—Observation. Ask "Do you feel sick to your stomach? Have you vomited?"

0   no nausea and no vomiting
1   mild nausea with no vomiting
2
3
4   intermittent nausea with dry heaves
5
6
7   constant nausea, frequent dry heaves and vomiting

TREMOR—Observation. Arms extended and fingers spread apart.

0   no tremor
1   not visible, but can be felt fingertip to fingertip
2
3
4   moderate, with patient's arms extended
5
6
7   severe, even with arms not extended

TACTILE DISTURBANCES—Observation. Ask "Have you any itching, pins and needles sensations, any burning, any numbness, or do you feel bugs crawling on or under your skin?"

0   none
1   very mild itching, pins and needles, burning or numbness
2   mild itching, pins and needles, burning or numbness
3   moderate itching, pins and needles, burning or numbness
4   moderately severe hallucinations
5   severe hallucinations
6   extremely severe hallucinations
7   continuous hallucinations

AUDITORY DISTURBANCES— Observation. Ask "Are you more aware of sounds around you? Are they harsh? Do they frighten you? Are you hearing anything that is disturbing to you? Are you hearing things you know are not there?"

0   not present
1   very mild harshness or ability to frighten
2   mild harshness or ability to frighten
3   moderate harshness or ability to frighten
4   moderately severe hallucinations
5   severe hallucinations
6   extremely severe hallucinations
7   continuous hallucinations

VISUAL DISTURBANCES—Observation. Ask "Does the light appear to be too bright? Is its color different? Does it hurt your eyes? Are you seeing anything that is disturbing to you? Are you seeing things you know are not there?"

0   not present
1   very mild sensitivity
2   mild sensitivity
3   moderate sensitivity
4   moderately severe hallucinations
5   severe hallucinations
6   extremely severe hallucinations
7   continuous hallucinations

HEADACHE, FULLNESS IN HEAD— Rate severity. Ask "Does your head feel different? Does it feel like there is a band around your head?" Do not rate for dizziness or light-headedness.

0   not present
1   very mild
2   mild
3   moderate
4   moderately severe
5   severe
6   very severe
7   extremely severe

Clinical Institute Withdrawal Assessment of Alcohol Scale—Revised (CIWA-Ar) *(continued)*

PAROXYSMAL SWEATS—Observation.

0   no sweat visible
1   barely perceptible sweating, palms moist
2
3
4   beads of sweat obvious on forehead
5
6
7   drenching sweats

AGITATION—Observation.

0   normal activity
1   somewhat more than normal activity
2
3
4   moderately fidgety and restless
5
6
7   paces back and forth during most of the
    interview, or constantly thrashes about

ANXIETY—Observation. Ask "Do you feel nervous?"

0   no anxiety, at ease
1   mildly anxious
2
3
4   moderately anxious, or guarded, so anxiety
    is inferred
5
6
7   equivalent to acute panic states as seen in
    severe delirium or acute schizophrenic
    reactions

ORIENTATION AND CLOUDING OF SENSORIUM—Observation. Ask "What day is this? Where are you? Who am I?"

0   oriented and can do serial additions
1   cannot do serial additions or is uncertain
    about date
2   disoriented for date by no more than
    2 calendar days
3   disoriented for date by more than
    2 calendar days
4   disoriented for place/or person

Total CIWA-Ar Score _____ (Maximum Possible Score 67)
Rater's Signature _____

The CIWA-Ar is not copyrighted and may be reproduced freely.

Sleep Disorder Scales

Pittsburgh Insomnia Rating Scale (PIRS)

Overview

The PIRS is a patient-completed measure of sleep problems that comes in two versions, a 65-item questionnaire and a 20-item questionnaire. Both versions are designed to assess the severity of insomnia experienced in the past week. The 20-item questionnaire may be particularly useful for tracking the impact of clinical interventions.

Availability and Conditions of Use

The copyright on the PIRS is owned by the University of Pittsburgh, which permits use of the instrument without charge only for noncommercial research and educational purposes. The PIRS questionnaires are downloadable from the Web Source shown below, from which complete administration/scoring instructions and methodological data are also available.

Source Reference. Moul DE, Pilkonis PA, Miewald JM, Carey TJ, Buysse DJ: "Preliminary Study of the Test-Retest Reliability and Concurrent Validities of the Pittsburgh Insomnia Rating Scale (PIRS)." *Sleep* 25 (Abstract Supplement):A246–A247, 2002.

Web Source. University of Pittsburgh Sleep Medicine Institute (http://www.sleep.pitt.edu/content.asp?id=1484&subid=2317).

Epworth Sleepiness Scale (ESS)

Overview

The ESS is a self-administered questionnaire in which the respondent is asked to rate, on a 4-point scale (0–3), his or her chances of dozing off in each of 8 different situations. The summed score provides a measure of impairment from a sleep disorder in terms of daytime fatigue.

Availability and Conditions of Use

The developer and copyright holder of the ESS, Dr. Murray Johns, permits use of the ESS by individual people (including clinicians and researchers) free of charge. The ESS is downloadable from the Web Source shown below, from which complete administration/scoring instructions and methodological data are also available.

Source Reference. Johns MW: "A New Method for Measuring Daytime Sleepiness: The Epworth Sleepiness Scale." *Sleep* 14:540–545, 1991.

Web Source. Official Web site of the Epworth Sleepiness Scale by Dr. Murray Johns (http://epworthsleepinessscale.com/1997-version-ess).

PTSD Checklist—Civilian Version (PCL-C)

Overview

The PCL is a standardized self-report rating scale for posttraumatic stress disorder (PTSD) comprising 17 items that correspond to the key symptoms of PTSD. Two versions of the PCL exist: 1) PCL-M is specific to PTSD caused by military experiences and 2) PCL-C is applied generally to any traumatic event.

The PCL can be easily modified to fit specific time frames or events. For example, instead of asking about "the past month," questions may ask about "the past week" or be modified to focus on events specific to a deployment.

How is the PCL completed?

- The PCL is self-administered.
- Respondents indicate how much they have been bothered by a symptom over the past month using a 5-point (1–5) scale, circling their responses. Responses range from 1 (*Not at All*) to 5 (*Extremely*).

How is the PCL scored?

1. Add up all items for a total severity score
   or
2. Treat response categories 3–5 (*Moderately* or above) as symptomatic and responses 1–2 (below *Moderately*) as nonsymptomatic, then use the following DSM criteria for a diagnosis:
   - Symptomatic response to at least 1 "B" item (Questions 1–5),
   - Symptomatic response to at least 3 "C" items (Questions 6–12), and
   - Symptomatic response to at least 2 "D" items (Questions 13–17).

Are results valid and reliable?

- Two studies of both Vietnam and Persian Gulf theater veterans show that the PCL is both valid and reliable. Additional references are available from the Deployment Health Clinical Center (DHCC).

What additional follow-up is available?

- All military health system beneficiaries with health concerns they believe are deployment related are encouraged to seek medical care.
- Patients should be asked, "**Is your health concern today related to a deployment?**" during all primary care visits.
- If the patient replies "**yes**," the provider should follow the Post-Deployment Health Clinical Practice Guideline (PDH-CPG) and supporting guidelines available through the DHCC and www.PDHealth.mil.

Source Reference. Weathers FW, Litz BT, Herman DS, et al: "The PTSD Checklist (PCL): Reliability, Validity, and Diagnostic Utility." Paper presented at the 9th Annual Conference of the International Society for Traumatic Stress Studies, San Antonio, TX, October 24–27, 1993. The PCL-C is a Government document in the public domain.

Web Source. U.S. Department of Veterans Affairs Mental Illness Research, Education and Clinical Centers (MIRECC) Web Site (http://www.mirecc.va.gov/index.asp).

PTSD Checklist—Civilian Version (PCL-C)

Client's name: _____

Instruction to patient: Below is a list of problems and complaints that veterans sometimes have in response to stressful life experiences. Please read each one carefully, put an "X" in the box to indicate how much you have been bothered by that problem *in the last month*.

No.	Response	Not at all (1)	A little bit (2)	Moderately (3)	Quite a bit (4)	Extremely (5)
1.	Repeated, disturbing *memories, thoughts, or images* of a stressful experience from the past?					
2.	Repeated, disturbing *dreams* of a stressful experience from the past?					
3.	Suddenly *acting* or *feeling* as if a stressful experience *were happening* again (as if you were reliving it)?					
4.	Feeling *very upset* when *something reminded* you of a stressful experience from the past?					
5.	Having *physical reactions* (e.g., heart pounding, trouble breathing, or sweating) when something reminded you of a stressful experience from the past?					
6.	Avoid *thinking about* or *talking about* a stressful experience from the past or avoid *having feelings* related to it?					
7.	Avoid *activities* or *situations* because they *remind you* of a stressful experience from the past?					
8.	Trouble *remembering important parts* of a stressful experience from the past?					
9.	Loss of *interest in things that you used to enjoy?*					
10.	Feeling *distant* or *cut off* from other people?					
11.	Feeling *emotionally numb* or being unable to have loving feelings for those close to you?					
12.	Feeling as if your *future* will somehow be *cut short?*					
13.	Trouble *falling* or *staying asleep?*					
14.	Feeling *irritable* or having *angry outbursts?*					
15.	Having *difficulty concentrating?*					
16.	Being *"super alert"* or watchful on guard?					
17.	Feeling *jumpy* or easily startled?					

The PCL-C is a Government document in the public domain.

Online Resources

Nursing, Psychiatry, and Psychopharmacology

Alzheimer's Association: http://www.alz.org

American Academy of Addiction Psychiatry: http://www.aaap.org

American Academy of Child and Adolescent Psychiatry:
 http://www.aacap.org

American Association of Neuroscience Nurses: http://www.aann.org

American Psychiatric Association: http://www.psych.org

American Psychiatric Nurses Association: http://www.apna.org

Anxiety and Depression Association of America: http://www.adaa.org

Attention Deficit Disorder Association: http://www.add.org

Children and Adults With Attention Deficit/Hyperactivity Disorder:
 http://www.chadd.org

International Bipolar Foundation: http://www.internationalbipolarfoundation.org

International Society of Psychiatric-Mental Health Nurses:
 http://www.ispn-psych.org

National Autism Association: http://nationalautismassociation.org

Mental Health America:
 http://www.mentalhealthamerica.net or www.nmha.org

National Alliance on Mental Illness: http://www.nami.org

National Institute of Mental Health: http://www.nimh.nih.gov

National Institute on Alcohol Abuse and Alcoholism: http://www.niaaa.nih.gov

National Institute on Drug Abuse: http://www.drugabuse.gov

National Sleep Foundation: http://www.sleepfoundation.org

National Suicide Prevention Lifeline:
 http://www.suicidepreventionlifeline.org; 1-800-273-TALK (8255)

Substance Abuse and Mental Health Services Administration (SAMHSA):
 http://www.samhsa.gov

Other Psychopharmacology Related

Cytochrome P450 enzymes: http://medicine.iupui.edu/clinpharm/ddis/table.aspx

Pharmacogenomics related to psychiatry: http://www.genomind.com

Psychopharmacology continuing education and resources: http://www.neiglobal.com

Index

*Page numbers printed in **boldface** type refer to tables or figures.*

Abbreviated Mental Test, 280
Abilify, Abilify Discmelt.
    See Aripiprazole
Abnormal Involuntary Movement Scale
    (AIMS), 425, **443–445**
Absorption of drugs, 18.
    See also Pharmacokinetics
Abuse history, **5**
Acamprosate, for alcohol dependence,
    191–194
Acetaminophen, interaction with black
    cohosh, 368
Acetylcholine
    in Alzheimer's dementia, 280
    in attention-deficit/hyperactivity
        disorder, 164
    in delirium, 272, 279
    pathways for, **26, 27**
    receptors for, **16–17**
    in sleep regulation, 225
Acetylcholinesterase inhibitors, for
    dementia, 276, 280, 284, 287,
    288, 295
    dosing of, 288
    in Lewy body dementia, 293
    side effects of, **285**
Actaea racemosa. See Black cohosh

Acute stress disorder (ASD), 33, 237,
    264
    diagnostic criteria for, 237, **240**
    medications for, 256
Adalat. *See* Nifedipine
Adderall, Adderall XR.
    See Dextroamphetamine/
    amphetamine
Addictive process, 185.
    See also Substance use disorders
ADHD. *See* Attention-deficit/
    hyperactivity disorder
Adjustment disorder
    with anxiety, **39**
    with depressed mood, 65
α_2-Adrenergic receptor agonists, 174
    for attention-deficit/hyperactivity
        disorder, **173**
α-Adrenergic receptors, **14**
β-Adrenergic receptors, **14**
Adult ADHD Self-Report Scale (Adult
    ASRS-v1.1), 157, 425, **455–457**
Advanced practice registered nurses
    (APRNs), 2
    culturally sensitive
        psychopharmacological
        treatment by, 379–399

Advanced practice registered nurses
    (APRNs) *(continued)*
    drug prescribing by
        (See Prescribing medications)
    essential skills of, 2
    holistic approach of, 2, 18, 20, 141,
        151, 324, 346, 347, 348, 380,
        381, 392, 393, 398
    number of patient visits to, 3
    online resources for, 469–470
    provision of mental health care by,
        2–3
    psychiatric assessment by, 3–7
        components of pre-prescribing
            assessment, 3, 4–5
        diagnostic tools for, 3, 6
        rating scales for, 423–468
Aggression/violence
    in alcohol intoxication, 310
    in anxiety disorders, 309
    in children and adolescents, 321
    in dementia, 275, 285, 287
    in elderly persons, 320
    medications for, 166, 285
    in phencyclidine intoxication, 312
    in posttraumatic stress disorder, 255
    psychiatric emergencies presenting
        with, 302, 303, 312, 313, 314,
        315
    in psychotic disorders, 152–153,
        308
    risk factors for, 314
    varenicline-induced, 197
Agitation
    in alcohol intoxication, 310
    antipsychotics for, 142
    in delirium, 273, 292
    in dementia, 287
    in depression, 64

drug-induced
    benzodiazepines, 319
    bupropion, 73, 75, 198
    cocaine, 312
    monoamine oxidase inhibitors,
        253
    selective serotonin reuptake
        inhibitors, 70–71, 253
    serotonin-norepinephrine
        reuptake inhibitors, 72
    vilazodone, 71
    in manic or hypomanic episode, 87
    psychiatric emergencies presenting
        with, 301–302, 304, 308
    in psychotic disorders, 131,
        152–153
    in serotonin syndrome, 80
Agoraphobia
    diagnostic criteria for panic disorder
        with or without, 33
    without history of panic disorder,
        33
AIMS (Abnormal Involuntary
    Movement Scale), 425, 443–445
Akathisia, antipsychotic-induced, 111,
    114, 147, 282, 305
Alcohol
    drug interactions with
        carbamazepine, 120
        disulfiram, 192, 207
        duloxetine, 49
        gabapentin, 109
        lithium, 120
        valproate, 120
    fetal alcohol syndrome due to, 209
    flushing syndrome due to, 387
    intoxication with, 310
    metabolic syndrome related to
        consumption of, 337–338

sensitivity of certain cultural groups
to, 387
withdrawal from, 203, **204–205**,
205, 310–311
benzodiazepines for, **204**, 287,
311
during pregnancy, 209
rating scale for, 425, 463–465
treatment of delirium due to,
287, 311
Alcohol abuse/dependence.
See also Substance use disorders
blood alcohol level: symptoms and
effects, 200, **200–201**
deaths from, 184
in elderly persons, 210
genetic factors in, 185
incidence of, 184
medications for, **191–194**
pharmacokinetics of, 200
neurobiology of, 188
during pregnancy, 209
presenting as psychiatric emergency,
310–311
prevalence of, 310
Aldoril. *See* Methyldopa
Alogia, 131
Alopecia, valproate-induced, 105
Alprazolam, **10**
for anxiety disorders, **43**, 47, 49
dose equivalencies for
benzodiazepines, 405–406,
407
dosing of, 49
interaction with fluoxetine, 48
overdose of, 49
prescribing considerations for, 47
Alzheimer's dementia, 42, 275, **276**.
See also Dementia

differentiating depression from, 65
herbal preparations for
ginkgo, 363
ginseng root, 360
gotu kola, 369
lemon balm, 370
medications for, **276**, 281–283,
287–292, **289**
acetylcholinesterase inhibitors,
276, 284, 287, 288, **289**
antipsychotics, 285–286, 287,
290
medical food: caprylidene, 287,
290
memantine, 284, 288
side effects of, **285**
neurobiology of, 279–280
Ambien, Ambien CR. *See* Zolpidem
Amenorrhea, antipsychotic-induced,
111
American Academy of Pediatrics, 176
American Association of Colleges of
Nursing, 2
American Heart Association, 176
American Psychiatric Association,
281
*Practice Guideline for the Treatment
of Patients With Bipolar
Disorder,* 92, 93–95, 96, 97,
117
*Practice Guideline for the Treatment
of Patients With Borderline
Personality Disorder,* 320
*American Psychiatric Association
Guideline Watch,* 255, 256
α-Amino-3-hydroxy-5-methyl-4-
isoxazolepropionic acid (AMPA)
receptors, 15
in schizophrenia, 139

γ-Aminobutyric acid (GABA)
in bipolar disorders, 90
in posttraumatic stress disorder, 244
receptors for, 15
benzodiazepine actions at,
40–41, 49
in sleep regulation, 225
in substance use disorders, 189
Amitriptyline, 11
dosing of, 261
indications for
depression with pain, 77
posttraumatic stress disorder,
246, 250, 261
interaction with topiramate, 193
pharmacodynamics and
pharmacokinetics of, 250
Amok, 391
Amotivation, 60, 131
AMPA (α-amino-3-hydroxy-5-methyl-
4-isoxazolepropionic acid)
receptors, 15
in schizophrenia, 139
Amygdala, 24
in fear conditioning, 37, 242, 245
in substance abuse, 189
Anabolic steroids, 10
Anafranil. See Clomipramine
Analytical worldview, 390
Anesthetics, interaction with valerian,
359
Anger, posttraumatic, 237
Angiotensin-converting enzyme
inhibitors, interaction with
lithium, 119
Anhedonia, 64, 67, 87, 131
Ankyrin 3 gene (ANK3), 419
Antabuse. See Disulfiram

Antacids, interaction with gabapentin,
109
Antibiotics, drug interactions with
buprenorphine, 195
carbamazepine, 106
Anticholinergic effects of drugs
antipsychotics, 111, 149, 290
in elderly persons, 51
meperidine, 292
mirtazapine, 74
monoamine oxidase inhibitors, 253
paroxetine, 42, 70
trazodone, 74
tricyclic antidepressants, 253
venlafaxine, 72
Anticoagulants
disulfiram interaction with, 193
herb interactions with
chamomile, 226
ginkgo, 364
passionflower, 367
Anticonvulsants. See also specific drugs
carbamazepine, 105–107
gabapentin, 109–110
indications for
bipolar disorder, 98–99,
104–110, 122, 123
acute mania, 91–93
in children and adolescents,
118
depressive episode, 93–95
maintenance treatment, 97
mixed states, 96
rapid cycling, 96
dementia, 285, 291
parasomnias, 232
posttraumatic stress disorder,
255

lamotrigine, 108–109, **109**
metabolic effects of, **344–345**
oxcarbazepine, 107
passionflower interaction with, 366
during pregnancy and breast-feeding,
    105, 107, 109, 110, 120–121
topiramate, 110
valproate, 104–105
Antidepressants, 68–78, **70–74**.
    See also specific drugs and classes
activation of bipolar disorder by, 95
augmentation of, 18
    lithium, 76, 83
    L-methylfolate, 8, 77–78, 83
    psychostimulants, 178
    second-generation
        antipsychotics, 76
bupropion, 75
for children, adolescents, and young
    adults, 50, 78, 79
informed consent for, 53, 79
delirium induced by, 273
dose equivalencies for, 406, **407**
drug interactions with, 40, 41, 81
    carbamazepine, 106
    cytochrome P450–related, 81,
        82
for elderly persons, 79
FDA warnings for, 41, 78, 79,
    258–259
indications for
    autism symptoms, 165, **166**
    in bipolar depression, 85, 91,
        93, 94–95, 97
    dementia, 277, 287, 290–291
    depressive disorders, 68–78,
        70–74
    in dementia, 284

mania precipitated by, 76, 80–81,
    83, 85, 94, 95
for medically compromised patients,
    79
metabolic effects of, **343–344**
mirtazapine, 75
monitoring treatment with, 53,
    80–81
monoamine oxidase inhibitors, 77
off-label use of, 69, 78, **166**
overdose of, 68
during pregnancy, 41, **46**, 52–53,
    67, 79
selective serotonin reuptake
    inhibitors, 67, 68–69
serotonin-norepinephrine reuptake
    inhibitors, 69, 75
serotonin syndrome and, 41, 48, 76,
    80, **254**
suicidality and, **11**, 41, **46**, 53, 69,
    75, 78, 208, 258–259
    in children and young adults,
        50, 53, 78, 79, 258–259
    in elderly persons, 51
switching between, 83, 406, **407**
time to efficacy of, 82
trazodone, 75
vilazodone, 69
for women, 79
Antidepressants, tricyclic (TCAs), 76–77.
    See also specific drugs
cytochrome P450 enzyme
    inhibition by, **82**
dosing of, **261**
drug interactions with, **253**
    disulfiram, **193**, 200
    methadone, **195**, 203
    paroxetine, **45**

Antidepressants, tricyclic (TCAs)
   (continued)
   indications for
      depressive disorders, 77
      parasomnias, 232
      posttraumatic stress disorder, 247,
         250–254, 257, 258, **261**
   interaction with passionflower, 366
   overdose of, 77, **254**, 258
   pharmacodynamics and
      pharmacokinetics of, **250–252**
   side effects of, 232, **253–254**, 258,
      344
   suicidality and, **11**
Antihistamines
   drug interactions with
      gabapentin, 109
      tricyclic antidepressants, **253**
   for insomnia, 226, 233
Antihypertensive agents, drug
      interactions with
   aripiprazole, 114
   olanzapine, 113
   quetiapine, 115
   risperidone, 113
   trazodone, 230
   tricyclic antidepressants, **253**
Antiparkinsonian agents, 111, 316
   interaction with tricyclic
      antidepressants, **253**
Antipsychotics, 141–149
   black box warnings for, **11**, 76, 111,
      112, 119, 150, 281, 286, 290,
      318, 333
   drug interactions with
      carbamazepine, 106, 143
      selective serotonin reuptake
         inhibitors, **253**
      tricyclic antidepressants, **253**

mechanism of action of, 111, 138,
   141, 281
patient education about, 152
pharmacokinetics and
   pharmacodynamics of,
   143–146, **144–146**, 281
prescribing considerations for,
   141–143
in psychiatric emergencies, 308,
   313, 315–316, **318**, 327
for psychotic disorders, 141–149
side effects of, 146–149, **318**
   anticholinergic effects, 149
   exacerbation of negative
      symptoms, 148–149
   extrapyramidal symptoms, 111,
      147, 282, 285–286
   hyperprolactinemia, 148
   metabolic effects, **342–343**
   neuroleptic malignant
      syndrome, 147
   sedation, 149
Antipsychotics: first-generation
   (FGAs), 111, 141.
   See also specific drugs
   for children and adolescents, 151,
      292, 322
   choice of, 141
   cost of, 111
   dose equivalencies for, **408**
   for elderly persons, 321
   indications for
      autism symptoms, **166**
      bipolar disorder, 92–93, **100**,
         110–111, 123
      delirium, 281–282, **282**, 286
         in children and adolescents,
            292
      dementia, 285–286, 287

psychiatric emergencies, 308,
315–316, **318**, 327
interaction with methadone, **195**
mechanism of action of, 111, 138,
141, 281
off-label uses of, **142, 166**
pharmacokinetics of, 111, **144–145**
during pregnancy and breast-
feeding, 111, 121, 149, 323
side effects of, 111, **318**, **342–343**
suicidality and, **11**
Antipsychotics: second-generation
(SGAs), 112–116, 141.
See also specific drugs
advantages of, 112, 122
aripiprazole, 114
for children and adolescents, 114,
117, 118, 150–151, 322
choice of, 141
cost of, 316
dose equivalencies for, **408–409**
dosing of, **100–101**, 285–286
indications for
antidepressant augmentation, 76
autism symptoms, **166**
bipolar disorder, 85, **100–101**,
112–116, 122, 123–124
acute mania, 92–93
in children and adolescents,
117, 118
depressive episode, 94, 95
maintenance treatment, 97
mixed states, 96
rapid cycling, 96
delirium, 281, **282**, 282–283,
286–287
dementia, 286, 287
personality disorders, 320
posttraumatic stress disorder, 255

psychiatric emergencies, 308,
315–316, **318**, 320
mechanism of action of, 141
off-label uses of, **142, 166**
olanzapine, 112–113
pharmacokinetics of, **145–146**
during pregnancy and breast-
feeding, 112, 121, 149, 323
quetiapine, 114–115
risperidone, 113
side effects of, 76, 112, 118, 122,
282, 283, **318**
in elderly dementia patients, 76,
112, 119, 150, 281, 286,
321, 333
extrapyramidal symptoms, 76,
113, 115, **282**, 290
metabolic syndrome, 76, 112,
113, 148, 333, **342**
sedation, 113, 114, 115, 122,
123, **282**, 283, 290
weight gain and metabolic
effects, 76, 92, 112, 113,
114, 115, 118, 148
suicidality and, **11**
ziprasidone, 115
Anxiety
causes of, 54–55
definition of, 31
in delirium tremens, 311
dementia and, 42, 287
drug-induced
bupropion, 75, **198**
gabapentin, 109
lamotrigine, 108
naltrexone, **191**
topiramate, 110
varenicline, **197**
herb-induced, 54–55

Anxiety *(continued)*
  herbal preparations for, 356–357
    ginkgo, 363
    gotu kola, 369
    kava, 362
    passionflower, 366
    schisandra, 365
    valerian, 359
  neurobiology of fear and, 37, 39, 40
  posttraumatic, 237
  presenting as psychiatric emergency, 309–310
Anxiety disorders, 31–55. *See also specific anxiety disorders*
  challenges in treatment of, 54
  classification of, 33
  clinical pearls related to, 54–55
  diagnostic criteria for, 33–39
    anxiety disorder due to general medical condition, 39
    generalized anxiety disorder, 38
    obsessive-compulsive disorder, 36–37
    panic disorder with or without agoraphobia, 33
    posttraumatic stress disorder, 238–239
    social phobia, 35
    specific phobia, 34
  due to general medical condition, 33, 39
  epidemiology of, 31, 32
  medications for, 40–50, 43–47
    antipsychotics, 142
    benzodiazepines, 49–50
    buspirone, 48
    choice of, 54
    diagnostic evaluation for, 54
    dose equivalencies for, 407
    dosing of, 42, 44–45
    duration of use of, 54
    FDA-approved indications and warnings for, 42, 43
    informed consent for, 42, 50, 54
    monitoring treatment with, 53–54
    off-label use of, 42, 50
    pharmacodynamics and pharmacokinetics of, 40–41
    prescribing considerations for, 46–47
    safety and precautions for use of, 41
    selective serotonin reuptake inhibitors, 42, 47–48
    serotonin-norepinephrine reuptake inhibitors, 48–49
    side effects of, 44–45, 53
      delirium, 273
  not otherwise specified, 33, 43
  overview of, 32–33
  prevalence of, 31, 32, 54
  rating scales for, 424, 427–432
  risk factors for, 55
  substance abuse and, 211
  substance-induced, 33
  symptoms of, 32
  treatment in special populations, 50–53
    cardiovascular impairment, 52
    children and adolescents, 50
    elderly persons, 51
    hepatic impairment, 52
    pregnant women, 52–53
    renal impairment, 52
Apathy, psychostimulants for, 177–178
Aplenzin. *See* Bupropion hydrobromide

Appetite
    assessment of, 4
    regulation of, 335–336
APRNs (advanced practice registered
    nurses), 2
Aricept. *See* Donepezil
Aripiprazole, 11, 114
    for children and adolescents, 114,
        151
    dose equivalencies for second-
        generation antipsychotics, 408
    dosing of, 101
    drug interactions with, 114
        fluoxetine, 114, 143, 146
    indications for
        antidepressant augmentation, 76
        autism symptoms, 151, 166
        bipolar disorder, 101, 112, 114,
            124
        acute mania, 92
        in children and adolescents,
            118
        depressive episodes, 95
        maintenance treatment, 97
        rapid cycling, 96
    mechanism of action of, 114
    off-label uses of, 142, 166
    pharmacokinetics of, 114, 143, 145
    side effects of, 114, 342
Armodafinil
    for attention-deficit/hyperactivity
        disorder, 175
    for hypersomnia, 231
ASD. *See* Acute stress disorder
Asenapine, 11, 115–116
    for bipolar disorder, 92–93, 101,
        112, 115–116
    dose equivalencies for second-
        generation antipsychotics, 409

    dosing of, 101, 116
    pharmacokinetics of, 115–116, 145
    side effects of, 342
Asperger's disorder, 163
Assessment
    culturally competent, 388, 389,
        393–394, 395–398
    before prescribing medications, 3–7
        history taking, 4–5
        laboratory evaluation, 6
        mental status examination, 5
    in psychiatric emergencies, 303,
        304–306
    psychiatric rating scales for,
        423–468
Ataque de nervios, 391
Ataxia, 15
    drug-induced
        benzodiazepines, 227, 228, 232,
            319
        carbamazepine, 107
        chlorpromazine, 318
        disulfiram, 191
        gabapentin, 109, 232
        lamotrigine, 108
        lithium, 103
        olanzapine, 318
        oxcarbazepine, 107
        topiramate, 110, 232
        valproate, 105
        zaleplon, 229
        zolpidem, 229
        passionflower-induced, 366
    in serotonin syndrome, 80
Ativan. *See* Lorazepam
Atomoxetine, 11, 12, 174
    for attention-deficit/hyperactivity
        disorder, 172
    for autism symptoms, 166

Atorvastatin, interaction with black
    cohosh, 368
Attention-deficit/hyperactivity disorder
    (ADHD), 155–157
    in adults, 156, 157
    areas of impairment related to, 156,
        158
    bipolar disorder and, 117, 120
    diagnostic criteria for, 160–161
    medications for, 165, 167–173,
        174–175, 178–179
    bupropion, 174–175
    clinical pearls related to,
        179–180
    combination of, 180
    dose equivalencies for, 408
    dosing of, 167–173, 175, 179
    duration of treatment with, 180
    modafinil, 175
    monitoring treatment with,
        175–176
    psychostimulants, 165, 174,
        178–179
    for autism with ADHD-like
        symptoms, 177
    during pregnancy, 178
    neurobiology of, 159, 164
    nomenclature for, 155
    psychiatric emergencies in, 321
    rating scales for, 425, 451–461
    symptoms of, 156, 157, 159, 179
Augmentation strategies, 18.
    See also specific drugs and classes
Autistic spectrum disorders, 158–159
    classification of, 158
    diagnostic criteria for
        Asperger's disorder, 163
        autistic disorder, 162
    management of, 159

medications to treat symptoms of,
    165, 166, 179, 180
    dosing of, 165, 166, 175
    monitoring treatment with,
        176–177
    in patients with ADHD-like
        symptoms, 177
    in specific patient groups, 177
    neurobiology of, 164–165
    neuroimaging in, 164
    prevalence of, 158
    symptoms of, 159
Axona. See Caprylidene

"Baby blues," 66
BAL (blood alcohol level), 200,
    200–201
Barbiturates, herb interactions with
    passionflower, 366
    valerian, 359
Bariatric surgery, 335
Basal ganglia, 24
Batten disease, 293
Behavioral assessment, 5
Behavioral Risk Factor Surveillance
    System (BRFSS), 60
Benadryl. See Diphenhydramine
Benzodiazepines, 49–50, 227.
    See also specific drugs
    abuse/dependence on, 41, 47, 49,
        53, 227
    as controlled substances, 9, 10
    dose equivalencies for, 405–406,
        407, 409
    drug interactions with, 41
        buprenorphine, 195
        carbamazepine, 106
        fluoxetine, 48
        methadone, 195

other central nervous system
depressants, 227
duration of use of, 41
for elderly persons, 116, 227, 321
flumazenil for reversal of, 311, 323
herb interactions with
kava, 362
passionflower, 366
indications for
alcohol withdrawal, **204**, 287,
311
anxiety disorders, 41, **43**, **47**, 49
in elderly persons, 51
fluoxetine augmentation of,
48
posttraumatic stress disorder,
255
bipolar disorder, 92, 93, 116
delirium, **282**, 287, 294
terminal, 293
insomnia, 227, **228**
neuroleptic malignant
syndrome, 147
parasomnias, 232
psychiatric emergencies,
309–310, 316, **319**
serotonin syndrome, 80
intoxication with, 311
monitoring treatment with, 53
pharmacodynamics and
pharmacokinetics of, 40–41,
47
during pregnancy and breast-
feeding, 53, 121, 227, 323
prescribing considerations for, 47
safety and precautions for use of, 41,
53, 116
side effects of, 41, 47, 53, 227, 232,
319

use in hepatic impairment, 52
withdrawal from, 41, 50, 203, 205,
204–205, 227, 287, 311
in neonate, 121
rebound insomnia and, 227
treatment of delirium due to,
287
Benztropine, 111, 316
Bioequivalent drug products, 7–8
Bipolar disorders, 85–124
age at onset of, 88, 119
bipolar I disorder, 86, 88
bipolar II disorder, 86, 88
in children and adolescents,
117–118
clinical pearls related to, 122–124
comorbidity with, 89, 121
course of, 86, 88
cyclothymic disorder, 86, 88–89
in elderly persons, 118–119
etiologies of, 91
functional impairment due to, 86,
87, 88
gender issues in, 121–122
genetic factors in, 89–90
inaccurate or delayed diagnosis of,
89
medications for, 85, 91, 97–117,
98–101
(*See also* Mood stabilizers)
anticonvulsants, 91, 104–110
carbamazepine, 105–107
gabapentin, 109–110
lamotrigine, 108–109, **109**
oxcarbazepine, 107
topiramate, 110
valproate, 104–105
antidepressants, 85, 91, 93,
94–95

Bipolar disorders,
  medications for *(continued)*
    antipsychotics
      first-generation, 91,
        110–111, **142**
      second-generation, 85, 91,
        112–116, **142**
    benzodiazepines, 91, 116
    calcium channel blockers, 116
    choice of, 91, 122
    dosing of, **98–101**
    lithium, 76, 85, 91, 102–103
    omega-3 fatty acids, 116–117
  metabolic syndrome and, 332
  neurobiology of, 89–91
  not otherwise specified, 86, 89
  overview of, 86–89
    depressive episode, 87–88
    hypomanic episode, 86–87
    manic episode, 86–87
    mixed episode, 88
  postpartum, 121
  prevalence of, 88
  with rapid cycling, 88, 96
  severity of, 88
  substance abuse and, 211
  suicidality and, 88
  treatment of, 91–97
    for acute mania, 91–93
    for depression, 93–95
    maintenance treatment, 97
    for mixed states, 95–96
    practice guidelines for, 92,
      93–95, 96, 97, 117
    psychotherapy, 91
    for rapid cycling, 96
    in special populations, 117–121
      children and adolescents,
        117–118

  elderly persons, 118–119
  medically compromised
    patients, 119–120
  pregnant or breast-feeding
    women, 120–121
Bipolar spectrum disorders, 85, 89, 95
Birth/developmental history, 4
  psychotic disorders and, 133,
    136–137
Black box warnings, 9, **11–12**
  for antidepressants, 41, 78, 79, 208
  for antipsychotics, 76, 111, 112,
    119, 150, 281, 286, 290, **318**,
    333
  for psychostimulants, **11–12**,
    167–171
  for varenicline, 208
Black cohosh (*Actaea racemosa;*
    Cimicifuga racemosa), **357**,
    367–368, 371
  adverse effects of, 368
  description of, 367
  efficacy of, 367–368
  herbal and drug interactions with,
    368
  mechanism of action of, 367
Blacking out, **391**
Bleeding, herb-induced
  black cohosh, 368
  ginkgo, 364
  St. John's wort, 358
Blood alcohol level (BAL), 200,
    200–201
Blood pressure changes
  drug-induced, **342–345**
    antidepressants, **343–344**
    antipsychotics, 111, 113, 115,
      121, 283, **318**, **342–343**
    benzodiazepines, **282**

buprenorphine, 195
carbamazepine, 107
clonidine, 173
clozapine, 12
disulfiram, 191
guanfacine, 173
methadone, 195
monoamine oxidase inhibitors,
    77, 247, **253, 254**, 258
mood stabilizers, **344–345**
oxcarbazepine, 107
prazosin, 232
psychostimulants, 230
tricyclic antidepressants, **253**
venlafaxine, **46, 48**, 258
ginseng-induced, 361
Body mass index (BMI), 334, 337, 338
Borderline personality disorder, 89,
    320
Brain. *See also* Neurobiology;
    Neuroimaging; Neurotransmitters;
    specific brain structures
"decade of the brain," 12, 184
neurotransmitters in, 12, **13–17**,
    26–27
reward circuit of, **26, 27**, 139, 146,
    185, 186, 188–189
structures and functions of, 12,
    24–25
Brain fog, **391**
Breast-feeding
medications and, 20, 263
    antipsychotics, 115, 121, 149,
        323
    benzodiazepines, 227, 323
    carbamazepine, 107, 121
    chlorpromazine, 111
    lamotrigine, 109, 121
    lithium, 103, 121

monoamine oxidase inhibitors,
    252
in psychiatric emergencies, 323
psychostimulants, 178
selective serotonin reuptake
    inhibitors, **252**
tricyclic antidepressants, 230,
    252
valproate, 105, 121
St. John's wort and, 358
Breathing-related sleep disorder, 222
BRFSS (Behavioral Risk Factor
    Surveillance System), 60
Brief psychotic disorder, 130, **131**,
    136
Brofaromine, for posttraumatic stress
    disorder, 246
Budeprion SR, Budeprion XL.
    See Bupropion
Buprenex. *See* Buprenorphine
Buprenorphine, for opioid dependence,
    195–196, 208, 211
Buprenorphine-naloxone, for opioid
    dependence, **195–196**, 208
Bupropion, **11**, 75
cytochrome P450 enzyme
    inhibition by, **82**, 174–175,
    198, 203
dosing of, **73**, 174, **199**
drug interactions with, **197**, 203
indications for
    antidepressant augmentation in
        posttraumatic stress
        disorder, **260–261**
    attention-deficit/hyperactivity
        disorder, 174–175
    autism symptoms, **166**
    bipolar depression, 95, 97
    depressive disorders, 67, **73**, 75

Bupropion,
    indications for *(continued)*
        nicotine dependence, 78,
            197–199
        selective serotonin reuptake
            inhibitor–induced sexual
            dysfunction, 42, 75
    mechanism of action of, 174, **197**
    during pregnancy, **197**, 208, 209
    side effects of, **73**, 75, 78, **197**, **198**,
        343
    suicidality and, 78, 208
Bupropion hydrobromide, 11, **73**, 75
BuSpar. *See* Buspirone
Buspirone
    dosing of, 44, 292
    drug interactions with, 48
    indications for
        anxiety disorders, **43**, **44**, **47**, 48
            in elderly persons, 51
        autism symptoms, **166**
        dementia, 292
    prescribing considerations for, 47
    side effects of, 44, 292
    use in medically compromised
        patients, 52, 292

CACNA1C gene, **418–419**
Caffeine
    for hypersomnia, 231
    insomnia due to, 233
    interaction with disulfiram, **193**,
        200
Calan. *See* Verapamil
Calcium channel blockers
    for bipolar disorder, 116
    interaction with carbamazepine,
        106
Campral. *See* Acamprosate

Caprylidene, for dementia, 287, 290
Carbamazepine, 105–107
    dosing of, **99**, 106, 291
    drug interactions with, 105, 106
        alcohol, 120
        antipsychotics, 106, 143
            aripiprazole, 114
            olanzapine, 113
            risperidone, 113
        bupropion, **198**, 203
        lamotrigine, 106, 108, **109**
        oral contraceptives, 120
        selective serotonin reuptake
            inhibitors, **253**
    indications for
        bipolar disorder, **99**, 105–107
            acute mania, 92–93
            in children and adolescents,
                118
            depressive episode, 94
            maintenance treatment, 97
            mixed states, 96
        dementia, 285, 291
        posttraumatic stress disorder,
            255
    interaction with black cohosh,
        368
    laboratory evaluation for use of,
        106, 291
    mechanism of action of, 106
    monitoring serum levels of, 106
    overdose of, 107
    pharmacokinetics of, 106
    during pregnancy and breast-
        feeding, 107, 120, 121
    side effects of, **12**, 106–107
Cardiovascular effects
    of drugs
        carbamazepine, 107

cocaine, 312
haloperidol, **282**, 290
lamotrigine, 108
lithium, 103, **282**
methadone, **195**
monoamine oxidase inhibitors,
    77, 247, **253**, **254**
psychostimulants, 176
second-generation
    antipsychotics, 113, 115,
    148, **282**
tricyclic antidepressants, 232,
    253, 258
of passionflower, 366
in serotonin syndrome, 80
Cardiovascular impairment
buspirone in, 52
metabolic syndrome as risk factor
    for, 332, 334
monoamine oxidase inhibitors in,
    252
psychostimulants in, 230
selective serotonin reuptake
    inhibitors in, 52
tricyclic antidepressants in, **252**
venlafaxine in, 258
ziprasidone in, 115
Cardizem. *See* Diltiazem
Carisoprodol, **10**
Cataplexy, 222
Catapres. *See* Clonidine
Catatonia, 131
Catechol O-methyltransferase gene
    (*COMT*), 185, **420**
CBT.
    See Cognitive-behavioral therapy
Centella asiatica. See Gotu kola
Centers for Disease Control and
    Prevention (CDC), 59, 60

Central nervous system (CNS)
    depressants
drug interactions with
    benzodiazepines, 227
    gabapentin, 109
    nonbenzodiazepine hypnotics,
        227
herb interactions with
    lemon balm, 370
    passionflower, 366
    valerian, 359
Central nervous system (CNS) effects
    of drugs. *See also* Cognitive effects
    of drugs; Dizziness; Headache;
    Sedation; Seizures; Tremor
bupropion, 75
buspirone, 44
selective serotonin reuptake
    inhibitors, 44
serotonin-norepinephrine reuptake
    inhibitors, 45
Cerebrovascular disease, disulfiram in,
    192
CerefolinNAC, 8
Chamomile
drug interactions with, 109, 226
for insomnia, 225–226
Chantix. *See* Varenicline
Chief complaint, 4
Childhood disintegrative disorder,
    158
Children and adolescents
anxiety disorders in, 50
    posttraumatic stress disorder,
        259, 263
bipolar disorder in, 117–118
delirium in, 292
dementia in, 293
depression in, 64, 79

Children and adolescents *(continued)*
neurodevelopmental disorders in,
155–180, 321
attention-deficit/hyperactivity
disorder, 155–157, **157**,
158, 160–161
autistic spectrum disorders,
158–159, **162–163**
medications for, 165–179,
166–173
neurobiology of, 159, 164–165
obesity in, 332
prescribing psychotropics for, 19
antianxiety medications, 50
anticonvulsants, 118
antidepressants, 50, 78, 79
suicide risk and, 50, 53, 78,
79, 258–259
antipsychotics
first-generation, 151, 292,
322
second-generation, 114, 117,
118, 150–151, 322
lithium, 103, 117–118
off-label uses, 19
psychiatric emergencies in,
321–322
sleep needs of, **217**
substance abuse in, 210
Chlordiazepoxide
for delirium, **282**
for delirium tremens, 311
dose equivalencies for
benzodiazepines, **407**
monitoring treatment with, 323
during pregnancy, 121, 323
Chlorpromazine, **11**
for children and adolescents, 151,
292, 322

dose equivalencies for first-
generation antipsychotics, **408**
dosing of, **100, 318**
in elderly persons, 111
indications for
acute mania, 92, **100,** 110, 123
autism symptoms, **166**
psychiatric emergencies, 308,
315, **318**
off-label uses of, 142, **166**
pharmacokinetics of, **144**
during pregnancy and breast-
feeding, 111, 149, 323
side effects of, **342**
Cimetidine, drug interactions with
bupropion, **198**
carbamazepine, 106
Cimicifuga racemosa.
See Black cohosh
Cingulate gyrus, **24**
Circadian rhythm sleep disorder, 222
Cisplatin, interaction with black
cohosh, 368
Citalopram, **11**
cytochrome P450 enzyme
inhibition by, **82**
dose equivalencies for selective
serotonin reuptake inhibitors,
407
dosing of, **70, 260,** 291
indications for
dementia, 287, 291
depressive disorders, 69, **70**
posttraumatic stress disorder,
246, **248, 260**
off-label use of, 69
pharmacodynamics and
pharmacokinetics of, 40, **248**
side effects of, **70,** 291, **343**

CIWA-Ar (Clinical Institute
Withdrawal Assessment of
Alcohol Scale, Revised), **204**, 405,
425, **459–461**
Clinical Antipsychotic Trials of
Intervention Effectiveness, 141
Clinical Institute Withdrawal
Assessment of Alcohol Scale,
Revised (CIWA-Ar), **204**, 205,
425, **459–461**
Clinical pearls, 20
for anxiety disorders, 54–55
for attention-deficit/hyperactivity
disorder and autism treatment,
179–180
for bipolar disorders, 122–124
for culturally sensitive
psychopharmacology, 399
for depressive disorders, 82–83
for herbal preparations, 371
for metabolic syndrome, 348
for neurocognitive disorders,
294–295
for psychiatric emergencies, 327
for psychotic disorders, 152–153
for sleep-wake disorders, 233–234
for substance use disorders, 212
for traumatic stress disorders, 265
Clomipramine, **11**
for autism symptoms, **166**
for obsessive-compulsive disorder,
77
for parasomnias, 232
Clonazepam
dose equivalencies for
benzodiazepines, **407**
dosing of, 49
indications for
acute mania, 93, 116

anxiety disorders, 47, 49
delirium, **282**
parasomnias, 232
passionflower interaction with, 366
prescribing considerations for, 47
Clonidine
for attention-deficit/hyperactivity
disorder, **173**
mechanism of action of, 174
for opiate withdrawal, **206**, 312
passionflower and, 366
Clorazepate, **407**
Clozapine, **11**, 283
for bipolar disorder, 95, 96
pharmacokinetics of, **145**
during pregnancy, 149
side effects of, **12**, 112, **342**
Clozaril. *See* Clozapine
CNS. *See* Central nervous system
Cocaine, **10**, 138, 185, 211, 310, 312
Codeine, **10**
Cogentin. *See* Benztropine
Cognex. *See* Tacrine
Cognitive assessment, **5**, 280
Cognitive-behavioral therapy (CBT)
for anxiety disorders in elderly
persons, 51
for posttraumatic stress disorder,
245–246, 263, 265
for stress management, 346
Cognitive effects of drugs
antipsychotics, 149
benzodiazepines, 227, **228**, 232,
319
carbamazepine, 107
clonazepam, 47
eszopiclone, **228**
lamotrigine, 108
lithium, 103

Cognitive effects of drugs *(continued)*
  paroxetine, 42
  topiramate, **191**
  zaleplon, **229**
  zolpidem, **229**
Cognitive impairment.
  See Neurocognitive disorders
Cognitive processing therapy, for
  posttraumatic stress disorder,
  265
Communication patterns, cultural,
  389–392
Community worldview, 392
Complementary and alternative
  therapies, 353–354
  for anxiety disorders in elderly
    persons, 51
  definition of, 354
  for depressive disorders, 77–78
  herbal preparations, 225–226,
    354–371, **356–357**
  prevalence of use of, 353
  types of, 51, 354
Computed tomography, **6**, 305
COMT gene, 185, **420**
Concerta. *See* Methylphenidate
Conduct disorder, 321
Confusion Assessment Method, 280
Confusion Rating Scale, 280
Consent for treatment
  of medications
    antidepressants in children and
      young adults, 53, 79
    in anxiety disorders, 42, 50, 54
    off-label use, 42, 50
    in psychiatric emergencies, 303
Consonar. *See* Brofaromine
Consortium to Establish a Registry for
  Alzheimer's Disease, 280

Constipation
  drug-induced
    antipsychotics, 111, 113, 115,
      149
    buprenorphine, **195**
    buprenorphine-naloxone, **195**
    buspirone, 292
    citalopram, 291
    duloxetine, 291
    gabapentin, 109
    lamotrigine, 108
    memantine, **285**
    methadone, **195**
    tricyclic antidepressants, 232,
      253
    valproate, 105
    varenicline, **198**
  herb-induced
    ginkgo, 364
    ginseng root, 361
    St. John's wort, 358
Controlled substances, 9, **10**
Cough preparations, **10**, 80, **194**
CPT (Current Procedural
  Terminology) coding, 347
Criminalization of the mentally ill,
  316
Crisis, psychiatric, 301, 303, 324.
  See also Psychiatric emergencies
Culturally sensitive
  psychopharmacology, 379–399
  clinical pearls related to, 399
  cultural language and
    communication patterns,
    389–392
  cultural language and concepts
    about illness and disease,
    390, **391**
  worldviews, 390, 392

culturally competent psychiatric
    assessment, 388, **389**,
    393–394, **395–398**
culturally competent therapeutic
    relationship, 387–388, **389**
drug metabolism and the
    cytochrome P450 system,
    385–386
factors guiding medication choice,
    384–385
genetic factors affecting
    pharmacodynamics and
    pharmacokinetics, 384
health care disparities, 379–380, 381
role of culture in relation to mental
    health, wellness, and illness,
    380–381
vs. stereotyping, 386–387
terminology related to, 382–385
    cultural competence, 382
    epigenetics, 384
    ethnic pharmacology, 384
    genetic polymorphisms, 383,
        384, 385
    genome, 384
    genotype, 383
    race and ethnicity, 382–383
Current Procedural Terminology
    (CPT) coding, 347
Cyclooxygenase-2 inhibitors,
    interaction with lithium, 119
Cyclothymic disorder, 86, 88–89
Cymbalta. *See* Duloxetine
Cyproheptadine, for serotonin
    syndrome, 80
Cytochrome P450 (CYP) enzyme
    system, 385–386, 411, **412–415**
    drug interactions related to, 40, 81,
        143

drug metabolism by, 385–386
    racial/ethnic differences in,
        387
    genetic polymorphisms of, 386,
        420–421
    herbal preparations and, 386
        black cohosh, 368
        ginkgo, 364
        ginseng root, 361
        gotu kola, 369
        kava, 362
        schisandra, 365
        St. John's wort, 355
    inducers of, **415**
    inhibitors of, **414**
    medications and, 385–386, 387
        antidepressants, 40, 81, **82**,
            174–175, **198**, 203,
            248–249, 386
        antipsychotics, 113, 114, 115,
            116, 143, **144–146**, 386
        armodafinil, 175
        atomoxetine, **172**, 174
        buprenorphine, **196**, 203
        carbamazepine, 106
        clonidine, **173**
        disulfiram, **193**, 200
        eszopiclone, **228**
        guanfacine, **173**, 174
        methadone, **196**, 203
        modafinil, 175
        psychostimulants, **167–169**,
            171, 174
        ramelteon, 226
        topiramate, **193**
        triazolam, **228**
        valproate, 104
        zaleplon, **229**
    substrates of, **412–413**

Dalmane. *See* Flurazepam
Daytrana Patch. *See* Methylphenidate,
    transdermal
DBH (dopamine-β-hydroxylase), 185
DEA. *See* U.S. Drug Enforcement
    Administration
"Decade of the brain," 12, 184
Deinstitutionalization, 302
Delirium, 272–274
    alcohol withdrawal, 287, 311
    clinical assessment of, 280
    clinical pearls related to, 294
    diagnostic criteria for, 320–321
    differential diagnosis of, 305, **307**
    drug-induced, 273
    in elderly persons, 272, 273, 321
    health care costs related to, 274
    life-threatening presentations of,
        278
    medications for, 281–283
        antipsychotics, **142**, 281–283,
            282, 286–287
        benzodiazepines, **282**, 287
        in children and adolescents, 292
        dosing of, 286–287
        in medically compromised
            patients, 292–293
        mood stabilizers, **282**
        side effects of, **282**
    neurobiology of, 272, 278–279
    nonpharmacological interventions
        for, 293–294, 321
    postoperative, 273, 279
    presenting as psychiatric emergency,
        305
    prevalence in hospitalized patients,
        273
    psychomotor subtypes of, 273
    risk factors for, 273, **274**

screening for, 280
symptoms of, 272
    persistent, 273, 286
    terminal, 292–293
Delirium Rating Scale, 280
Delirium Symptom Interview, 280
Delirium tremens, 310–311
Delusional disorder, 130–131, **131**,
    135
Delusions, 131, 152
    in delirium, 292
    in dementia, 287, 293
Dementia, 274–278
    age-related prevalence of, 274
    Alzheimer's, 275, **276**
        (*See also* Alzheimer's dementia)
    causes of, 275
    in children, 293
    clinical assessment of, 280
    clinical pearls related to, 294–295
    course of, 274
    diagnosis of, 278
    differentiation from delirium, **307**
    in elderly persons, 274, 275, **276**,
        293, 320
    frontotemporal, **276**
    herbal preparations for
        ginkgo, 363
        ginseng root, 360
        gotu kola, 369
        lemon balm, 370
    HIV, 277
    Huntington's, **277**
    incidence of, 274
    Lewy body, 275, **276**, 293
    medical food for: caprylidene, 287,
        290
    in medically compromised patients,
        293

medications for, 276–277, 284–286
  acetylcholinesterase inhibitors,
      276, 280, 284, **285**,
      287–288, **289**
  anticonvulsant mood stabilizers,
      285, 291
  antidepressants, 284, 290–291
  antipsychotics, **142**, 285–286,
      287, 290
    risks in elderly patients, 76,
        112, 119, 150, 281,
        286, 290, **318**, 321,
        333
  benzodiazepines, 292
  buspirone, 292
  dosing of, 287–292, **289**
  memantine, 284, **285**, 287, 288
  neurobiology of, 279–280
  nonpharmacological treatment of,
      285, 293–294, 295
  parkinsonism and, 275
  screening for, 280
  symptoms of, 274, 275, **276–277**,
      284, 287
  vascular, 275, **276**
Demerol. *See* Meperidine
Depacon. *See* Valproate
Depade. *See* Naltrexone
Depakene. *See* Valproate
Depakote, Depakote ER.
  See Valproate
Deplin. *See* L-Methylfolate
Depression, drug-induced
  acamprosate, **191**
  benzodiazepines, 227, 232
  bupropion, **198**
  gabapentin, 109
  melatonin, 226
  varenicline, **197**, 208

Depressive disorders, 59–83
  bipolar depression, 87–88
    treatment of, 93–95, 112
  in children and adolescents, 64, 79
  clinical pearls related to, 82–83
  in cyclothymic disorder, 88
  dementia and, 284, 287
  electroconvulsive therapy for, 293
  diagnosis of, 59–60
  diagnostic criteria for
    dysthymic disorder, **63–64**
    major depressive disorder
      recurrent, **62**
      single episode, **61**
  differentiation from delirium, **307**
  folate deficiency and, 77
  herbal preparations for, **356–357**
    schisandra, 365
    St. John's wort, 355
  insulin resistance, diabetes and, 333
  medications for, 68–78, **70–74**
    (*See also* Antidepressants)
    augmentation of
      lithium, 76, 83
      L-methylfolate, 8, 77–78, 83
      second-generation
        antipsychotics, 76
    bupropion, 75
    dose equivalencies for, **407**
    drug interactions with, 40, 41, 81
    FDA warnings for, 78
    mirtazapine, 75
    monitoring treatment with, 80–81
    monoamine oxidase inhibitors, 77
    psychostimulants, 177–178
    selective serotonin reuptake
      inhibitors, 67, 68–69
    serotonin-norepinephrine
      reuptake inhibitors, 69, 75

Depressive disorders,
    medications for *(continued)*
        serotonin partial agonist and
            reuptake inhibitor:
            vilazodone, 69
        switching between, 83, 407
        trazodone, 75
        tricyclic antidepressants, 76–77
    neurobiology of, 66, 67
    overview of, 60–67, 81
        depressive disorder not otherwise
            specified, 65
        dysthymic disorder, 63–64, 65
        major depressive disorder, 61,
            62, 64–65
        mood disorder due to general
            medical conditions (with
            depressive features), 65
        postpartum depression, 66–67
        premenstrual dysphoric disorder,
            66
    prevalence of, 59
    protective factors for, 60
    psychotherapy for, 81
    with psychotic features, 61, 62, 64,
        76
    rating scales for, 424, 427–430,
        433–438
    risk factors for, 60
    substance abuse and, 211
    suicidality and, 60, 64, 81
    after traumatic exposure, 237
    treatment in special populations, 79
        children, adolescents, and young
            adults, 79
        elderly and medically
            compromised patients, 79
        women, 79

treatment-resistant, 67, 68, 83
Dermatological effects
    of drugs, 12
        carbamazepine, 12, 106, 107
        disulfiram, 191
        first-generation antipsychotics,
            111
        lamotrigine, 12, 104, 108, 123
        lithium, 103
        modafinil, 175
        oxcarbazepine, 107
        valproate, 105
        ziprasidone, 115
    of herbal preparations
        black cohosh, 368
        ginkgo, 364
        gotu kola, 369
        kava, 362
        lemon balm, 371
        schisandra, 365
        St. John's wort, 358
Desipramine, 11, 261
Desvenlafaxine, 11
    for anxiety disorders, 45
    for depressive disorders, 69, 72
    dose equivalencies for serotonin-
        norepinephrine reuptake
        inhibitors, 407
    dosing of, 45, 72
    side effects of, 45, 72, 333, 343
Desyrel. *See* Trazodone
Detoxification, 203, 204–207, 205.
    See also Withdrawal from drugs
    from alcohol or benzodiazepines,
        203, 204–205, 205
    from opioids, 203, 205, 206–207
Developmental history, 4
    psychotic disorders and, 136–137

Dexedrine, Dexedrine Spansules ER.
    See Dextroamphetamine
Dexmethylphenidate, **11**
    for attention-deficit/hyperactivity
        disorder, **168–169**
Dextroamphetamine, **10, 11,** 174
    for attention-deficit/hyperactivity
        disorder, **169**
    dose equivalencies for
        psychostimulants, **408**
    for hypersomnia, 230
Dextroamphetamine/amphetamine,
    10, 174
    dose equivalencies for
        psychostimulants, **408**
    dosing of, **170**
    extended-release, **171**
    indications for
        attention-deficit/hyperactivity
            disorder, **170–171**
        autism symptoms, **166**
        hypersomnia, 230
DHA (docosahexaenoic acid), for
    bipolar disorder, 116–117
Diabetes mellitus.
    See also Glycemic dysregulation
    depression and, 333
    in metabolic syndrome, 334
    schizophrenia and, 332
    second generation antipsychotic–
        induced, 113, 148
    use of disulfiram in, **192**
Dialectical behavioral therapy
    for anxiety disorders in elderly
        persons, 51
    for borderline personality disorder,
        89
    for stress management, 346

Diarrhea
    drug-induced
        acamprosate, **191**
        acetylcholinesterase inhibitors,
            285
        carbamazepine, 106
        lithium, 76, 103
        selective serotonin reuptake
            inhibitors, **253**
        serotonin-norepinephrine
            reuptake inhibitors, 257
        valproate, 105
    herb-induced
        ginkgo, 364
        ginseng root, 361
        valerian, 360
    in serotonin syndrome, 80
Diazepam, **10**
    for anxiety disorders, **43, 47,** 359
    dose equivalencies for
        benzodiazepines, 405–406, **407**
    interaction with buspirone, 48
    for parasomnias, 232
    prescribing considerations for, **47**
Dietary supplements, 8–9.
    See also Nutrition/diet
    herbal preparations, 225–226,
        354–371, **356–357**
    for metabolic syndrome, 340–341
Digoxin, interaction with trazodone, 230
Dilantin. *See* Phenytoin
Dilaudid. *See* Hydromorphone
Diltiazem, for mania, 116
Diphenhydramine
    dose equivalencies for
        nonbenzodiazepine hypnotics,
            409
    for insomnia, 226, 233

Discontinuation of drugs, 18.
    See also Withdrawal from drugs
    lamotrigine, 108
    lithium, 102
    selective serotonin reuptake
        inhibitors, 41, 42, 46, 254
    valproate, 104
    venlafaxine, 45, 46, 48
Distractibility
    in attention-deficit/hyperactivity
        disorder, 156, 157, 159
    in mania/hypomania, 86
Distribution of drugs, 18.
    See also Pharmacokinetics
Disulfiram
    for alcohol dependence, 191–194
    drug interactions with, 193, 200
    alcohol, 192, 207
    pharmacokinetics of, 200
Diuretics, interactions with lithium,
        102, 119
Divalproex sodium. *See* Valproate
Dizziness
    drug-induced
        antipsychotics, 76, 111, 113,
            114, 115, 149
        benzodiazepines, 227, 228, 232,
            282, 319
        bupropion, 75
        buspirone, 48
        carbamazepine, 106
        doxepin, 230
        eszopiclone, 228
        gabapentin, 109, 232
        lamotrigine, 108
        lithium, 103
        methadone, 195
        mirtazapine, 75
        naltrexone, 191

    oxcarbazepine, 107
    serotonin-norepinephrine
        reuptake inhibitors, 48, 69
    topiramate, 109, 232
    trazodone, 75, 230
    valproate, 105
    zolpidem, 229
    herb-induced
        black cohosh, 368
        ginkgo, 364
        lemon balm, 371
        passionflower, 366
        St. John's wort, 358
        valerian, 226
Docosahexaenoic acid (DHA), for
        bipolar disorder, 116–117
Dolophine. *See* Methadone
Donepezil, 285, 288, 289
Dopamine, 12, 67
    antipsychotic effects on, 141, 146,
        148
    in attention-deficit/hyperactivity
        disorder, 164
    in bipolar disorders, 90
    in brain reward circuit, 26, 146,
        186, 188–189
    in delirium, 272
    pathways for, 26, 138–139
    receptors for, 15, 148
    in schizophrenia, 138–139
    in sleep regulation, 225
    in substance use disorders, 185,
        186, 188–189, 212
Dopamine agonists
    interaction with second-generation
        antipsychotics, 113, 114
    for neuroleptic malignant
        syndrome, 147
Dopamine-β-hydroxylase (DBH), 185

Dopamine receptor gene (*DRD2*), 420
Dose equivalencies for psychotropic
   drugs, 405–406, 407–409
Doxepin, 11
   dose equivalencies for
      nonbenzodiazepine hypnotics,
      409
   for insomnia, 227, 230
DRD2 gene, 420
Drug interactions.
   See specific drugs and classes
Dry mouth
   drug-induced
      antipsychotics, 111, 113, 115,
         149
      buspirone, 292
      citalopram, 291
      doxepin, 230
      duloxetine, 291
      eszopiclone, 228
      gabapentin, 232
      mirtazapine, 75
      topiramate, 232
      trazodone, 75, 230
      tricyclic antidepressants, 253
   St. John's wort–induced, 358
DSM-IV-TR
   anxiety disorders in
      acute stress disorder, 237, 240
      anxiety disorder due to general
         medical condition, 38
      classification of, 33
      generalized anxiety disorder, 38
      obsessive-compulsive disorder,
         36–37
      panic disorder with or without
         agoraphobia, 33
      posttraumatic stress disorder,
         237, 238–239

      social phobia, 35
      specific phobia, 34
   attention-deficit/hyperactivity
      disorder in, 160–161
   autistic spectrum disorders in, 158,
      164
      Asperger's disorder, 163
      autistic disorder, 162
   bipolar disorders in, 85, 86,
      88–89
   delirium in, 320–321
   depressive disorders in
      dysthymic disorder, 63–64
      major depressive disorder,
         recurrent, 62
      major depressive disorder, single
         episode, 61
   personality disorders in, 317
   psychotic disorders in, 133
      brief psychotic disorder, 136
      delusional disorder, 130, 135
      psychotic disorder due to general
         medical condition, 137
      schizoaffective disorder, 134
      schizophrenia, 132–133
      schizophreniform disorder, 134
   sleep disorders in, 221
   substance use disorders in, 310
      substance abuse, 188
      substance dependence, 187
      substance intoxication, 190
      substance withdrawal, 190
Duloxetine, 11
   cytochrome P450 enzyme
      inhibition by, 82
   dose equivalencies for serotonin-
      norepinephrine reuptake
      inhibitors, 406, 407
   dosing of, 45, 72, 291

Duloxetine *(continued)*
  drug interactions with, 49
    aripiprazole, 114
  indications for
    anxiety disorders, **43, 45, 46,** 48
    dementia, 284, 291
    depressive disorders, 69, **72**
  interaction with smoking, 48
  prescribing considerations for, **46, 49**
  side effects of, **45, 46, 72,** 291, **343**
  use in hepatic or renal impairment,
    49, 52
Dyslipidemia, 331, 334–335
  alcohol consumption and, 337–338
  drug-induced, **342–345**
    second-generation
      antipsychotics, 113, 118,
      148, **342**
Dyssomnias, 220–222, **221**
  breathing-related sleep disorder, 222
  circadian rhythm sleep disorder, 222
  hypersomnias, 222
    medications for, 230–231
    narcolepsy, 222
    primary, 222
  not otherwise specified, 222
  primary insomnia, 220
    medications for, 225–230,
    228–229
Dysthymic disorder, **63–64,** 65
Dystonia, 111, 113, 115, 147, **318**

Ebstein's anomaly, lithium-induced,
    103, 120
Ecological worldview, 392
Ecstasy (3,4-methylenedioxymeth-
    amphetamine), **10,** 80
Edema, drug-induced
  gabapentin, 109

  lithium, 103
  olanzapine, 113
  oxcarbazepine, 107
Edinburgh Postnatal Depression Scale
  (EPDS), 66, 424, **436–437**
Educational history, 4
Effexor, Effexor XR. *See* Venlafaxine
Eicosapentaenoic acid (EPA), for
  bipolar disorder, 116–117
Elavil. *See* Amitriptyline
Elderly persons
  aggression in, 320–321
  anxiety disorders treatment in, 51
  assessment of psychiatric symptoms
    in, 19
  bipolar disorder treatment in,
    118–119
  delirium in, 272, 273, 321
  dementia in, 274, 275, **276,** 293,
    320
  depression in, 64–65
    treatment of, 79
  dosing in, 19
  drug interactions in, 150
  inadvertent drug abuse in, 19
  medication compliance in, 51
  nonresponse to paroxetine in, 42, 51
  pharmacokinetics in, 51, 150
  polypharmacy in, 51, 79, 150, 177,
    210
  prescribing psychotropics for, 19
    antipsychotics, 111, 150, 321
    risks of second-generation
      antipsychotics, 76, 112,
      119, 150, 281, 286,
      318, 321, 333
    benzodiazepines, 116, 227, 321
    doxepin, 230
    lithium, 103

psychostimulants, 177–178
trazodone, 230
psychiatric emergencies in, 320–321
sleep needs of, 217
St. John's wort in, 358
substance abuse treatment in, 210
suicide in, 210, 314, 320
Electrocardiogram
baseline, for medication use, 6
lithium, 76, 102
psychostimulants, 176
tricyclic antidepressants, 232
in psychiatric emergencies, 305
Electroconvulsive therapy, 147, 293
Electroencephalogram, 6, 216
Emergency situations.
See Psychiatric emergencies
Emotional memory, 37
Emotional symptoms, cultural and
psychiatric language for, 391
Emsam. *See* Selegiline, transdermal
Energy drinks, 231
Enuresis, imipramine for, 77
EPA (eicosapentaenoic acid), for
bipolar disorder, 116–117
EPDS (Edinburgh Postnatal Depression
Scale), 66, 424, 436–437
Epigenetics, 384
Epinephrine
in posttraumatic stress disorder, 243
in substance use disorders, 189
Epworth Sleepiness Scale (ESS), 215,
426, 462
EPS. *See* Extrapyramidal symptoms
Equetro. *See* Carbamazepine
Escitalopram, 11
for children and adolescents, 78
cytochrome P450 enzyme
inhibition by, 82

dose equivalencies for selective
serotonin reuptake inhibitors,
407
dosing of, 44, 70, 260
indications for
anxiety disorders, 43, 44, 46
posttraumatic stress disorder,
246, 248, 260
dementia, 287
depressive disorders, 69, 70
interaction with antipsychotics,
143
pharmacodynamics and
pharmacokinetics of, 40, 248
prescribing considerations for, 46
side effects of, 44, 70, 343
suicidality and, 46
Eskalith. *See* Lithium
ESS (Epworth Sleepiness Scale), 215,
426, 462
Eszopiclone
dose equivalencies for
nonbenzodiazepine hypnotics,
409
for insomnia, 228
Ethnic psychopharmacology, 384
Ethnicity, 382
Ethnopharmacology, 384, 386, 399.
See also Culturally sensitive
psychopharmacology
Evaluation and Management services,
coding for, 347
Excretion of drugs, 18–19.
See also Pharmacokinetics
Exelon. *See* Rivastigmine
Exercise, 341
Exposure therapy, for anxiety disorders,
51, 246, 265
Extensive metabolizers, 385, 387, 420

Extrapyramidal symptoms (EPS),
    antipsychotic-induced, 111, 147,
    282, **282**, 285–286, **318**
    rating scale for, 425, 447–449
    second-generation antipsychotics,
        76, 113, 115, **282**, 290, **318**
    treatment of, 111

Falling-out, **391**
Family psychiatric history, **4**
Fanapt. *See* Iloperidone
Fatigue
    psychostimulants for, 177–178
    wakefulness-promoting agents for,
        231
FDA. *See* U.S. Food and Drug
    Administration
Fear, 31, 32. *See also* Anxiety
    neurobiology of, 37, 39, **40**,
        241–243
    posttraumatic stress disorder and,
        237, 241–243
Feeding behavior, regulation of,
    335–336
Fentanyl, **10**
Fetal alcohol syndrome, 209
FGAs. *See* Antipsychotics: first-
    generation
Fight-or-flight response, 37, 243
Flumazenil, for benzodiazepine reversal,
    311, 323
Fluoxetine, **11**
    for children and adolescents, 78
    cytochrome P450 enzyme
        inhibition by, **82**
    dose equivalencies for selective
        serotonin reuptake inhibitors,
        407
    dosing of, **44**, **48**, **70**, **260**

drug interactions with, 48
    aripiprazole, 114, 143, 146
    carbamazepine, 106
    duloxetine, 49
    methadone, 203
    risperidone, 113
    tricyclic antidepressants, **253**
indications for
    anxiety disorders, **43**, **44**, **46**, 48
    posttraumatic stress disorder,
        246, **249**, **260**
    autism symptoms, **166**
    depressive disorders, 68–69, **70**
    premenstrual dysphoric
        disorder, 79
    during venlafaxine
        discontinuation, 48
    off-label use of, 69, **166**
    pharmacodynamics and
        pharmacokinetics of, 18, 40,
        46, 48, 143, **249**
    prescribing considerations for, **46**
    side effects of, **44**, **46**, **70**, **343**
Fluphenazine, **11**
    dose equivalencies for first-
        generation antipsychotics, **408**
    pharmacokinetics of, **144**
    side effects of, **342**
Flurazepam
    dose equivalencies for
        benzodiazepine hypnotics, **409**
    for insomnia, **228**
Flushing syndrome, alcohol-induced, 387
Fluvoxamine, **11**
    cytochrome P450 enzyme
        inhibition by, **82**
    dose equivalencies for selective
        serotonin reuptake inhibitors,
        407

dosing of, 44, 46, 47, 71
drug interactions with
aripiprazole, 114
carbamazepine, 106
clozapine, 253
haloperidol, 253
olanzapine, 113
ramelteon, 227
indications for
anxiety disorders, 43, 44, 46, 47,
69
posttraumatic stress disorder,
246, 249
autism symptoms, 166
depressive disorders, 69, 71
pharmacodynamics and
pharmacokinetics of, 40,
249
prescribing considerations for, 46
side effects of, 44, 71, 344
use in cardiovascular impairment,
52
Focalin, Focalin XR.
See Dexmethylphenidate
Folate deficiency, depression and, 77
Fornix, 24
Frontotemporal dementia, 276

GABA. See γ-Aminobutyric acid
Gabapentin, 109–110
dosing of, 99
drug interactions with, 109, 110
indications for
bipolar disorder, 93, 99,
109–110, 123
dementia, 285
parasomnias, 232
mechanism of action of, 109
during pregnancy, 110

side effects of, 109–110, 232, 334,
344
Galactorrhea, antipsychotic-induced,
111, 122
Galantamine, 285, 288, 289
Gastrointestinal effects
of drugs
acamprosate, 191
acetylcholinesterase inhibitors,
285
aripiprazole, 114
buprenorphine, 195
buprenorphine-naloxone, 195
bupropion, 73, 75, 198
buspirone, 44, 292
carbamazepine, 106
gabapentin, 109
lamotrigine, 109
lithium, 76, 103
melatonin, 226
methadone, 195
mirtazapine, 74
naltrexone, 191
olanzapine, 113
oxcarbazepine, 107
psychostimulants, 176
second-generation
antipsychotics, 76
selective serotonin reuptake
inhibitors, 42, 44, 46,
70–71, 253, 291
serotonin-norepinephrine
reuptake inhibitors, 45, 46,
72, 257, 291
topiramate, 110
trazodone, 74, 230
valproate, 105
varenicline, 198
vilazodone, 71

Gastrointestinal effects *(continued)*
  of herbal preparations
    black cohosh, 368
    ginkgo, 364
    ginseng root, 361
    gotu kola, 369
    kava, 362
    lemon balm, 371
    passionflower, 366
    schisandra, 365
    St. John's wort, 258
    valerian, 226, 360
  in serotonin syndrome, 80
Gated calcium channel gene
  (CACNA1C), **418–419**
Gender
  anxiety disorders and, 31, **32**
    posttraumatic stress disorder,
      236, 239, 259
  bipolar disorder and, 121–122
  depression and, 60
Generalized anxiety disorder, 33
  diagnostic criteria for, **38**
  epidemiology of, **32**
  medications for, **43**
    in elderly persons, 51
Generic drugs, 7
  selective serotonin reuptake
    inhibitors, 68, **70**, 82
Genetic factors
  in bipolar disorders, 89–90
  in psychotic disorders, 135–136
  in substance use disorders, 185
Genetic markers, 18, 185
Genetic polymorphisms, 383, 384,
  385
Genetic testing, 18
Genome, 384
Genotype, 383, 387

psychopharmacogenetics, 18, 417,
  418–421
Geodon. *See* Ziprasidone
Ghrelin, 335
Ginkgo (*Ginkgo biloba*), **356**, 363–364
  adverse effects of, 364
  description of, 363
  efficacy of, 363
  herbal and drug interactions with,
    364
  mechanism of action of, 363
Ginseng root (*Panax ginseng*), **356**,
  360–361
  adverse effects of, 361
  description of, 360
  efficacy of, 360
  herbal and drug interactions with,
    361
  mechanism of action of, 360
Glucophage. *See* Metformin
Glutamate
  in Alzheimer's dementia, 280
  in autistic spectrum disorders, 165
  in bipolar disorders, 90
  in posttraumatic stress disorder, 244
  receptors for, **15**
  in schizophrenia, 139–140
  in sleep regulation, 225
  in substance use disorders, 189
Glycemic dysregulation, 331.
  See also Diabetes mellitus
  alcohol consumption and, 337–338
  drug-induced, **342–345**
    desvenlafaxine, 333
    mirtazapine, 333
    second generation antipsychotics,
      113, 115, 118, 148, **318**
    ginseng-induced, 361
    schizophrenia and, 333

Gotu kola (*Centella asiatica*), 357,
     369–370
   adverse effects of, 370
   description of, 369
   efficacy of, 369
   herbal and drug interactions with,
     369
   mechanism of action of, 369
Grapefruit juice, drug interactions with
   methadone, 195
   psychostimulants, 169–171, 174
   triazolam, 228
Guanfacine, 174
   for attention-deficit/hyperactivity
     disorder, 173
Guilt feelings, 64, 87, 237

Halcion. *See* Triazolam
Haldol. *See* Haloperidol
Half-life of drugs, 18.
   See also Pharmacokinetics
   antipsychotics
     first-generation, 143, 144–145
     second-generation, 113, 114,
       115, 145–146, 283
   benzodiazepines, 47, 49, 52, 121,
     228
   bupropion, 73
   caffeine, 231
   clonidine, 173
   diphenhydramine, 226
   in elderly persons, 51
   guanfacine, 173
   lamotrigine, 108
   lithium, 102
   mirtazapine, 74
   nonbenzodiazepine hypnotics, 228,
     229
   phenelzine, 251

   psychostimulants, 167, 169, 170
   ramelteon, 226
   selective serotonin reuptake
     inhibitors, 40, 44, 46, 48,
       70–71, 248–249
   serotonin-norepinephrine reuptake
     inhibitors, 40, 72, 250
   trazodone, 74, 230
   tricyclic antidepressants, 250–251,
     252
   vilazodone, 71
Hallucinations, 131, 152
   in delirium, 273, 292
   in delirium tremens, 311
   in dementia, 275, 287, 293
Haloperidol, 11
   for children and adolescents, 151
   dose equivalencies for first-
     generation antipsychotics, 108
   for elderly persons, 321
   indications for
     acute mania, 92, 93, 110
     autism symptoms, 166
     delirium, 281–282, 282, 286, 292
       in children and adolescents,
         292
     dementia, 290
     psychiatric emergencies, 315,
       316, 318, 321
   interaction with selective serotonin
     reuptake inhibitors, 253
   interaction with valerian, 359
   intravenous, 282
   off-label uses of, 142, 166
   pharmacokinetics of, 143, 144
   during pregnancy, 149, 323
   side effects of, 282, 318, 343
Hamilton Anxiety Scale (Ham-A), 424,
     431–432

Hamilton Rating Scale for Depression.
    See 17-Item Hamilton Rating
    Scale for Depression (Ham-D-17)
Headache
    drug-induced
        buprenorphine-naloxone, 195
        bupropion, 75, 198
        buspirone, 48, 292
        carbamazepine, 106
        eszoplicone, 228
        lamotrigine, 108
        lithium, 103
        melatonin, 226
        methadone, 195
        mirtazapine, 75
        monoamine oxidase inhibitors,
            253
        naltrexone, 191
        oxcarbazepine, 107
        prazosin, 232
        psychostimulants, 176, 178, 230
        second-generation
            antipsychotics, 76
        selective serotonin reuptake
            inhibitors, 46, 69, 253,
            291
        serotonin-norepinephrine
            reuptake inhibitors, 69,
            257, 291
        trazodone, 75
        valproate, 105
        varenicline, 198
    herb-induced
        black cohosh, 368
        ginkgo, 364
        ginseng root, 361
        valerian, 226, 360
    in premenstrual dysphoric disorder,
        66

Health care disparities, 379–380, 381
Healthy People initiative, 332, 346
Heart pain/broken heart, 391
Helplessness, 237, 238, 240, 315
Hematological effects
    of drugs
        carbamazepine, 12, 106, 107
        clozapine, 12
        lamotrigine, 108
        tricyclic antidepressants, 254
        valproate, 105
    herb-induced bleeding
        black cohosh, 368
        ginkgo, 364
        St. John's wort, 358
Hepatic effects
    of drugs
        atomoxetine, 12
        buprenorphine, 195
        carbamazepine, 106, 107, 291
        monoamine oxidase inhibitors,
            254
        naltrexone, 192
        nefazodone, 12, 78
        tacrine, 288
        valproate, 105, 291
    of herbal preparations
        black cohosh, 368
        gotu kola, 369
        kava, 361, 362
        passionflower, 367
Hepatic impairment
    bupropion in, 197
    buspirone in, 52, 292
    disulfiram in, 192
    duloxetine in, 49, 52
    lorazepam in, 52
    naltrexone in, 192
    ramelteon in, 227

selective serotonin reuptake
inhibitors in, **252**
topiramate in, **192**
tricyclic antidepressants in, **252**
venlafaxine in, 258
Herbal preparations, 354–371,
356–357
anxiety induced by, 54–55
black cohosh, 367–368, 371
clinical pearls related to, 371
dosing of, **356–357**
drug interactions with, 120
gabapentin, 109
ginkgo, 363–364
ginseng root, 360–361
gotu kola, 369–370
for insomnia, 225–226, 233
kava, 361–362
lemon balm, 370–371
medication history for, 4, 81, 371
passionflower, 365–367
schisandra, 364–365
St. John's wort, 354–358, 371
use in elderly persons, 51
valerian, 358–360, 371
Heroin abuse/dependence, **10**, 185,
202, 310
blood-borne infections and, 311
intoxication due to, 311
withdrawal from, **206–207**, 312
Hippocampus, **24**, 37
Histamine
in delirium, 272
pathways for, **27**
receptors for, **16**
in sleep regulation, 225
History taking, **4**
in psychiatric emergencies, 303, 305
HIV dementia, 277

Holistic approach, 2, 18, 20, 141, 151,
324, 346, 347, 348, 380, 381,
392, 393, 398
Homicidal ideation, 131
in children, 321
as psychiatric emergency, 303, 308,
315, 324
varenicline-induced, **197**
Hopelessness, 60, **63**, 65, 237, 314,
314, **315**
HPA axis. *See* Hypothalamic-pituitary-
adrenal axis
5-HT. *See* Serotonin
5HT2C gene, **418**
Human Rights Watch, 316
Huntington's dementia, 277
Hwa-byung, **391**
Hydrochlorothiazide, interaction with
topiramate, **193**
Hydrocodone, **10**, 110
Hydromorphone, **10**, 202
Hydroxyzine
dose equivalencies for
nonbenzodiazepine hypnotics,
409
for insomnia, **206**, 226
Hyperactivity
in attention-deficit/hyperactivity
disorder, 156, **157**, 159
in delirium, 273
medications for, **166**
psychostimulant-induced, 230
Hyperammonemia, valproate-induced,
105
Hypericum perforatum. See St. John's wort
Hyperprolactinemia, drug-induced
ramelteon, 227
second-generation antipsychotics,
113, 148

Hypersomnia, 222
    medications for, 230–231
Hypertension
    alcohol consumption and, 337–338
    in delirium tremens, 311
    drug-induced, 342–345
        psychostimulants, 230
        tricyclic antidepressants, 253
        venlafaxine, 46, 48, 258
    ginseng-induced, 361
    in metabolic syndrome, 331
Hypertensive crisis, monoamine
        oxidase inhibitor–induced, 77,
        247, 253, 254, 258
Hyperthermia
    in delirium tremens, 311
    in serotonin syndrome, 80
    topiramate-induced, 192
Hypomania, 86–87, 88.
    See also Bipolar disorders
    St. John's wort–induced, 358
Hyponatremia, drug-induced
    carbamazepine, 106
    oxcarbazepine, 107
    venlafaxine, 258
Hypotension, drug-induced
    antipsychotics, 111, 113, 115, 121,
        283, 318
    benzodiazepines, 282
    buprenorphine, 195
    carbamazepine, 107
    clonidine, 173
    clozapine, 12
    disulfiram, 191
    guanfacine, 173
    methadone, 195
    monoamine oxidase inhibitors, 253
    oxcarbazepine, 107
    prazosin, 232

tricyclic antidepressants, 253
Hypothalamic-pituitary-adrenal (HPA)
        axis
    in bipolar disorders, 91
    in delirium, 272, 278–279
    in metabolic syndrome, 336
    in posttraumatic stress disorder,
        243
Hypothalamus, 24, 335

Iloperidone, 11
    dose equivalencies for second-
        generation antipsychotics, 408
    pharmacokinetics of, 145
    side effects of, 342
Imipramine, 11
    dosing of, 261
    indications for
        enuresis, 77
        parasomnias, 232
        posttraumatic stress disorder,
            246, 250, 261
    pharmacodynamics and
        pharmacokinetics of, 250
Impulsivity
    in attention-deficit/hyperactivity
        disorder, 156, 157, 159
    in borderline personality disorder,
        320
    medications for, 166
Inattention
    in attention-deficit/hyperactivity
        disorder, 156, 157
    medications for, 166
    in psychotic disorders, 131
Incarcerated persons, treatment of
    psychiatric emergencies in,
        316–317
Inderal. See Propranolol

Informed consent
for medication use
antidepressants in children and
young adults, 53, 79
in anxiety disorders, 42, 50, 54
off-label use, 42, 50
in psychiatric emergencies, 303
Insomnia. *See also* Sleep-wake disorders
in delirium tremens, 311
drug-induced
(*See* Sleep effects, of drugs)
herbal preparations for, 225–226
chamomile, 225–226
valerian, 225–226, **356**, 358–360
lemon balm and, 370
medications for, 225–230, **228–229**
antidepressants, **74**, 77, 227,
230
antihistamines, 226, 233
benzodiazepines, 227
dose equivalencies for, 409
melatonergic hypnotics, 226–227
nonbenzodiazepine hypnotics,
227
nonpharmacological interventions
for, 233
primary, 220
Insulin resistance, 336
alcohol consumption and, 337–338
depression and, 333
drug-induced
second generation
antipsychotics, 148
valproate, 122
schizophrenia and, 333
Insurance coverage for medications,
346–347
Interpersonal and social rhythm
therapy, 91

Interpersonal therapy, 51
Intoxication, 189, 305
with alcohol, 310
with benzodiazepines, 311
diagnostic criteria for, **190**
with opioids, 311
with phencyclidine, 312–313
with psychostimulants, 312
Intuniv, Intuniv ER.
See Guanfacine
Invega, Invega Sustenna.
See Paliperidone
Irritability
in anxiety disorders, 32
in autistic spectrum disorders, 159,
177, 179
medications for, 150, 151, **166**,
179
in bipolar disorders, 80, 86, 87, 117
in depressive disorders, **63**, 64, 66
drug-induced
carbamazepine, 107
serotonin-norepinephrine
reuptake inhibitors, 69
after traumatic exposure, 237
valerian-induced, 360
Isocarboxazid, **11**
Isoniazid, interaction with black
cohosh, 368
Isoptin. *See* Verapamil
17-Item Hamilton Rating Scale for
Depression (Ham-D-17), 424,
433–435

Jet lag, 222, 226

Kainate receptors, **15**
in schizophrenia, 139
Kapvay ER. *See* Clonidine

Kava, **356**, 361–362
  adverse effects of, 361, 362
  description of, 361
  efficacy of, 362
  herbal and drug interactions with,
    362
  gabapentin, 109
  mechanism of action of, 361–362
Ketamine, **10**, 140
Ketoconazole, interaction with
  aripiprazole, 114
Kindling, 37, 244
Klonopin. *See* Clonazepam

Laboratory evaluation
  during alcohol withdrawal, **205**
  for dementia, 278
  for medication use, **6**
    carbamazepine, 106, 291
    disulfiram, **194**
    lithium, 76, 102, 103
    naltrexone, **194**
    olanzapine, 113
    psychostimulants, 176, 230
  for metabolic syndrome, 338–339,
    339, 347
  during opiate withdrawal, **207**
  in psychiatric emergencies, 305
  during sedative-hypnotic
    withdrawal, **205**
  for sleep disorders, 216
Lafora disease, 293
Lamictal. *See* Lamotrigine
Lamotrigine, 108–109
  discontinuation of, 108
  dosing and titration of, **99**, 108, **109**
  drug interactions with, 108
    carbamazepine, 106, 108, **109**
    valproate, 104, 108, **109**

indications for
  bipolar disorder, **99**, 108–109,
    123
  acute mania, 93
  in children and adolescents,
    118
  with comorbid cocaine
    abuse, 211
  depressive episode, 93–95
  maintenance treatment, 94,
    97
  mixed states, 96
  rapid cycling, 96
  posttraumatic stress disorder,
    255
  mechanism of action of, 108
  pharmacokinetics of, 108
  during pregnancy and breast-
    feeding, 109, 120, 121
  side effects of, **12**, 108, 334, **344**
Language and communication patterns,
  cultural, 389–392
Latuda. *See* Lurasidone
Legal/criminal history, **5**
Lemon balm (*Melissa officinalis*), **357**,
  370–371
  adverse effects of, 371
  description of, 370
  efficacy of, 370
  herbal and medication interactions
    with, 370
  mechanism of action of, 370
Leptin, 335, 336
Levodopa, drug interactions with
  aripiprazole, 114
  bupropion, **198**, 203
  olanzapine, 113
  risperidone, 113
Levothroid. *See* Levothyroxine

Levothyroxine, 103
Lewy body dementia, 275, **276**, 293
Lexapro. *See* Escitalopram
Librium. *See* Chlordiazepoxide
Limbic system, **25**
  in bipolar disorder, 90
  in emotional processing, 242, 243
  in posttraumatic stress disorder,
    242, 244
  in premenstrual dysphoric disorder,
    66
  in schizophrenia, 140
  serotonin pathways in, **13**, **27**
  in substance abuse, 186
Lipid changes, 331, 334–335
  alcohol consumption and, 337–338
  drug-induced, **342–345**
    second-generation antipsychotics,
      113, 118, 148, **342**
Lipitor. *See* Atorvastatin
Lisdexamfetamine, **11**, 174
  for attention-deficit/hyperactivity
    disorder, **171**
  dose equivalencies for
    psychostimulants, **408**
Lithium, 102–103
  discontinuation of, 102
  dosing of, **98**, 102
  drug interactions with, 102, 119
    alcohol, 120
    topiramate, 110, **193**
  indications for
    antidepressant augmentation,
      76, 83
    bipolar disorder, 76, **98**,
      102–103, 122–123
      acute mania, 91, 92, 93
      in children and adolescents,
        103, 117–118

    depressive episode, 93–95
    in elderly persons, 103
    maintenance treatment, 97,
      102
    mixed states, 96
    rapid cycling, 96
    delirium, **282**
  laboratory evaluation for use of, 76,
    102, 103
  mechanism of action of, 102
  for medically compromised patients,
    103
  monitoring serum levels of,
    102–103
  pharmacokinetics of, 102
  during pregnancy and breast-
    feeding, 103, 120–121
  side effects of, 103, 334, **344**
  toxicity of, 102, 103
Lithobid. *See* Lithium
Locus coeruleus, **24**, **25**
Lorazepam, **10**
  for alcohol/benzodiazepine
    withdrawal, **204**, 205
  dose equivalencies for
    benzodiazepines, **407**
  for elderly persons, 321
  indications for
    acute mania, 93, 116
    anxiety disorders, **43**, **47**, 49
    delirium, **282**
      terminal, 293
    psychiatric emergencies,
      309–310, 316, **319**
  passionflower interaction with, 366
  during pregnancy, 121, 323
  prescribing considerations for, 47
  side effects of, **319**
  use in hepatic impairment, 52

Loxapine, 11
for acute mania, 110
dose equivalencies for first-
generation antipsychotics, 408
off-label uses of, 142
pharmacokinetics of, 144
Loxitane. *See* Loxapine
LSD (lysergic acid diethylamide), 10,
137
Lunesta. *See* Eszopiclone
Lurasidone, 11
dose equivalencies for second-
generation antipsychotics, 408
side effects of, 342
Luther, Martin, 31
Luvox, Luvox CR. *See* Fluvoxamine
Lyrica. *See* Pregabalin
Lysergic acid diethylamide (LSD), 10,
137

Magnesium supplementation, 340
Magnetic resonance imaging (MRI), 6
in autistic spectrum disorders, 164
functional
of anxiety responses, 39
in autistic spectrum disorders,
164
in psychiatric emergencies, 305
Major depressive disorder (MDD),
61–62, 64–65.
See also Depressive disorders
Manerix. *See* Moclobemide
Mania, 86–87, 88.
See also Bipolar disorders
antidepressant-precipitated, 76,
80–81, 83, 85, 94, 95
herb-induced
ginseng root, 361
St. John's wort, 358

rating scales for, 424, 439–445
symptoms of, 86–87
treatment of, 91–93
MAO. *See* Monoamine oxidase
MAOIs. *See* Monoamine oxidase
inhibitors
Marijuana, 10, 137, 310
Massage therapy, 51, 233, 354
MDD (major depressive disorder),
61–62, 64–65.
See also Depressive disorders
Medical conditions
anxiety disorder due to, 33, 39
delirium in patients with, 273, 279,
292–293
dementia in patients with, 293
mood disorder due to (with
depressive features), 65
presenting as psychiatric
emergencies, 304–305, 306,
322
sleep disorder due to, 223
symptom overlap between anxiety
disorders and, 32
treatment of bipolar disorder in
patients with, 119–120
use of psychotropics in patients
with, 19–20
agents for alcohol and opioid
dependence, 192
antianxiety medications, 52
antidepressants, 79
antipsychotics, 150, 292–293
mood stabilizers, 103, 120
psychostimulants, 177–178
Medical foods, 8
caprylidene for dementia, 287,
290
Medical/surgical history, 4

Medication history, 4, 81, 233
Medline Plus, 209
Melatonin, 226
Melatonin receptor antagonist,
    226–227. *See also* Ramelteon
Melissa officinalis. See Lemon balm
Memantine, for dementia, 284, **285,** 288
Memory impairment
    in dementia, 275, **276–277**
    drug-induced
        benzodiazepines, 227, **228,** 232
        eszopiclone, **228**
        lamotrigine, 108
        lithium, 103
        zaleplon, **229**
        zolpidem, **229**
    in psychotic disorders, 131
Menopausal symptoms, black cohosh
    for, 367–368
Mental health nursing, 1–3
    culturally sensitive, 379–399
Mental illness
    metabolic syndrome and, 332–333,
        348
    monoamine hypothesis of, 12
    role of culture in, 380–381
    stigma of, 379–380, 383, 388
Mental status examination, 5
    in psychiatric emergencies, 303
Meperidine, **10,** 80, 292
Metabolic syndrome, 331–348.
    See also Dyslipidemia; Glycemic
        dysregulation; Hypertension;
        Weight changes
    alcohol consumption and, 337–338
    bipolar disorder and, 332
    clinical pearls related to, 348
    core features of, 331, 334–336,
        335

costs of, 332
drugs associated with, 333, 338,
    342–345, 348
    assessing risks and benefits of,
        346–347
    mood stabilizers, 333–334
    second-generation
        antipsychotics, 76, 112,
            113, 148, 333
factors associated with, 336–338
    among mentally ill persons,
        332–333, 348
    monitoring for, 338–339, **339,**
        347
    overview of, 331–334
    prevalence of, 332
    psychoeducation about, 338, 341,
        348
    risk factors for, 332
    schizophrenia and, 332
    smoking and, 337
    stress and, 336–337
    treatment of, 339–347, **340**
        diet/nutrition, 340–341
        exercise, 341
        identifying patient's readiness to
            change, 341, 346
        metformin, 339–340
        stress management, 346
        supporting patient self-efficacy,
            346
Metabolism of drugs, 18–19, 21.
    See also Pharmacokinetics
Metadate CR, Metadate ER.
    See Methylphenidate
Metformin
    for drug-induced weight gain,
        339–340
    interaction with topiramate, **193**

Methadone, 10
    drug interactions with, 195, 203
    mechanism of action of, 195, 202
    for opioid dependence, 195–196,
        208
    pharmacokinetics of, 203
    during pregnancy, 209
Methadose. See Methadone
Methamphetamine, 10, 185
Methotrexate, interaction with black
    cohosh, 368
N-Methyl-D-aspartate (NMDA)
    receptor antagonist.
    See Memantine
N-Methyl-D-aspartate (NMDA)
    receptors, 15
    in posttraumatic stress disorder,
        244
    in schizophrenia, 139–140
Methyldopa, interaction with black
    cohosh, 368
3,4-Methylenedioxymethamphetamine
    (Ecstasy), 10, 80
Methylenetetrahydrofolate reductase
    gene (MTHFR), 419
L-Methylfolate, 8, 77–78, 83
Methylin, Methylin ER.
    See Methylphenidate
Methylphenidate, 10, 11
    dose equivalencies for
        psychostimulants, 408
    dosing of, 167–168
    extended-release, 167–168
    indications for
        attention-deficit/hyperactivity
            disorder, 167–168
        autism symptoms, 166
        hypersomnia, 230
    transdermal, 167

Milnacipran, 344
Mini Mental State Examination, 280
Minipress. See Prazosin
Mirtazapine, 11
    cytochrome P450 enzyme
        inhibition by, 82
    dosing of, 74
    indications for
        antidepressant augmentation in
            posttraumatic stress
            disorder, 260
        bipolar depression, 95
        depressive disorders, 74, 75
        selective serotonin reuptake
            inhibitor–induced sexual
            dysfunction, 42
    interaction with methadone, 203
    side effects of, 74, 75, 333, 344
Misoprostol, 164
Moclobemide, for posttraumatic stress
    disorder, 246
Modafinil, 10
    for attention-deficit/hyperactivity
        disorder, 174, 175
    for hypersomnia, 231
    side effects of, 175, 231
Models of illness and disease, 390, 391
Monoamine hypothesis of mental
    illness, 12
Monoamine oxidase (MAO), 185
    kava inhibition of, 362
    St. John's wort inhibition of, 355
Monoamine oxidase inhibitors
    (MAOIs), 77
    dietary restrictions for use of, 77,
        247, 253, 258, 261
    drug interactions with, 48, 77, 253
        bupropion, 198, 203
        methadone, 195

indications for
depressive disorders, 77
posttraumatic stress disorder, 247,
251–254, 257, 258, 261
overdose of, 254
passionflower interaction with, 366
pharmacodynamics and
pharmacokinetics of, 251, 252
serotonin syndrome and, 80
side effects of, 77, 247, 253–254, 258
suicidality and, 11
Montreal Cognitive Assessment, 280
Mood stabilizers, 102–116.
See also specific drugs and classes
advantages and limitations of, 122
anticonvulsants, 98–99, 104–110
carbamazepine, 105–107
gabapentin, 109–110
lamotrigine, 108–109, 109
oxcarbazepine, 107
topiramate, 110
valproate, 104–105
for autism symptoms, 165
for bipolar disorder, 98–101,
102–116
acute mania, 91–93
depressive episodes, 93–94
maintenance treatment, 97
mixed states, 95–96
rapid cycling, 96
for children and adolescents,
117–118
for delirium, 281
for elderly persons, 119
first-generation antipsychotics,
110–111
indications for
delirium, 282
dementia, 285

lithium, 98, 102–103
for medically compromised patients,
103, 120
metabolic effects of, 333–334,
344–345
for posttraumatic stress disorder, 255
during pregnancy and breast-
feeding, 120–121
second-generation antipsychotics,
100–101, 112–116
aripiprazole, 114
olanzapine, 112–113
quetiapine, 114–115
risperidone, 113
ziprasidone, 115
Morphine, 110, 202
MRI. *See* Magnetic resonance imaging
MTA (Multimodal Treatment of
Attention Deficit Hyperactivity
Disorder) trial, 156–157
MTHFR gene, 419
Multimodal Treatment of Attention
Deficit Hyperactivity Disorder
(MTA) trial, 156–157
Muscarinic receptors, 16
Music therapy, 51, 233, 354

Naloxone
buprenorphine-naloxone for opioid
dependence, 195–196, 208
for opioid overdose, 311
Naltrexone
extended-release injectable, 191–194
interaction with opioids, 192, 207
for opioid dependence, 191–194
Namenda. *See* Memantine
Narcan. *See* Naloxone
Narcolepsy, 222
medications for, 230–231

Nardil. *See* Phenelzine
National Health and Nutrition
  Examination Survey (NHANES),
  333
National Institute of Mental Health,
  210
  Clinical Antipsychotic Trials of
    Intervention Effectiveness, 141
  Multimodal Treatment of Attention
    Deficit Hyperactivity Disorder
    trial, 156–157
National Institute on Drug Abuse, 184
National Library of Medicine, 209
National Sleep Foundation, 216
Natural model of illness and disease,
  391
Nausea/vomiting.
  See Gastrointestinal effects
Navane. *See* Thiothixene
Nefazodone, **11, 12,** 78, **82, 228**
Nembutal. *See* Pentobarbital
Neural tube defects, drug-induced
  carbamazepine, 107, 120
  valproate, 105, 120
Neuroanatomy, 12, **24**
Neurobiology
  of attention-deficit/hyperactivity
    disorder, 159, 164
  of autistic spectrum disorders,
    164–165
  of bipolar disorders, 89–91
  of delirium, 272, 278–279
  of depression, 67
  of fear and anxiety, 37, 39, **40**
  of posttraumatic stress disorder,
    241–245
  of premenstrual dysphoric disorder,
    66
  of schizophrenia, 137–141

of sleep, 225, 232
of substance abuse and dependence,
  186–189
Neurocognitive disorders, 271–295,
  281–286, **282, 285**
  clinical assessment of, 280
  clinical pearls related to, 294–295
  delirium, 272–274, **274**
  dementia, 274–278, **276–277**
  medications for psychiatric symptoms
    of, 281–286, **282, 285**
  dosing guidelines for, 286–292,
    289
  neurobiology of, 278–280
  nonpharmacological interventions
    for, 285, 293–294, 295, 321
  treatment in special populations,
    292–293
Neurodevelopmental disorders,
  155–180
  attention-deficit/hyperactivity
    disorder, 155–157, **157, 158**
  autistic spectrum disorders,
    158–159
  diagnostic criteria for
    Asperger's disorder, **163**
    attention-deficit/hyperactivity
      disorder, **160–161**
    autistic disorder, **162**
  medications for, 165–179, **166–173**
  neurobiology of, 159, 164–165
  psychiatric emergencies in, 321
Neuroimaging, **6**
  in autistic spectrum disorders, 164
  in bipolar disorders, 90
  in dementia, 278
  of neural circuitry of fear, 37, 39
  in psychiatric emergencies, 305
  in schizophrenia, 140

Neuroleptic malignant syndrome
(NMS), 80, 113, 115, 147, **282**,
290, **318**
Neurontin. *See* Gabapentin
Neuropeptide Y, 335
Neurotransmitters, 12.
See also specific neurotransmitters
in Alzheimer's dementia, 280
in attention-deficit/hyperactivity
disorder, 164
in autistic spectrum disorders, 165
in bipolar disorders, 90
in delirium, 272, 279
in depression, 67
in fear/stress response, 243
pathways of, **26–27**
in posttraumatic stress disorder,
243–245
in premenstrual dysphoric disorder,
66
receptors for, **13–17**
in schizophrenia, 138–140
in sleep regulation, 225
in substance use disorders, 185,
186, 188–189
NHANES (National Health and
Nutrition Examination Survey),
333
Nicotine. *See also* Smoking/tobacco use
dependence on, 184, 231
medications for, 78, **197–199**
pharmacokinetics of, 203
during pregnancy, **197**, 208,
209
neurobiology of, 188
for hypersomnia, 231
Nicotine replacement therapies,
197–199, 208
Nicotinic receptors, 17

Niemann-Pick disease, 293
Nifedipine, for mania, 116
Nightmare disorder, 222–223
medications for, 231–232
Nimodipine, for mania, 116
Nimotop. *See* Nimodipine
Nizoral. *See* Ketoconazole
NMDA receptors.
See N-Methyl-D-aspartate
receptors
NMS (neuroleptic malignant
syndrome), 80, 113, 115, 147,
282, 290, **318**
Nonbenzodiazepine hypnotics, 227,
228, 229
dose equivalencies for, **409**
Nonsteroidal anti-inflammatory drugs,
interaction with lithium,
102, 119
Noradrenergic and specific serotonergic
antidepressant. *See* Mirtazapine
Norepinephrine, 12, 67
in attention-deficit/hyperactivity
disorder, 164
in bipolar disorders, 90
pathways for, **26, 27**
in posttraumatic stress disorder,
243, 245
receptors for, **14**
in sleep regulation, 225
Norepinephrine-dopamine reuptake
inhibitor, 67, 75.
See also Bupropion
Nortriptyline, **11**
dosing of, **261**
pharmacodynamics and
pharmacokinetics of, **251**
for posttraumatic stress disorder,
246, **251, 261**

Nurse-patient relationship
    culturally competent, 387–389,
        389, 394, 398
    in psychiatric emergencies, 302
Nutrition/diet
    caffeine in, 231
    dietary supplements, 8–9, 354
        herbal preparations, 225–226,
            354–371, 356–357
        for metabolic syndrome, 340–341
    drug interactions with grapefruit
        juice
        methadone, 195
        psychostimulants, 169–171, 174
        triazolam, 228
    medical foods, 8
        caprylidene for dementia, 287,
            290
    monoamine oxidase inhibitor
        interactions with tyramine in,
        77, 247, 253, 258, 261
    omega-3 fatty acids for bipolar
        disorder, 116–117
    psychoeducation about, 341
    U.S. Department of Agriculture
        Choose My Plate Web site,
        341
Nuvigil. See Armodafinil

Obesity, 148, 331, 332, 346.
    See also Weight changes
Obsessive-compulsive disorder (OCD),
    33
    diagnostic criteria for, 36–37
    epidemiology of, 32
    medications for, 43, 69, 71, 77, 166
        in elderly persons, 51
Obstetrical factors, psychotic disorders
    and, 136–137

Occupational history, 4
OCD. See Obsessive-compulsive disorder
Oculogyric crisis, 147
Off-label drug use
    of antidepressants, 69, 78, 166
    of antipsychotics, 141, 142, 166
    in anxiety disorders, 42
    in autism, 166, 179
    in children and adolescents, 19
    documenting discussion with
        patient about, 42
    informed consent for, 42, 50
    of psychostimulants, 166
Olanzapine, 11, 112–113
    for children and adolescents, 151,
        322
    dose equivalencies for second-
        generation antipsychotics, 409
    dosing of, 100, 286, 290, 318
    drug interactions with, 113
    indications for
        bipolar disorder, 100, 112–113,
            123
        acute mania, 92, 93
        in adolescents, 118
        maintenance treatment, 97
        rapid cycling, 96
    delirium, 282, 283, 286
    dementia, 290
    posttraumatic stress disorder, 255
    psychiatric emergencies, 315, 318
    laboratory evaluation for use of, 113
    mechanism of action of, 112, 283
    off-label uses of, 142
    pharmacokinetics of, 113, 143, 145,
        283
    during pregnancy, 323
    side effects of, 112, 113, 318, 339,
        342

Olanzapine-fluoxetine combination, **11**
  for bipolar disorder
    depressive episodes, 94, 95, **100**,
      112
    rapid cycling, 96
  dosing of, **100**
Oleptro. *See* Trazodone
Omega-3 fatty acids, for bipolar
  disorder, 116–117, 118
Online resources, 469–470
Opioid system, in posttraumatic stress
  disorder, 244
Opioids/opiates
  abuse and dependence on
    blood-borne infections and,
      311
    deaths due to, 184
    detoxification from, 203, 205,
      206–207
    medications for, **191–196**
    "street value" of, 208
  as controlled substances, **10**, 202
  delirium induced by, 273
  drug interactions with
    gabapentin, 109
    naltrexone, **192**, 207
  overdose of, 184
  pharmacokinetics of, 202–203
  withdrawal from, 203, 205,
    206–207, 312, 366
Oral contraceptives, **4**
  conception while taking, 67
  drug interactions with
    carbamazepine, 106, 120
    lamotrigine, 108
    oxcarbazepine, 120
    topiramate, 110, 120
Orap. *See* Pimozide
Orphan Drug Amendments, 8

Outside Forces model of illness and
  disease, **391**
Overdose of drugs
  alprazolam, 49
  antidepressants, 68
    monoamine oxidase inhibitors,
      254
    selective serotonin reuptake
      inhibitors, 68, 257
    tricyclic antidepressants, 76–77,
      254, 258
    venlafaxine, 41, 258
  benzodiazepines, 311, 323
  carbamazepine, 107
  opioids, 184
Oxazepam
  for anxiety, 366
  for delirium, **282**
  dose equivalencies for
    benzodiazepines, **407**
Oxcarbazepine, 107
  for bipolar disorder, **98**, 107, 123
    acute mania, 92
    in children and adolescents,
      118
    depressive episodes, 95
    maintenance treatment, 97
  dosing of, **98**, 107
  interaction with oral contraceptives,
    106, 120
  mechanism of action of, 107
  during pregnancy, 107
  side effects of, 107, 123
Oxycodone, **10**, 202
OxyContin. *See* Oxycodone

P-YMRS (Parent Version of the Young
  Mania Rating Scale), 424,
  439–441

Package inserts for medications, 42
Pain
    olanzapine-induced, 113
    tricyclic antidepressants for, 77
Paliperidone, 11
    dose equivalencies for second-
        generation antipsychotics,
        408
    pharmacokinetics of, 145
Pamelor. *See* Nortriptyline
Panax ginseng. See Ginseng root
Pancreatic effects
    of drugs
        carbamazepine, 107
        valproate, 105
    of passionflower, 367
Panic disorder
    diagnostic criteria for, 33
    epidemiology of, 32
    medications for, 43
        dose equivalencies for, 407
        in elderly persons, 51
Parapectolin, 10
Parasomnias, 221, 222–223
    medications for, 231–232
Parent Version of the Young Mania
    Rating Scale (P-YMRS), 424,
    439–441
Parkinsonism
    antipsychotic-induced, 147
    dementia and, 275
    medications for, 111, 316
        interaction with tricyclic
            antidepressants, 253
Paroxetine, 11
    cytochrome P450 enzyme
        inhibition by, 82
    discontinuation syndrome with, 42,
        46

dose equivalencies for selective
    serotonin reuptake inhibitors,
    407
dosing of, 44, 70, 260
drug interactions with
    aripiprazole, 114
    duloxetine, 49
    methadone, 203
    risperidone, 113
    tricyclic antidepressants, 45, 253
indications for
    anxiety disorders, 42, 43, 44, 46
    posttraumatic stress disorder,
        246, 248, 252, 258,
        260
    bipolar depression, 94, 97
    depressive disorders, 68–69, 70
    nonresponse of elderly persons to,
        42, 51
    off-label use of, 69
    pharmacodynamics and
        pharmacokinetics of, 40, 248
    during pregnancy, 46, 52–53, 79
    prescribing considerations for, 46
    side effects of, 42, 44, 46, 70, 344
Passionflower (*Passiflora incarnata),*
    357, 365–367
    adverse effects of, 367
    description of, 365–366
    efficacy of, 366
    herbal and drug interactions with,
        366–367
    mechanism of action of, 366
Past psychiatric history, 4
Patient Health Questionnaire: Somatic,
    Anxiety, and Depressive
    Symptoms (PHQ-SADS), 424,
    427–430
Paxil, Paxil CR. *See* Paroxetine

PCL-C (PTSD Checklist—Civilian Version), 426, **463–464**
PCP (phencyclidine), 137, 140, 312–313
Pentobarbital, 366
Perceptual disturbances, 131, 152
in delirium, 273, 292
in delirium tremens, 311
in dementia, 275, 287, 293
Periactin. *See* Cyproheptadine
Periodic limb movements of sleep, 222
Perphenazine, **11**
for acute mania, 110
dose equivalencies for first-generation antipsychotics, **408**
off-label uses of, **142**
pharmacokinetics of, **144**
Personality disorders, 317
borderline personality disorder, 89, 320
psychiatric emergencies in patients with, 317, 320
Personalized medicine, 417, **418–421**
Pervasive developmental disorders. *See* Neurodevelopmental disorders
Pexeva. *See* Paroxetine
Peyote, **10**
Pharmacodynamics, 19, 21
of antipsychotics, 143
of benzodiazepines, 40–41
genetic factors affecting, 384
of monoamine oxidase inhibitors, **251**
of psychostimulants, 174
of selective serotonin reuptake inhibitors, 40, **248–249**
of serotonin-norepinephrine reuptake inhibitors, 40, **250**
of tricyclic antidepressants, 250–251

Pharmacogenetics, 18, 417, **418–421**
Pharmacokinetics, 18–19, 21.
See also Cytochrome P450 enzyme system
of alcohol, 200
of antipsychotics, 111, 143–146, **144–146**, 281
aripiprazole, 114
asenapine, 115–116
olanzapine, 113, 283
quetiapine, 283
risperidone, 113, 282–283
ziprasidone, 115
of carbamazepine, 106
in children, 19
of disulfiram, 200
in elderly persons, 19, 51, 150
genetic factors affecting, 384
of lamotrigine, 108
of lithium, 102
of methadone, 203
of monoamine oxidase inhibitors, **251–252**
of nicotine replacement therapies, 203
of psychostimulants, 174
of selective serotonin reuptake inhibitors, 40, **248–249**, 252
of serotonin-norepinephrine reuptake inhibitors, 40, **250**
of tricyclic antidepressants, **250–252**
of valproate, 104
of varenicline, 203
Phencyclidine (PCP), 137, 140, 312–313
Phenelzine, **11**
dosing of, **261**
for posttraumatic stress disorder, 246, **261**

Phenobarbital, drug interactions with
bupropion, 198, 203
selective serotonin reuptake
inhibitors, 253
Phenytoin, drug interactions with
bupropion, 198, 203
trazodone, 230
PHQ-SADS (Patient Health
Questionnaire: Somatic, Anxiety,
and Depressive Symptoms), 424,
427–430
Physical activity, 341
Pimozide, 11
for children and adolescents, 151
off-label uses of, 142
pharmacokinetics of, 144
Pioglitazone, interaction with
topiramate, 193
Piper methysticum. See Kava
PIRS (Pittsburgh Insomnia Rating
Scale), 215–216, 426, 462
Pittsburgh Insomnia Rating Scale
(PIRS), 215–216, 426, 462
Pituitary, 24, 25
PMDD (premenstrual dysphoric
disorder), 65, 66, 79
medications for, 66, 68, 70, 71, 166
PMHNs (psychiatric mental health
nurses), culturally sensitive
treatment by, 380–399
Polycystic ovarian syndrome, valproate-
induced, 122
Polypharmacy, 20, 51, 79, 150, 177, 210
Polysomnography, 6, 216
Polyuria and polydipsia, lithium-
induced, 76, 282
Poor metabolizers, 385, 386, 387
Postpartum disorders
bipolar disorder, 88, 121

depression, 29, 61, 62, 64, 66–67,
68, 79
rating scale for, 66, 424, 437–438
psychosis, 20, 136
Posttraumatic stress disorder (PTSD),
33, 235–265
in children and adolescents, 259, 263
clinical features of, 237, 245, 246,
264
clinical pearls related to, 265
combat-related, 236, 237, 246, 259
course of, 241
delayed-onset, 241
diagnostic criteria for, 237, 238–239
medications for, 245–259
alpha- and beta-blockers, 232,
256, 262
antidepressants, 246–247
efficacy of, 247
monoamine oxidase
inhibitors, 247,
251–254, 257, 258,
261
pharmacodynamics and
pharmacokinetics of,
248–252
selective serotonin reuptake
inhibitors, 246,
248–249, 252–254,
257, 260, 263
serotonin-norepinephrine
reuptake inhibitors, 247,
250, 257–258, 261
tricyclic antidepressants, 247,
250–254, 257, 258, 261
benzodiazepines, 255
dosing of, 259, 260–262
FDA-approved indications and
warnings for, 258–259

mood stabilizers and
anticonvulsants, 255
during pregnancy and breast-
feeding, 263
pretreatment assessment and
monitoring of, 264
safety and efficacy of, 257–258
second-generation
antipsychotics, 255
metabolic syndrome and, 336–337
neurobiology of, 244–245
fear and response to threat,
241–243
nomenclature for, 236
overview of, 236
prevalence of, 236
psychiatric comorbidity with, 241,
246
rating scales for, 264, 425,
467–468
risk factors for, 239, 241, 259
traumatic events precipitating, 237
treatment approach to, 245
pharmacotherapy, 245–259
psychotherapy, 245–246, 263,
264–265
in specific populations, 259, 263
in women, 236, 239, 259
*Practice Guideline for the Treatment of
Patients With Bipolar Disorder,* 92,
93–95, 96, 97, 117
*Practice Guideline for the Treatment of
Patients With Borderline Personality
Disorder,* 320
Prazosin
dosing of, **262**
for parasomnias, 231–232
for posttraumatic stress disorder,
232, 256, **262**

Prefrontal cortex, **24**, **25**
Pregabalin, **10**
Pregnancy. *See also* Breast-feeding;
Postpartum disorders
autistic spectrum disorders related
to exposures in, 164
bipolar disorder in, 120–121
effects of untreated mental illness in,
20
medications in, 20, 263
acamprosate, **192**
antidepressants, 67, 79
bupropion, **197**, 208, 209
monoamine oxidase
inhibitors, **252**
selective serotonin reuptake
inhibitors, 41, **46**,
52–53, 79, **252**
serotonin-norepinephrine
reuptake inhibitors, 53
tricyclic antidepressants,
252
antipsychotics, 111, 112, 115,
121, 149, 323
benzodiazepines, 53, 121, 227,
323
buprenorphine, **195**
buprenorphine-naloxone, **195**
carbamazepine, 107, 120
disulfiram, **192**
doxepin, 230
gabapentin, 110
lamotrigine, 109, 120
lithium, 103, 120–121
methadone, 209
misoprostol, 164
naltrexone, **192**
nicotine replacement therapies,
208

Pregnancy,
    medications in *(continued)*
        oxcarbazepine, 107
        psychostimulants, 178
        risk categories for, 21, **22**
        thalidomide, 164
        topiramate, 110, **192**
        trazodone, 230
        valproate, 105, 120, 164
        varenicline, **197**
    psychiatric emergencies in, 322–323
    psychotic disorders related to
        exposures in, 133, 136
    St. John's wort in, 358
    substance use disorders in, 209
    testing for, 305
Premenstrual dysphoric disorder
    (PMDD), 65, 66, 79
    medications for, 66, 68, **70, 71, 166**
Prescribing medications
    antianxiety drugs, **46–47**
    antipsychotics, 141–143
    for children and adolescents, 20
        (See also Children and
        adolescents)
    clinical judgment and rationale for,
        3, 7, 20
    controlled substances, 9, **10**
    decision not to prescribe, 7
    for elderly persons, 20
        (See also Elderly persons)
    for medically compromised patients,
        20–21
        (See also Medical conditions)
    negotiating patient demands for, 6–7
    for pregnant women, 21
        (See also Pregnancy)
    psychiatric assessment before, 3–7,
        4–6

    in psychiatric emergencies,
        315–316, **318–319**, 325
    special considerations in, 19–21
Prescription drug abuse, 183–184, 310
Priapism, trazodone-induced, 230, 232
Pristiq. *See* Desvenlafaxine
Procardia. *See* Nifedipine
Prolactin elevation, drug-induced
    ramelteon, 227
    second generation antipsychotics,
        113, 148
Propranolol
    dosing of, **262**
    for posttraumatic stress disorder,
        256, **262**
    for tremor, 103
Provigil. *See* Modafinil
Prozac, Prozac Weekly. *See* Fluoxetine
Psychiatric emergencies, 301–327
    aftercare planning and, 302, **326**
    approach to crisis intervention in,
        303–304, 324–325, **326**
    causes of increase in, 302
    clinical pearls related to, 327
    common presentations of, 303
    confidentiality and consent for
        treatment in, 303
    definition of, 303
    differential diagnosis of, 304–306
        delirium, 305, **307**
        medical conditions, 304–305, **306**
    ensuring security in, 302, 304, 313,
        315, **326**
    incidence of, 302
    models of response in, 302
    patient seclusion and restraint in,
        308, 323, 325, **326**
    prioritizing symptom management
        in, 305

psychiatric disorders with acute
manifestations, 308–315,
309
agitation/aggression, 301–302,
304, 308, 313, **314, 315**
anxiety, 309–310
psychosis, 308–309
substance intoxication and
withdrawal, 310–313
alcohol, 310–311
benzodiazepines, 311
opiates, 311–312
phencyclidine, 312–313
psychostimulants, 312
suicidal ideation, threats, and
attempts, 313–315, **315**
psychotropic medications used in,
315–316, **318–319,** 325
settings for patient presentation to,
301–302
therapeutic alliance in, 302
treatment in special populations,
316–323
children and adolescents,
321–322
elderly persons, 320–321
incarcerated persons, 316–317
medically compromised patients,
322
patients with personality
disorders, 317, 320
pregnant or breast-feeding
women, 322–323
substance users, 322
treatment monitoring in, 323
Psychiatric mental health nurses
(PMHNs), culturally sensitive
treatment by, 380–399
Psychiatric nursing, 1–3

Psychiatric rating scales, 423–468
Abnormal Involuntary Movement
Scale (AIMS), 425, **443–445**
Adult ADHD Self-Report Scale
(Adult ASRS-v1.1), 157, 425,
455–457
Clinical Institute Withdrawal
Assessment of Alcohol Scale,
Revised (CIWA-Ar), **204,** 205,
425, **459–461**
Edinburgh Postnatal Depression
Scale (EPDS), 66, 424,
436–437
Epworth Sleepiness Scale (ESS),
215, 426, 462
Hamilton Anxiety Scale (Ham-A),
424, **431–432**
17-Item Hamilton Rating Scale for
Depression (Ham-D-17), 424,
433–435
Patient Health Questionnaire:
Somatic, Anxiety, and
Depressive Symptoms
(PHQ-SADS), 424, **427–430**
Pittsburgh Insomnia Rating Scale
(PIRS), 215–216, 426, 462
PTSD Checklist—Civilian Version
(PCL-C), 426, **463–464**
Vanderbilt ADHD Diagnostic
Parent Rating Scale
(VADPRS), 157, 425,
447–450
Vanderbilt ADHD Diagnostic
Teacher Rating Scale
(VADTRS), 157, 425,
451–454
Parent Version of the Young Mania
Rating Scale (P-YMRS), 424,
439–441

Psychomotor activation/agitation.
     See also Agitation
     in attention-deficit/hyperactivity
          disorder, 156, **157**
     in bipolar disorder, 87
     in delirium, 273
     in depressive disorders, 64, 87
     in psychotic disorders, 131
     in serotonin syndrome, 80
Psychopharmacogenetics, 18, 417,
     418–421
Psychostimulants, 174
     abuse/dependence on, 138,
          167–171, 176, 179, 230, 312
     black box warnings for, **11–12**,
          167–171
     as controlled substances, 9, **10**, 176
     dose equivalencies for, **408**
     dosing of, **167–171**, 175, 179
     grapefruit juice interactions with,
          169–171, 174
     indications for
          attention-deficit/hyperactivity
               disorder, 165, **167–171**,
               174, 178–179
          autism symptoms, 165, **166**
          autism with ADHD-like
               symptoms, 177
          depression, fatigue, or apathy in
               elderly or medically
               compromised patients,
               177–178
          hypersomnia, 230
     intoxication with, 312
     laboratory evaluation for use of,
          176, 230
     mechanisms of action of, **167–171**,
          174
     monitoring treatment with, 175–176

off-label uses of, **166**
     pharmacokinetics of, 174
     precautions for use in bipolar
          disorder, 120
     during pregnancy and breast-
          feeding, 178
     side effects of, 176, 230
          growth effects, 179
     use in special populations, 177–178
Psychotherapy, 2
     for anxiety disorders in elderly
          persons, 51
     for bipolar disorders, 91
     for dementia, 293
     for depressive disorders, 81
     for posttraumatic stress disorder,
          245–246, 263, 264–265
     for stress management, 346
Psychotic disorders, 129–153.
     See also Schizophrenia
     algorithms for treatment of, 141
     antipsychotic agents for, 141–149
          (*See also* Antipsychotics)
     patient education about, 152
     pharmacokinetics and
          pharmacodynamics of,
          143–146, **144–146**
     prescribing considerations for,
          141–143
     side effects of, 146–149
     brief, 130, **131, 136**
     clinical pearls related to, 152–153
     comorbidity with, 133
     definition of psychosis, 130, 308
     dementia and, 285, 287
     depression with psychotic features,
          61, 62, 64, 76
     diagnostic criteria for, 133
          brief psychotic disorder, **136**

delusional disorder, 130, **135**
psychotic disorder due to general
   medical condition, **137**
schizoaffective disorder, **134**
schizophrenia, **132–133**
schizophreniform disorder, **134**
differentiation from delirium, **307**
etiology of, 133, 135–137
family history of, 130
neurobiology of, 137–141
overview of, 130–133, **131**, 151
pathophysiology of schizophrenia,
   137–141
postpartum, 20, **136**
presenting as psychiatric emergency,
   308–309
prevalence of, 130–131
risk factors for, 133, 135–137
shared, 133
substance-induced, 133, 137, 138
suicide and, 314
symptoms of, 131, 308
treatment in special populations,
   149–151
   children and adolescents,
      150–151
   elderly persons, 150
   medically compromised patients,
      150
   pregnant or breast-feeding
      women, 149
PTSD. *See* Posttraumatic stress disorder
PTSD Checklist—Civilian Version
   (PCL-C), 426, **463–464**

QTc interval prolongation
   drug-induced
      antipsychotics, 115, **282**, 290
      methadone, **195**

passionflower-induced, 367
use of tricyclic antidepressants in
   patients with, 232
Quetiapine, **11**, 114–115
for children and adolescents, 151
dose equivalencies for second-
   generation antipsychotics, **409**
dosing of, **101**, 286–287, 290
drug interactions with, 115
indications for
   antidepressant augmentation, 76
   bipolar disorder, **101**, 112,
      114–115, 124
   acute mania, 92, 93
   in children and adolescents,
      118
   depressive episode, 94, 95, 112
   maintenance treatment, 97
   mixed states, 96
   rapid cycling, 96
   delirium, **282**, 283, 286–287
   dementia, 290
mechanism of action of, 114, 283
off-label uses of, **142**
pharmacokinetics of, **146**, 283
side effects of, 114, 115
Quinidine, interaction with
   aripiprazole, 114

Race, 382. *See also* Culturally sensitive
   psychopharmacology
Ramelteon
   dose equivalencies for
      nonbenzodiazepine hypnotics,
      409
   for insomnia, 226–227
Raphe nucleus, **24**, **25**
Rash. *See* Dermatological effects
Rating scales. *See* Psychiatric rating scales

Razadyne ER, Razadyne ER.
  See Galantamine
Readiness to change model, 341, 346
Relational worldview, 390
Relaxation techniques, 51, 233
REM sleep behavior disorder, 223
  medications for, 232
Remeron, Remeron SolTab.
  See Mirtazapine
Reminyl. *See* Galantamine
Renal effects of drugs
  carbamazepine, 107
  of lithium, 76
  in serotonin syndrome, 80
  topiramate, 107
Renal impairment
  acamprosate in, 192, 194
  bupropion in, 197
  buspirone in, 52, 292
  disulfiram in, 192
  duloxetine in, 52
  naltrexone in, 192
  selective serotonin reuptake
    inhibitors in, 252
  topiramate in, 192, 232
  tricyclic antidepressants in, 252
  venlafaxine in, 258
Respiratory depression, drug-induced
  buprenorphine, 195
  diazepam, 47
  methadone, 195
Restless legs syndrome, 222
Restoril. *See* Temazepam
Restraint of patients, 308, 323, 325, 326
Rett's disorder, 158
ReVia. *See* Naltrexone
Rheumatrex. *See* Methotrexate
Rifampin, interaction with zolpidem,
  229

Risperdal, Risperdal Consta, Risperdal
  M-Tab. *See* Risperidone
Risperidone, 11, 113
  for children and adolescents, 150,
    322
  dose equivalencies for second-
    generation antipsychotics,
    408–409
  dosing of, 100, 286, 290, 318
  drug interactions with, 113
    topiramate, 110
  indications for
    autism symptoms, 166
    bipolar disorder, 100, 112, 113,
      123
    acute mania, 92, 93
    in children and adolescents,
      118
    depressive episodes, 95
    maintenance treatment, 97
    delirium, 282, 282–283, 286
    dementia, 290
    posttraumatic stress disorder, 255
    psychiatric emergencies, 315, 318
  mechanism of action of, 113, 282
  off-label uses of, 142, 166
  pharmacokinetics of, 113, 146,
    282–283
  during pregnancy, 323
  side effects of, 282, 283, 318, 342
Ritalin, Ritalin LA, Ritalin SR.
  See Methylphenidate
Rivastigmine, 285, 288, 289
Romazicon. *See* Flumazenil
Rozerem. *See* Ramelteon

Saphris. *See* Asenapine
Sarafem. *See* Fluoxetine
Savella. *See* Milnacipran

Schisandra (*Schisandra chinensis*), **356,**
  364–365
  adverse effects of, 365
  description of, 364–365
  efficacy of, 365
  herbal and drug interactions with,
    365
  mechanism of action of, 365
Schizoaffective disorder, 130, **131, 134**
Schizophrenia, **131.**
  See also Psychotic disorders
  agitation/aggression in, 152–153
  antipsychotic agents for, 141–149
    (*See also* Antipsychotics)
    patient education about, 152
    pharmacokinetics and
      pharmacodynamics of,
      143–146, **144–146**
    prescribing considerations for,
      141–143
    side effects of, 146–149
  clinical pearls related to, 152–153
  diagnostic criteria for, **132–133**
  dopamine hypothesis of, 138–139
  hypofrontality in, 140
  metabolic syndrome and, 332
  neuroimaging in, 140
  pathophysiology of, 137–141
  premature death in, 332, 333
  prevalence of, 130
  substance abuse and, 211
  suicidality and, 314
Schizophreniform disorder, 130, **131,**
  134
Scientific model of illness and disease,
  391, **391**
Seclusion and restraint of patients, 308,
  323, 325, **326**
Secobarbital, 366

Seconal. *See* Secobarbital
Sedation
  drug-induced
    antipsychotics, 111, 123, 149,
      282, 290, **318**
    second-generation, 113, 114,
      115, 122, 123, **282,**
      283, 290, **318**
    benzodiazepines, 47, 49, 116,
      228, 319
    buprenorphine, **195**
    buspirone, **44**
    carbamazepine, 106, 107
    diphenhydramine, 226
    gabapentin, 109, 110, 232
    lithium, 103
    methadone, **195**
    mirtazapine, 74, 75
    oxcarbazepine, 107
    selective serotonin reuptake
      inhibitors, **44, 70**
    serotonin-norepinephrine
      reuptake inhibitors, 45, 69,
      72, 258
    topiramate, 110, 232
    trazodone, 74, 75, 230, 291
    tricyclic antidepressants, 230,
      232, **253**
    valproate, 105
    zaleplon, **229**
    zolpidem, **229**
  passionflower-induced, 366
Sedative-hypnotics, 226–230,
  228–229
  antihistamines, 226
  benzodiazepines, 49–50, 227
    (*See also* Benzodiazepines)
    interaction with gabapentin, 109
  melatonergic hypnotics, 226–227

Sedative-hypnotics *(continued)*
  nonbenzodiazepine hypnotics, 227
    dose equivalencies for, **409**
    withdrawal from, 203, **204–205**,
      205
Seizures
  in delirium tremens, 311
  drug-induced
    buprenorphine, **195**
    bupropion, **73**, **75**, 175, **197**
    carbamazepine, 107
    clozapine, **12**
    lithium, 103
    olanzapine, 113
    quetiapine, 115
    risperidone, 113
    venlafaxine, 258
  ginkgo-induced, 364
  during lamotrigine withdrawal, 108
  in serotonin syndrome, 80
Selective serotonin reuptake inhibitors
    (SSRIs), 12.
  See also specific drugs
  augmentation of
    bupropion, 75
    mirtazapine, 75
    in posttraumatic stress disorder,
      260
    second-generation
      antipsychotics, 76
    trazodone, 75
  benefits of, 68
  cost of, 68, 82
  cytochrome P450 enzyme
    inhibition by, **82**
  discontinuation syndrome with, 41,
    42, **46**, **254**
  dose equivalencies for, 406, **407**
  dosing of, **44**, **70–71**, **260**

drug interactions with, 40, 41, **253**,
  257
  buprenorphine, **195**
  methadone, **195**
generic forms of, 68, 82
indications for
  anxiety disorders, 41, 42, **43**, **44**,
    46, 47–48
  duration of use of, 54
  in elderly persons, 51
  posttraumatic stress disorder,
    246, 247, **248–249**,
    252–254, 257, 258,
    260
  autism symptoms, **166**
  dementia, 287, 290–291
  depressive disorders, 66, 67,
    68–69, **70–71**
  postpartum depression, 68
  premenstrual dysphoric
    disorder, 66, 68
interaction with St. John's wort, 358
mechanism of action of, 67
monitoring treatment with, 53
off-label use of, 69, **166**
overdose of, 68, 257
pharmacodynamics and
  pharmacokinetics of, 40,
  248–249, **252**
during pregnancy, 41, **46**, 52–53,
  79
safety and precautions for use of, 41,
  53
serotonin syndrome and, 41, 48, 80,
  254
side effects of, 42, **44**, 53, 69, **70–71**,
  253–254, 257, **343–344**
suicidality and, **11**, 41
use in cardiovascular impairment, 52

Selegiline, 11
   cytochrome P450 enzyme
      inhibition by, 82
   transdermal, 77
Selenium supplementation, 340
Self-medication model of substance
   abuse, 184, 212
Septum, 24, 25
Seroquel, Seroquel XR.
   See Quetiapine
Serotonin (5-HT), 12
   in Alzheimer's dementia, 280
   in autistic spectrum disorders, 165
   in bipolar disorders, 90
   in delirium, 272
   in depression and anxiety, 67, 68
   pathways for, 26, 27
   in posttraumatic stress disorder,
      244–245
   in premenstrual dysphoric disorder,
      66
   receptors for, 13–14
   in sleep regulation, 225
   in substance use disorders, 189
Serotonin-norepinephrine reuptake
   inhibitors (SNRIs).
   See also specific drugs
   cost of, 75, 82
   cytochrome P450 enzyme
      inhibition by, 82
   dose equivalencies for, 406, 407
   dosing of, 45, 72
   indications for
      anxiety disorders, 41, 43, 45, 46,
         48–49
      duration of use, 54
      in elderly persons, 51
      posttraumatic stress disorder,
         247, 250, 257–258

dementia, 284, 291
depressive disorders, 67, 69, 72,
   75
interaction with methadone, 195
interaction with St. John's wort, 358
mechanism of action of, 67
monitoring treatment with, 53
pharmacodynamics and
   pharmacokinetics of, 40, 250
during pregnancy, 53
safety and precautions for use of, 41,
   53
serotonin syndrome and, 80
side effects of, 45, 46, 53, 69, 72,
   257–258, 343
suicidality and, 11
Serotonin partial agonist and reuptake
   inhibitor, 69. *See also* Vilazodone
Serotonin receptor gene (*5HT2C*), 418
Serotonin syndrome, 41, 48, 76, 80,
   195, 208, 254, 355
Serotonin transporter gene (*SLC6A4*),
   418
Sertraline, 11
   in children and adolescents, 46
   cytochrome P450 enzyme
      inhibition by, 82
   dose equivalencies for selective
      serotonin reuptake inhibitors,
      407
   dosing of, 44, 46, 47, 71, 260
   drug interactions with
      methadone, 203
      zolpidem, 229
   indications for
      anxiety disorders, 43, 44, 46, 47
      posttraumatic stress disorder,
         246, 248, 252, 258, 260
      autism symptoms, 166

Sertraline,
  indications for *(continued)*
    depressive disorders, 68–69, 71
    premenstrual dysphoric
      disorder, 79
  off-label use of, 69, **166**
  pharmacodynamics and
    pharmacokinetics of, 40, **248**
  prescribing considerations for, **46**
  side effects of, **44**, 46, 71, **344**
  switching to duloxetine from, 406
Sexual effects of drugs
  antipsychotics, 111, 122
  buspirone, **44**
  monoamine oxidase inhibitors, **253**
  selective serotonin reuptake inhibitors,
    42, **44**, **46**, 69, **70–71**, **253**
  serotonin-norepinephrine reuptake
    inhibitors, **45, 72**
  trazodone, 230, 232
  vilazodone, **71**
Sexual history, 4
SGAs. *See* Antipsychotics: second-
  generation
Shift work sleep disorder, 222, 231
Silenor. *See* Doxepin
Sinequan. *See* Doxepin
SLC6A4 gene, **418**
Sleep apnea, 222, 231
Sleep effects
  of drugs
    acamprosate, **191**
    aripiprazole, 114
    buprenorphine-naloxone, **195**
    bupropion, **73**, 75, **198**
    caffeine, 233
    monoamine oxidase inhibitors,
      253
    oxcarbazepine, 107

    psychostimulants, 176, 230
    selective serotonin reuptake
      inhibitors, **70–71, 253**
    serotonin-norepinephrine
      reuptake inhibitors, **72**
    sertraline, **46**
    varenicline, **198**
    vilazodone, **71**
  of herbal preparations
    ginseng root, 361
    lemon balm, 370
    passionflower, 366
    valerian, 359, 360
Sleep hygiene, 223, **224–225**, 233
Sleep in America poll, 216
Sleep paralysis, 223
Sleep terror disorder, 223
  medications for, 231–232
Sleep-wake disorders, 215–234
  anxiety and, 32
  clinical pearls related to, 233–234
  depression and, 64, 65, 87
  effects of, **217**
  evaluation of, 4, 216, **218–219**
  medications for, 216, 225–232
    for hypersomnia, 230–231
    initiation of, 233
    for insomnia, 74, 77, 225–230,
      228–229
    for parasomnias, 231–232
    precautions for use of, 233, 234
  mortality risk and, 216
  neurobiology of sleep, 225, 232
  nonpharmacological interventions
    for, 233
  overview of, 215–216
  prevalence of, 216
  rating scales for, 215
  sleep cycle, 217

sleep needs across the life span,
    217
stages of sleep, 217, 220, **220**
types of, 220–223, **221**
    dyssomnias, 220–222
    parasomnias, 222–223
    sleep disorder due to general
        medical condition, 223
Sleepwalking disorder, 223
    medications for, 232
Smoking/tobacco use, 184.
    See also Nicotine
    deaths related to, 184
    drug interactions with
        duloxetine, 48
        olanzapine, 113
    medications for cessation of, 78,
        197–199
    pharmacokinetics of, 203
    during pregnancy, **197**, 208, 209
    metabolic syndrome and, 337
SNRIs. *See* Serotonin-norepinephrine
    reuptake inhibitors
Social history, **4**
    psychotic disorders and, 137
Social phobia, 33
    diagnostic criteria for, **35**
    epidemiology of, **32**
    medications for, **43**
Society of Critical Care Medicine, 281
Soma. *See* Carisoprodol
Somatostatin, in Alzheimer's dementia,
    279, 280
Sonata. *See* Zaleplon
Specific phobia, 33
    diagnostic criteria for, **34**
    epidemiology of, **32**
SSRIs. *See* Selective serotonin reuptake
    inhibitors

St. John's wort (*Hypericum perforatum*),
    80, 354–358, **356**, 371
    adverse effects of, 358
    black cohosh and, 368
    description of, 354
    efficacy in depression, 355
    for elderly persons, 358
    herbal and drug interactions with,
        355, 358
    mechanism of action of, 355
    during pregnancy and breast-
        feeding, 358
STEP-BD (Systematic Treatment
    Enhancement Program for Bipolar
    Disorder), 91, 94
Stereotyping, 386–387
Stevens-Johnson syndrome, **12**
    carbamazepine and, 106, 107
    ginkgo and, 364
    lamotrigine and, 108, 123
    modafinil and, 175
Strattera. *See* Atomoxetine
Stress
    anxiety disorders and, 54–55
    bipolar disorder and, 91
    brain regulation of, **24–25**, **27**, 37
    cultural concepts and, 381, 384, 388
    delirium and, 278
    herbal preparations for
        ginkgo, 363
        ginseng, 360
        schisandra, 364
    metabolic syndrome and, 336–337
    postpartum depression and, 66
    sleep disturbances and, **218**, **225**,
        233
    substance use disorders and, 184
    traumatic stress disorders, 235–265
Stress management, **225**, 346

Stroke, 65, 178, 332
 antidepressants and, 252, 254
 cocaine intoxication and, 312
 delirium and, 278, 281
 metabolic syndrome and, 332, 334
Suboxone. *See* Buprenorphine-naloxone
Substance Abuse and Mental Health
  Services Administration, 208
Substance-induced disorders
 anxiety disorder, 33, 54
 psychosis, 133, 137, 138
 sleep disorder, 221
Substance use/abuse history, 5
Substance use disorders, 183–212.
 See also specific substances of abuse
 addictive process in, 185
 anxiety and, 54
 benzodiazepine abuse/dependence,
  41, 47, 49, 53, 227, 311
 clinical pearls related to, 212
 deaths from, 184
 detoxification from, 203, 205
  alcohol/benzodiazepine
   withdrawal protocol,
   204–205
  opioid withdrawal protocol,
   206–207
 diagnostic criteria for, 310
  substance abuse, 188
  substance dependence, 187
  substance intoxication, 190
  substance withdrawal, 190
 genetic factors in, 185
 health consequences of, 184, 185
 among incarcerated persons, 317
 intoxication due to, 189, 190,
  310–313
 medications for, 190

in alcohol/abuse dependence,
 191–194
dosing of, 191–199, 209
FDA-approved indications and
 warnings for, 208
in nicotine dependence, 197–199
in opioid abuse/dependence,
 191–196
side effects and precautions for
 use of, 191–199, 207–208
neurobiology of, 186–189
overview of, 186
pharmacokinetics of alcohol and
 alcoholism treatment, 200–201
pharmacokinetics of nicotine and
 smoking cessation treatment,
 203
pharmacokinetics of opiates and
 addiction treatment, 202–203
during pregnancy, 209
prescription drug abuse, 183–184,
 310
presenting as psychiatric emergency,
 305, 310–313, 322
 alcohol, 310–311
 benzodiazepines, 311
 cocaine, 312
 opiates, 311–312
 phencyclidine, 312–313
prevalence of, 310
psychiatric comorbidity with, 185,
 208, 211, 212
psychostimulant abuse/dependence,
 138, 167–171, 176, 179, 230,
 312
self-medication model of, 184, 212
societal perspectives on, 313
suicide and, 314

treatment in special populations,
209–211
children and adolescents, 210
elderly persons, 210
patients with comorbid
psychiatric illness, 211
pregnant women, 209
withdrawal from, 189, **190**, 203,
205, 310–313
Subutex. *See* Buprenorphine
Suicidal ideation or behavior
bipolar disorder and, 88
in children and adolescents, 321
depressive disorders and, 60, 64, 81,
88
in elderly persons, 210, 314, 320
epidemiology of, 314
among incarcerated persons, 317
interventions for, 315
medication-related
acamprosate, **192**
antidepressants, **11**, 41, **46**, 53,
69, 75, 78, 208, 258–259
in children and young adults,
50, 53, 78, 79,
258–259
in elderly persons, 51
atomoxetine, **172**
bupropion, **198**
lamotrigine, 108
valproate, 105
varenicline, **197**, 208
as psychiatric emergency, 303,
313–315
risk factors for, 314, **314, 315**
schizophrenia and, 314
*The Surgeon General's Vision for a
Healthy and Fit Nation,* 341

Sweating
in anxiety disorders, 32
in delirium tremens, 311
drug-induced
buprenorphine, **195**
clomipramine, 232
imipramine, 232
methadone, **195**
valerian-induced, 360
Switching between psychotropic
medications, dose equivalencies
for, 405–406, **407–409**
Symbyax. *See* Olanzapine-fluoxetine
combination
Synthroid. *See* Levothyroxine
Systematic Treatment Enhancement
Program for Bipolar Disorder
(STEP-BD), 91, 94

Tachycardia
in anxiety disorders, 32
drug-induced
carbamazepine, 107
second-generation antipsychotics,
113, 115, 283
tricyclic antidepressants, **253**
passionflower-induced, 367
in serotonin syndrome, 80
Tacrine, 288
Tagamet. *See* Cimetidine
Tardive dyskinesia, 111, 113, 118, 147,
290
TCAs. *See* Antidepressants, tricyclic
Tegretol. *See* Carbamazepine
Temazepam
dose equivalencies for
benzodiazepine hypnotics, **409**
for insomnia, **228**

Tenex. *See* Guanfacine
Teratogenicity.
    See Pregnancy, medications in
Terminology
    cultural, 382–385
    pharmacological, 18–19
Testosterone, **10**, 227
Texas Medication Algorithm Project, 141
Thalamus, **24, 25**
Thalidomide, 164
Therapeutic alliance
    culturally competent, 387–389,
        389, 394, 398
    in psychiatric emergencies, 302
Therapeutic equivalence evaluation
    codes, 8
Thioridazine, **11, 144**
Thiothixene, **11**
    for acute mania, 110
    dose equivalencies for first-
        generation antipsychotics, **408**
    off-label uses of, **142**
    pharmacokinetics of, **144**
Thorazine. *See* Chlorpromazine
Thyroid effects of lithium, 76, 103,
    121, **282**
Thyroid medications, 103
    interaction with lemon balm, 370
Titration of drug dosage, 18
Tofranil. *See* Imipramine
Topamax. *See* Topiramate
Topiramate, 110
    dosing of, **99, 194**
    drug interactions with, 110
        carbamazepine, 106
        oral contraceptives, 110, 120
    indications for
        alcohol dependence, **191–194**,
            208

bipolar disorder, 93, 95, **99**,
    110, 123
    in children and adolescents,
        118
    parasomnias, 232
    mechanism of action of, 110
    during pregnancy, 110
    side effects of, 110, 232, **344**
Tourette syndrome, 151
Transtheoretical Model of Change, 341,
    346
Tranxene. *See* Clorazepate
Tranylcypromine, **11**
Traumatic stress disorders,
    235–265
    acute stress disorder, 33, 237, **240**,
        256, 264
    clinical pearls related to, 265
    neurobiology of, 244–245
        fear and response to threat,
            241–243
    posttraumatic stress disorder,
        235–265, **238–239**
    prevalence of, 236
    spectrum of, 237
    treatment approach to, 245–263
        medications, 245–259,
            248–254, 260–262
        pharmacotherapy, 245–246,
            263, 265
        pretreatment assessment and
            monitoring, 264
        in specific populations, 259,
            263
Trazodone, **11**
    dose equivalencies for
        nonbenzodiazepine hypnotics,
            409
    dosing of, 74, 230, 291

indications for
antidepressant augmentation in
posttraumatic stress
disorder, 260
dementia, 291
depressive disorders, 74, 75
insomnia, 227, 230
interaction with prazosin, 232
during pregnancy, 230
side effects of, 74, 75, 230
Tremor, 15
in anxiety disorders, 32
in delirium tremens, 311
drug-induced
antipsychotics, 147
gabapentin, 109
lamotrigine, 108
lithium, 76, 103
oxcarbazepine, 107
selective serotonin reuptake
inhibitors, 253
topiramate, 110
valproate, 105
in Lewy body dementia, 275
propranolol for, 103
Tresall. See Methotrexate
Triazolam
dose equivalencies for
benzodiazepine hypnotics, 409
for insomnia, 228
interaction with fluoxetine, 48
Trifluoperazine, 11
pharmacokinetics of, 145
side effects of, 343
Trihexyphenidyl, 111
Trilafon. See Perphenazine
Trileptal. See Oxcarbazepine
Triptans, 80
Tubizid. See Isoniazid

Twin studies
of bipolar disorders, 90
of psychotic disorders, 130
Tylenol. See Acetaminophen

Urinary retention, drug-induced
antipsychotics, 111, 149
tricyclic antidepressants, 232, 253
U.S. Department of Agriculture
Choose My Plate Web site, 341
U.S. Drug Enforcement
Administration (DEA), 53
Controlled Substances Schedules, 9,
10, 202
U.S. Food and Drug Administration
(FDA), 7–9
approved indications and
warnings
for antianxiety medications, 42,
43
for antidepressants, 78
for posttraumatic stress disorder
medications, 258–259
for substance abuse medications,
208
black box warnings for psychotropic
drugs, 9, 11–12
antidepressants, 41, 78, 79,
258–259
antipsychotics, 76, 111, 112,
119, 150, 281, 286, 290,
318
psychostimulants, 11–12,
167–172
varenicline, 208
dietary supplements and, 8–9
drug oversight by, 7
generic drugs and, 7
medical foods and, 8

U.S. Food and Drug Administration
    (FDA) *(continued)*
  pregnancy risk categories for
    medications, 21, 22
  therapeutic equivalence evaluation
    codes, 8

VADPRS (Vanderbilt ADHD
    Diagnostic Parent Rating Scale),
    157, 425, 447–450
VADTRS (Vanderbilt ADHD
    Diagnostic Teacher Rating Scale),
    157, 425, 451–454
Valerian (*Valeriana officinalis*), 356,
    358–360, 371
  adverse effects of, 360
  description of, 358
  efficacy of, 359
  herbal and drug interactions with,
    359
  gabapentin, 109
  for insomnia, 225–226, 359
  lemon balm and, 370
  mechanism of action of, 358
  side effects of, 226
Valium. *See* Diazepam
Valproate, 104–105
  discontinuation of, 104
  dosing of, 98, 291
  drug interactions with, 104
    alcohol, 120
    carbamazepine, 106
    lamotrigine, 104, 108, 109
    topiramate, 110
  formulations of, 102
  indications for
    bipolar disorder, 98, 104–105,
      123
    acute mania, 91–93

  in children and adolescents,
    118
  depressive episode, 94, 95
  maintenance treatment, 97
  mixed states, 96
  rapid cycling, 96
  delirium, 282
  dementia, 285, 291
  posttraumatic stress disorder,
    255
  mechanism of action of, 102
  monitoring serum levels of, 105
  pharmacokinetics of, 104
  during pregnancy and breast-
    feeding, 105, 121, 164
  side effects of, 105, 122, 334, 345
Vanderbilt ADHD Diagnostic Parent
    Rating Scale (VADPRS), 157,
    425, 447–450
Vanderbilt ADHD Diagnostic Teacher
    Rating Scale (VADTRS), 157,
    425, 451–454
Varenicline, for nicotine dependence,
    197–199
Vascular dementia, 275, 276
Venlafaxine, 11
  augmentation of, 261
  cytochrome P450 enzyme
    inhibition by, 82
  discontinuation syndrome with, 45,
    46, 48
  dose equivalencies for serotonin-
    norepinephrine reuptake
    inhibitors, 407
  dosing of, 45, 48, 72, 261
  drug interactions with
    methadone, 203
    monoamine oxidase inhibitors,
      258

indications for
anxiety disorders, **43, 45, 46,** 48
posttraumatic stress disorder,
246, **250,** 257–258,
261
bipolar depression, 95
depressive disorders, 69, **72**
overdose of, 41, 258
pharmacodynamics and
pharmacokinetics of, **250**
prescribing considerations for, **46**
side effects of, **45, 46,** 48, **72,**
257–258, **343**
Verapamil, for bipolar disorder, 116
Viibryd. *See* Vilazodone
Vilazodone, **11**
for depression, 69
dose equivalencies for selective
serotonin reuptake inhibitors,
407
dosing of, **71**
mechanism of action of, 69
side effects of, **71**
Violence. *See* Aggression/violence
Vistaril. *See* Hydroxyzine
Visual disturbances, drug-induced
antipsychotics, 111, 149
benzodiazepines, **282**
carbamazepine, 106, 107
gabapentin, 109
lamotrigine, 108
lithium, 103
oxcarbazepine, 107
psychostimulants, 230
topiramate, 110, **192**
tricyclic antidepressants, 232, **253**
valproate, 105
Vivitrol. *See* Naltrexone, extended-
release injectable

Vyvanse. *See* Lisdexamfetamine

Waist circumference, 331, 334, **335,**
337, 338
Wakefulness-promoting agents, 231
Warfarin, ginkgo interaction with, 364
Weight changes
black cohosh–induced, 368
in depressive disorders, 64, 87
drug-induced, 342–345
antipsychotics, 148, 150
first-generation, 111,
342–343
second-generation, 76, 92,
112, 113, 114, 115,
118, 148, 339, **342**
bupropion, **343**
carbamazepine, 106
clomipramine, 232
duloxetine, **45**
gabapentin, 109, 334, **344**
imipramine, 232
lamotrigine, 334, **344**
lithium, 76, 334, **344**
metformin for treatment of,
339–340
milnacipran, **344**
mirtazapine, 74, 75, 333, **344**
monoamine oxidase inhibitors,
253
psychoeducation about, 338
selective serotonin reuptake
inhibitors, 44, 70–71, **253,**
343–344
serotonin-norepinephrine
reuptake inhibitors, **72,**
343
topiramate, 110, **191, 344**
trazodone, 74, 75

Weight changes,
    drug induced (continued)
    tricyclic antidepressants, 253, 344
    valproate, 334, 345
    vilazodone, 71
    in premenstrual dysphoric disorder,
        66
Wellbutrin, Wellbutrin SR,
    Wellbutrin XL.
    See Bupropion
Withdrawal from drugs.
    See also Discontinuation of drugs
    alcohol, 203, 204–205, 205,
        310–311
        benzodiazepines for, 287, 311
        during pregnancy, 209
        rating scale for, 425, 463–465
        treatment of delirium due to,
            287, 311
    benzodiazepines, 41, 50, 203,
        204–205, 205, 227, 311
        in neonate, 121
        rebound insomnia and, 227
        treatment of delirium due to,
            287
    caffeine, 231
    diagnostic criteria for, 190
    in elderly persons, 320
    presenting as psychiatric emergency,
        305, 310–313
    substances of abuse, 189, 190
        cocaine, 312
        opiates, 203, 205, 206–207,
            312, 366
        phencyclidine, 313
Worldviews, 390, 392

Worthlessness, feelings of, 64, 87

Xanax, Xanax XR. See Alprazolam

YMRS. See Young Mania Rating Scale
Young Mania Rating Scale (YMRS),
    424, 439
    Parent Version (P-YMRS), 424,
        439–441

Zaleplon, 409
Ziprasidone, 11, 115
    administering with food, 115
    for bipolar disorder, 101, 112, 115
        acute mania, 92–93
        depressive episodes, 95
        maintenance treatment, 97
        mixed states, 96
    dose equivalencies for second-
        generation antipsychotics, 408
    dosing of, 101
    mechanism of action of, 115
    pharmacokinetics of, 115, 146
    during pregnancy and breast-
        feeding, 115
    side effects of, 115, 342
Zoloft. See Sertraline
Zolpidem, 10
    dose equivalencies for
        nonbenzodiazepine hypnotics,
        409
    for insomnia, 229
    passionflower interaction with, 366
Zyban. See Bupropion
Zyprexa, Zyprexa Relprevv, Zyprexa
    Zydis. See Olanzapine